AF578225

PROGRESS IN CLINICAL AND BIOLOGICAL RESEARCH

1983 TITLES

Vol 115: **Prevention of Hereditary Large Bowel Cancer,** John R.F. Ingall, Anthony J. Mastromarino, *Editors*

Vol 116: **New Concepts in Thyroid Disease,** Roberto J. Soto, Gerardo Sartorio, Ismael de Forteza, *Editors*

Vol 117: **Reproductive Toxicology,** Donald R. Mattison, *Editor*

Vol 118: **Growth and Trophic Factors,** J. Regino Perez-Polo, Jean de Vellis, Bernard Haber, *Editors*

Vol 119: **Oncogenes and Retroviruses: Evaluation of Basic Findings and Clinical Potential,** Timothy E. O'Connor, Frank J. Rauscher, Jr., *Editors*

Vol 120: **Advances in Cancer Control: Research and Development,** Paul F. Engstrom, Paul N. Anderson, Lee E. Mortenson, *Editors*

Vol 121: **Progress in Cancer Control III: A Regional Approach,** Curtis Mettlin, Gerald P. Murphy, *Editors*

Vol 122: **Advances in Blood Substitute Research,** Robert B. Bolin, Robert P. Geyer, George J. Nemo, *Editors*

Vol 123: **California Serogroup Viruses,** Charles H. Calisher, Wayne H. Thompson, *Editors*

Vol 124: **Epilepsy: An Update on Research and Therapy,** Giuseppe Nisticò, Raoul Di Perri, H. Meinardi, *Editors*

Vol 125: **Sulfur Amino Acids: Biochemical and Clinical Aspects,** Kinya Kuriyama, Ryan J. Huxtable, Heitaroh Iwata, *Editors*

Vol 126: **Membrane Biophysics II: Physical Methods in the Study of Epithelia,** Mumtaz A. Dinno, Arthur B. Callahan, Thomas C. Rozzell, *Editors*

Vol 127: **Orphan Drugs and Orphan Diseases: Clinical Realities and Public Policy,** George J. Brewer, *Editor*

Vol 128: **Research Ethics,** Kåre Berg, Knut Erik Tranøy, *Editors*

Vol 129: **Zinc Deficiency in Human Subjects,** Ananda S. Prasad, Ayhan O. Çavdar, George J. Brewer, Peter J. Aggett, *Editors*

Vol 130: **Progress in Cancer Control IV: Research in the Cancer Center,** Curtis Mettlin, Gerald P. Murphy, *Editors*

Vol 131: **Ethopharmacology: Primate Models of Neuropsychiatric Disorders,** Klaus A. Miczek, *Editor*

Vol 132: **13th International Cancer Congress,** Edwin A. Mirand, William B. Hutchinson, Enrico Mihich, *Editors.* Published in 5 Volumes: Part A: **Current Perspectives in Cancer.** Part B: **Biology of Cancer (1).** Part C: **Biology of Cancer (2).** Part D: **Research and Treatment.** Part E: **Cancer Management**

Vol 133: **Non-HLA Antigens in Health, Aging, and Malignancy,** Elias Cohen, Dharam P. Singal, *Editors*

See pages following the index for previous titles in this series.

ETHOPHARMACOLOGY:

PRIMATE MODELS OF NEUROPSYCHIATRIC DISORDERS

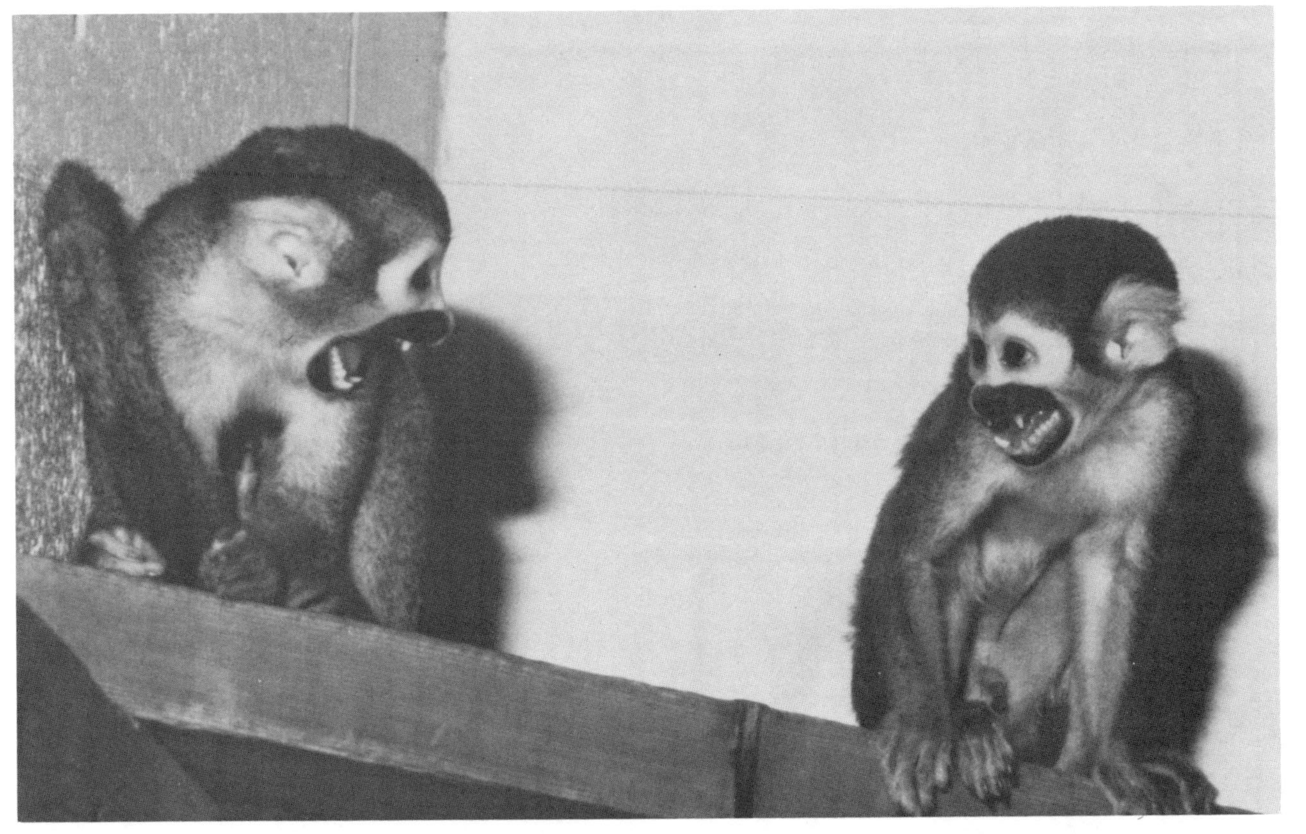

Frontispiece. Vocal displays by male squirrel monkeys *(Saimiri sciureus)*. Photograph by C. Miczek. (*See* Miczek and Gold, this volume, pages 137–155.)

ETHOPHARMACOLOGY:
PRIMATE MODELS OF NEUROPSYCHIATRIC DISORDERS

Proceedings of the Symposium on Primate Ethopharmacology held under the auspices of the IX Congress of the International Primatological Society in Atlanta, Georgia, August 1982

Editor
KLAUS A. MICZEK
Department of Psychology
Tufts University
Medford, Massachusetts

ALAN R. LISS, INC. • NEW YORK

Address all Inquiries to the Publisher
Alan R. Liss, Inc., 150 Fifth Avenue, New York, NY 10011

Printed in the United States of America.

Library of Congress Cataloging in Publication Data

Symposium on Primate Ethopharmacology (1982 :
Atlanta, Ga.)
Ethopharmacology, primate models of neuropsychiatric disorders.

(Progress in clinical and biological research ; v. 131)
Includes index.
1. Psychiatry, Comparative--Congresses.
2. Psychology, Pathological--Animal models--Congresses.
3. Psychopharmacology--Congresses. 4. Primates--Behavior--Congresses. I. Miczek, Klaus A.
II. International Primatological Society. Congress (9th : 1982 : Atlanta, Ga.) III. Title. IV. Series.
[DNLM: 1. Mental disorders--Chemically induced--Congresses. 2. Psychotropic drugs--Pharmacodynamics--Congresses. 3. Behavior, Animal--Drug effects--Congresses. 4. Disease models, Animal--Congresses.
5. Primates--Congresses. WI PR668E v.131 / QV 77 S9897e 1982]
RC455.4.C6S95 1982 615′.78 83-12002
ISBN 0-8451-0131-5

Contents

Contributors

Lillian Bailey, Department of Pharmacology and the Research Institute of Pharmaceutical Sciences, School of Pharmacy, University of Mississippi, University, MS 38677 **[293]**

H.F. Baker, Division of Psychiatry, Clinical Research Center, Harrow, Middlesex, England **[101]**

John A. Bedford, Department of Pharmacology and the Research Institute of Pharmaceutical Sciences, School of Pharmacy, University of Mississippi, University, MS 38677 **[293]**

Douglas M. Bowden, Department of Psychiatry and Behavioral Sciences, University of Washington, Seattle, WA 98195 **[157]**

Gary L. Brammer, Department of Psychiatry, University of California Los Angeles, School of Medicine, Los Angeles, CA 90024, Nonhuman Primate Research Laboratory, Veterans Administration Medical Center, Sepulveda, CA 91343, and Neurobiochemistry Laboratory, Veterans Administration Brentwood Medical Center, Los Angeles, CA 90073 **[185, 313]**

L.D. Byrd, Yerkes Regional Primate Research Center and Departments of Pharmacology and Psychology, Emory University, Atlanta, GA 30322 **[1]**

Thomas J. Crowley, Department of Psychiatry, University of Colorado School of Medicine, Denver, CO 80262 **[255]**

John M. Davis, Department of Research, Illinois State Psychiatric Institute, Chicago, IL 60612 **[33]**

Mark F. Dubach, Regional Primate Research Center and Department of Anthropology, University of Washington, Seattle, WA 98195 **[157]**

Michael H. Ebert, Laboratory of Clinical Science, National Institute of Mental Health, Bethesda, MD 20014 **[199]**

Michael S. Eison, Department of Experimental Psychology, University of Cambridge, Cambridge, England **[79]**

Lisa H. Gold, Department of Psychology, Tufts University, Medford, MA 02155 **[137]**

James L. Howard, Department of Pharmacology, Wellcome Research Laboratories, Research Triangle Park, NC 27709 **[307]**

Susan D. Iverson, Department of Experimental Psychology, University of Cambridge, Cambridge, England **[79]**

Gary W. Kraemer, Wisconsin Psychiatric Research Institute and Primate Laboratory, University of Wisconsin, Madison, WI 53706 **[199]**

The boldface number in brackets indicates the opening page number of that contributor's article.

C. Raymond Lake, Departments of Psychiatry and Pharmacology, Uniformed Services University of the Health Sciences, School of Medicine, Bethesda, MD 20014 **[199]**

Melvin Lyon, Psychopharmacological Research Laboratory, Sct. Hans Mental Hospital, DK-4000 Roskilde, Denmark **[79]**

Michael T. McGuire, Department of Psychiatry, University of California Los Angeles, School of Medicine, Los Angeles, CA 90024, and Nonhuman Primate Research Laboratory, Veterans Administration Medical Center, Sepulveda, CA 91343 **[185, 313]**

William T. McKinney, Department of Psychiatry, University of Wisconsin, Madison, WI 53706 **[199]**

Klaus A. Miczek, Department of Psychology, Tufts University, Medford, MA 02155 **[xi,137]**

Erik B. Nielsen, Psychopharmacological Research Laboratory, Sct. Hans Mental Hospital, DK-4000 Roskilde, Denmark **[79]**

Gerald T. Pollard, Department of Pharmacology, Wellcome Research Laboratories, Research Triangle Park, NC 27709 **[307]**

Michael J. Raleigh, Department of Psychiatry, University of California Los Angeles, School of Medicine, Los Angeles, CA 90024, Nonhuman Primate Research Laboratory, Veterans Administration Medical Center, Sepulveda, CA 91343, and Neurobiochemistry Laboratory, Veterans Administration Brentwood Medical Center, Los Angeles, CA 90073 **[185, 313]**

Martin Reite, Department of Psychiatry, University of Colorado School of Medicine, Denver, CO 80262 **[219]**

R.M. Ridley, Division of Psychiatry, Clinical Research Center, Harrow, Middlesex, England **[101]**

E.N. Sassenrath, Behavioral Sciences Laboratory, Department of Psychiatry, School of Medicine, University of California, Davis, CA 95616 **[277]**

R. Francis Schlemmer, Department of Research, Illinois State Psychiatric Institute, Chicago, IL 60612 **[33]**

Robert Short, Department of Psychiatry, University of Colorado School of Medicine, Denver, CO 80262 **[219]**

E.O. Smith, Yerkes Regional Primate Research Center and Departments of Anthropology and Biology, Emory University, Atlanta, GA 30322 **[1]**

Marvin C. Wilson, Department of Pharmacology and the Research Institute of Pharmaceutical Sciences, School of Pharmacy, University of Mississippi, University, MS 38677 **[293]**

Preface

The behavioral analysis of drug action has been in the domain of psychopharmacology. The introduction of the term ethopharmacology emphasizes the contribution of ethology to the way in which we look at behavior and its underlying mechanisms. Indeed, it is mainly the ethological method of observation that has attracted researchers to study the behavioral processes that are the target of drug action. Intimate familiarity with the behavioral repertoire of a species and its functional significance enables reliable and exquisitively sensitive analysis of subtle, unusual, and potentially pathological effects of drugs.

Pharmacological manipulation in concert with physiological, biochemical, *and* behavioral analyses may be the most fruitful interdisciplinary approach to the study of species-typical as well as atypical, disordered behavior.

In recent years, the behavioral analysis has become the weakest link in the neurosciences. The rich and fascinating repertoire of primate behavior demands the development of sophisticated quantitative methodologies. The contributions to this volume exemplify the most successful integrations of pharmacological and behavioral research methodologies, often paired with physiological measurements. The multiple authors of most chapters represent experts from anthropology, endocrinology, neurochemistry, physiology, pharmacology, psychology, and psychiatry, each contributing the unique methodological and conceptual features of their speciality. Their efforts stand in sharp contrast to the current trend toward more specialization.

Have the authors succeeded in developing novel and satisfactory models of psychosis, depression, hallucination, drug abuse, violence, or other disorders? If the answer may not always be completely positive, it certainly can be stated that most promising research strategies have been developed that are bound to reshape our thinking not only about the existing animal models, but also about the disorders themselves.

The production of the present volume incorporated the use of the emerging word processing technology. Each contribution was edited as a computer file and moved in this format to the publisher and typesetter. While the editor, production manager, and typesetters had to struggle with the current Babel of software and hardware conventions, the potential benefits to the rapid, efficient, and high-quality communication of scientific information were apparent.

The volume emerged from a symposium that was held under the auspices of the IX. Congress of the International Primatological Society in Atlanta, Georgia, in August 1982. The hospitable arrangements made by Dr. Fred King and his staff from the Yerkes Regional Primate Research Center were greatly appreciated.

The symposium and the preparation of this volume were supported in part by donations from the following organizations: CIBA-GEIGY Corp., Summit, New Jersey, and Merck Sharp & Dohme, West Point, Pennsylvania.

Klaus A. Miczek

Ethopharmacology: Primate Models of Neuropsychiatric Disorders, pages 1–31

Studying the Behavioral Effects of Drugs in Group-Living Nonhuman Primates

E.O. Smith and L.D. Byrd

Yerkes Regional Primate Research Center (E.O.S., L.D.B.), Departments of Anthropology and Biology (E.O.S.), and Departments of Pharmacology and Psychology (L.D.B.), Emory University, Atlanta, Georgia 30322

INTRODUCTION

Studies of the behavioral effects of drugs traditionally have emphasized isolated animal preparations. Such an approach has provided orderly, systematic data, and experiments with individual animals in isolation have been quite useful in characterizing drugs with respect to their behavioral effects and in predicting the effects of drugs on human behavior. In recent years, highly sophisticated techniques have also evolved for studying and quantitating the behavior of animals living together in groups normally characteristic of species in the wild. Through careful application of ethological techniques, one can now describe and quantitate drug-induced changes in behavior in group-living nonhuman primates. The availability of techniques for studying the behavior of nonhuman primates living in groups under seminatural conditions offers an alternative paradigm for studying the behavioral effects of drugs that can enhance our understanding of drug effects on human and animal behavior and permit an assessment of the generality of effects observed in experiments with individual animals. Moreover, the dynamic network of relationships characteristic of primate societies can be of substantial value in revealing the effects of drugs that may be less readily identifiable or measurable in isolated, individual subjects. Group-living nonhuman primates display a wide range of complex behaviors, many of which involve dynamic interactions with other members of the group. Studying the behavior of group-living nonhuman primates to determine the effects of drugs that act on the central nervous system is especially appropriate, therefore, because of parallels between human and nonhuman primates and some types of group or social behaviors (Raleigh and McGuire, 1980; Sassenrath and Chapman, 1976). Furthermore, the extent to which drug-induced behavioral changes may be influenced by group dynamics can be ascertained (see McGuire et al., 1982, for a complete discussion of some of the strengths and weaknesses of this approach). van Hooff (1972:4.10) has noted:

> An approach which compares the different effects of various pharmacological influences on a broad spectrum of natural responses appears to offer the best guarantee against premature and simplistic generalizations. . . . The benefits to interdisciplinary contacts will clearly be mutual, since pharmacological procedures may also be a valuable tool in unraveling the organization of behavior.

A number of investigators have undertaken research to determine the effects of drugs in groups of primates, and the results of several studies are summarized in Table I. The studies demonstrate that the behavior of group-living nonhuman primates can be of value in revealing experimentally induced alterations of behavior mediated via the central nervous system. Furthermore, the studies indicate that the type of response to a drug may vary with the context or social setting, and that specific drugs can differentially affect various behaviors exhibited in the social setting. These factors substantiate our view that it is desirable and advantageous to study drug effects in nonhuman primates living in relatively natural groups because of the more direct relevance to the use of drugs in human societies.

As can be seen, however, the studies summarized typically have not utilized groups that approximate those found in natural settings (cf. Burgess et al., 1980; Crowley et al., 1974) nor, with minor exceptions (Burgess et al., 1980; Raleigh and McGuire, 1980), with groups housed outdoors, although some chronic administrations have taken place in large social groups (Sassenrath and Chapman, 1976). The research paradigm that we have developed is based upon a study group that approximates the typical "macaque-like" pattern of social organization, with the group consisting of multiple adult males, adult females, and young of various ages, and with all members housed outdoors in a semi-free-ranging environment.

METHODOLOGICAL CONSIDERATIONS

Stumptail macaques (*Macaca arctoides*) (Fooden, 1967, 1976) were chosen as subjects for our studies for several reasons: 1) This species reproduces well in captivity and does not exhibit seasonal mating; i.e., there is little change in the reproductive behavior of the group during a 12-month period (Trollope, 1978; Trollope and Blurton Jones, 1970, 1975). Although some have suggested the presence of birth peaks (Estrada and Estrada, 1976, 1981), stumptail macaques maintain a relatively constant pattern of mating behavior during the year and do not conform to the well-defined seasonal pattern characteristic of many macaques. 2) Stumptail macaques exhibit a well-organized dominance hierarchy that remains relatively stable over time (Bernstein, 1980; Bernstein and Guilloud, 1965; Boelkins, 1967; Gouzoules, 1975; Rhine, 1972, 1973; Rhine and Kronenwetter, 1972; Weisbard and Goy, 1976). 3) The behavioral repertoire of stumptail macaques living in heterogeneous groups has been studied extensively and is well documented (e.g., Bertrand, 1969; Blurton Jones and Trollope, 1968; Chevalier-Skolnikoff, 1974). The behavioral classifications that have been developed are quite appropriate to the study of drug effects. 4) Stumptail macaques have been used successfully in previous psychopharmacological research and a good foundation of basic information is available (e.g., Bellarosa et al., 1980; Evans, 1975; Lovell et al., 1980; Schlemmer, 1977; Wilson et al., 1977a,b).

Our study group consists of 39 animals, varying in age from newborn to old adult (Table II), and approximates what one would expect in a natural group in the wild (Bertrand, 1969). In the experiments to be described, adult males, weighing between 14.1 and 22.6 kg and ranging in age from 5 to 11.5 years, were selected as subjects to receive drug treatments. To avoid confounding influences due to age, only fully adult males (i.e., animals with fully developed canines, temporal musculature and body mass, and sexual maturity) were used. The males were distributed in rank throughout the dominance hierarchy of the group and included the highest-ranking and the lowest-ranking monkeys in the group.

The group of 39 animals is housed in a 28.4 × 32.7 m outdoor enclosure at the Yerkes Regional Primate Research Center Field Station near Lawrenceville, Georgia (Fig. 1). Positioned along one side of the chain link enclosure is (1) a 4.4 × 12.2 m animal housing unit and (2) an animal capture and isolation unit (Smith, 1981). Easy access to the animals is accomplished by previously entraining the daily movement of the subjects into the capture unit. Experimental animals now enter the capture/isolation unit whenever the door leading into the unit from the outdoor animal enclosure is opened (see Smith, 1981, for details). The capture/isolation unit was designed and fabricated so as to ensure that animals could be manipulated easily and a drug injection protocol could be instituted. Located adjacent to the animal enclosure, the unit consists of a series of tunnels linked together with sliding doors that terminate in a small animal cage with an opening through which the animal can extend an arm for an injection (Fig. 2). The unit is connected to the animal enclosure by two openings so that the animal's path is unidirectional. Target animals—i.e., those to receive drug treatment—receive training via operant conditioning techniques so they will present an arm without coercion and voluntarily accept intramuscular injection in the manner described by Byrd (1973, 1977). Following training, target animals readily accept saline or drug injections on a regular basis without the use of force or aversive stimulation. The ability to ensure regular access to animals in a group without the use of physical force or stress is an important dimension of our research.

During the course of a study, all animals are restricted to the outdoor enclosure on a prescribed daily schedule, weather permitting. While in the outdoor compound, each member of the group can be observed from a tower located 4.27 m above one side of the enclosure (Fig. 3). Data characterizing the behavior of individual animals are collected and stored in a digital format using a commercially available, microprocessor-based data collection device, the Datamyte 900* (Smith and Begeman, 1980). Upon completion of each data collection period, the data are transferred to a PDP 11/23 computer for permanent storage and for data processing. The Datamyte and similar digital encoding devices have revolutionized observational studies by making it possible to record data almost as fast as the behavior occurs or is observed, to record data without having to interrupt direct observation of the experimental subject, and to record data in a format that is compatible with a wide variety of computers so that the observational data can be dumped or transferred directly without an intervening treatment or transformation.

In our studies, subjects are typically observed and data recorded during 15-minute test periods at preselected post-injection times using the focal-animal technique described by Altmann (1974). The focal-animal sampling technique is particularly appropriate for this type of study since it is designed to record all occurrences of behavioral actions and interactions of a specific monkey during each sampling period. A complete chronological record of the focal animal's actions is obtained as well as the actions directed toward him by others. For example, a focal-animal sample on animal A provides a record of interactions where A is either the initiator or recipient of the behavior. This means that during A's observation periods and B's observation periods, all interactions between A and B are recorded; data from either observation period or both may be used to estimate rates of interaction. An illustrative example of the data format and the information comprising each entry are shown in Fig. 4.

*The Datamyte Model 900 is manufactured by Electro/General Corporation, 14960 Minnetonka Industrial Road, Minnetonka, MN 55343.

TABLE I. Reports of Studies of Drug Effects in Groups of Nonhuman Primates

Drug	Species	Group size	Reference	Comments
Sedative-hypnotics				
Ethanol	*Macaca mulatta*	4 adult males	Peretti and Lewis (1969)	Dramatic changes in aggressive behavior in lowest-ranking animal. Lowest-ranking animal exhibited the highest mean daily ethanol consumption. Dominance hierarchy reorganized ($\overline{X}$ daily intake/animal = 19.41 cc).
Ethanol	*M. mulatta*		Cressman and Cadell (1971)	Produced significant increase in play behavior.
Ethanol	*M. mulatta*	2 groups: 3 infant males; 3 infant males and 1 infant female	Kraemer et al. (1981)	Peer separation paradigm; decreased separation-induced despair at low doses, but at high doses alcohol exacerbated the despair response as compared to placebo (1–3 g/kg/day) for three 4-week periods.
Ethanol	*M. nemestrina*	30 individuals	Crowley et al. (1974)	Five males as subjects–produced ataxia without motor slowing, regressive play-fighting typical of juveniles, and substantial increase in ratio of heterosexual-to-autosexual behaviors (0.5–2.0 ml/kg).
Pentobarbital sodium	*M. nemestrina*	30 individuals	Crowley et al. (1974)	Five males as subjects–reduced submissive behaviors and increased dominance-to-submission ratio (0.25–1.0 mg/kg).
Methaqualone	*M. mulatta*	2 males, 6 females	Claus et al. (1980)	Two males and one mid-ranking female drugged. Increase in affiliative acts. Males engaged in previously unrecorded sexual behavior. Female increased in aggressive behavior (10 mg/kg).
Methaqualone	*M. mulatta*	1 male, 2 females	Claus et al. (1981)	Simultaneous administration to all subjects. Five separate experiments. Increase in affiliative behavior from experiment to experiment (10 mg/kg).
Diazepam	*M. mulatta*	4 juveniles	Grove et al. (1977)	Increased proportion of food obtained by submissive animals in both tests between pairs of animals and when drugs were administered to all group members. Similar effects were noted when only the dominant animal of the pair was tested (2.5 mg/kg).
Diazepam	*M. mulatta*	2 males, 2 females	Lovell et al. (1980)	Similar to Lovell et al. (1980) with *d*-amphetamine (2.5 mg/kg).

(continued)

TABLE I. Reports of Studies of Drug Effects in Groups of Nonhuman Primates (continued)

Drug	Species	Group size	Reference	Comments
Stimulants				
Cocaine	*Saimiri sciureus*	4 groups: 6–9 animals per group	Miczek and Yoshimura (1982)	Increased rate, but not duration, of locomotion; increased frequency of stationary posture; reduced incidence of sitting; head-checking increased. Antagonist results similar to those for *d*-amphetamine (10 mg/kg).
Amphetamine	*M. mulatta*	6 juvenile males	Miller et al. (1973)	Increased frequency of social interactions (0.25 mg/kg).
d-Amphetamine	*Callithrix jacchus*	6 adolescents	Scraggs and Ridley (1978)	Dose-dependent increase in small head movements (checking), an almost total suppression of other activities including eating, grooming, playing, object manipulation and social interaction, but little change in amount of movement (2–8 mg/kg).
d-Amphetamine	*C. jacchus*	6 adolescents	Scraggs and Ridley (1979)	Results similar to Scraggs and Ridley (1978). Found head-checking is blocked in a dose-dependent manner by haloperidol, but not by propranolol, aceperone, or diazepam (*d*-amphetamine: 4.0 mg/kg; haloperidol: 0.03–0.18 mg/kg).
d-Amphetamine	*C. jacchus*	6 adolescents	Baker and Ridley (1979)	Chronic administration in increasing doses over 27 days. Head-checking increased, locomotion declined, social contact was reduced, and inactivity increased. Administration of haloperidol (0.01 mg/kg) was given in combination. Destructive self-grooming was eliminated (*d*-amphetamine: 4.0 mg/kg; haloperidol: 0.01 mg/kg).
d-Amphetamine	*Cercopithecus aethiops*	3 male-female pairs	Kjellberg and Randrup (1972)	Reduction in grooming, sexual behavior, and vocalization (0.05–0.37 mg/kg).
d-Amphetamine	*C. aethiops*	1 male, 2 females	Schiørring (1972)	Observed stereotyped self-grooming, "staring" into space, decrease in sexual behavior, and a change in the rank order of the females (0.1–0.15 mg/kg).
d-Amphetamine	*C. aethiops*	3 groups: 1 male and 2 females each	Schiørring (1977)	Disrupted total social interactions. Stereotyped mutual grooming. Rank order changes between females under treatment (0.2 mg/kg).

d-Amphetamine	*C. aethiops*	3 groups of 3 individuals: 1 adult male; 2 adult females	Schiørring (1979)	Disruption of normal social patterns; grooming relations significantly altered. Rank reversal between two females in one of the three groups. Increased stereotyped behavior, social isolation, and long periods of visual fixation noted in all groups. Normal social interaction disrupted at even low doses (0.1–0.7 mg/kg).
d-Amphetamine	*C. aethiops*	2 mother-infant pairs	Schiørring and Hecht (1979)	Individual variability noted but general disruption of normal social contact. Mothers did not engage in ventro-ventral contact with infants nor respond to infant distress calls. Administration to the infants resulted in general disruption of interactions with mother and abolition of distress calling (0.1–0.2 mg/kg).
d-Amphetamine	*S. sciureus*	2 groups: 8 adult males; 4 adult males	Poignant and Avril (1978)	Administered to one or two animals in two groups. Reduced levels of social interaction, increase in number of solitary behaviors (locomotion, self-grooming, feeding, drinking) (0.6 mg/kg p.o.).
d-Amphetamine	*S. sciureus*	4 groups: 6–9 animals per group	Miczek et al. (1981)	Experiment I: Nine adult males used; decreased affiliative responses to familiar group members; decreased attack and threat toward intruding conspecifics; increased frequency of stereotyped movements (3×0.5 mg/kg over 24 hr). Experiment II: Six juvenile animals used; increased time spent away from mother when no unfamiliar male was present (0.3–1.0 mg/kg).
d-Amphetamine	*S. sciureus*	4 groups: 6–9 animals per group	Miczek and Yoshimura (1982)	Amphetamine administered three times in 24-hr period, then chlorpromazine, haloperidol, physostigmine, or vehicle. Increased rate, but not duration, of locomotion; increased frequency of stationary posture; reduced sitting posture; increased head-checking movements. Increase in locomotor frequency antagonized by chlorpromazine, haloperidol, and physostigmine. Chlorpromazine and physostigmine increased duration of locomotion. All antipsychotics increased duration of stationary posture (amphetamine: 1.0 mg/kg; chlorpromazine:0.25–1.0 mg/kg; haloperidol: 0.25–0.50 mg/kg; physostigmine: 0.04–0.08 mg/kg).
d-Amphetamine	*M. mulatta*	3 males, 3 females	Bellarosa et al. (1980)	Increased vocalization, self-grooming, play, social grooming, and aggression (low doses). Higher doses decreased most forms of social interaction. Increased food-getting behavior in subordinate animals when entire group was drugged (0.125–2.0 mg/kg).
d-Amphetamine	*M. mulatta*	2 groups: 3 males, 6 females	Haber (1979)	Increase in submission from low-ranking animals; increase in aggression from high-ranking animals. Increase in percent time spent in proximity to close associates (1.5–2.0 mg).

(continued)

TABLE I. Reports of Studies of Drug Effects in Groups of Nonhuman Primates (continued)

Drug	Species	Group size	Reference	Comments
d-Amphetamine	*M. mulatta*	2 groups: 3 males, 6 females	Haber et al. (1977)	Similar results to Haber (1979).
d-Amphetamine	*M. mulatta*	2 groups: 3 males, 6 females	Haber et al. (1979)	Similar results to Haber (1979).
d-Amphetamine	*M. mulatta*	2 males, 2 females	Lovell et al. (1980)	Low-ranking animals were able to obtain preferred food items when higher-ranking subjects were drugged (0.125–2.0 mg/kg).
d-Amphetamine	*M. mulatta*	2 groups: 22–24 individuals	Burgess et al. (1980)	Significant decrease was observed in nearest neighbor distance and increase in percent touching. Drugged three males (2.0 mg/kg).
d-Amphetamine	*M. mulatta*	4 juveniles	Grove et al. (1977)	Effects on food competition in paired animals. Extensive food capture by least dominant animal when either both subjects were drugged or when only the dominant animal was drugged. When administered to the entire group, submissive animals obtained all food. Dominance status of subjects influenced drug effect (0.5 mg/kg).
d-Amphetamine	*M. mulatta*	14 animals: 3 male-male pairs; 3 female-female pairs; 1 male-female pair	Thierry et al. (1981)	Simultaneous injection to both members of each pair. Significant reduction in social interaction (0.2 mg/kg).
d-Amphetamine	*M. mulatta*	8 juvenile males	Miller (1976)	Acute administration to one individual at a time. Affiliative behavior abolished under treatment; agonistic behavior increased 2.5 times (1.0 mg/kg).
d-Amphetamine	*M. arctoides*	3 males, 3 females	Nail et al. (1980)	Similar results to Lovell et al. (1980) (0.07–1.0 mg/kg).
d-Amphetamine	*M. arctoides*	2 males, 1 female	Miller and Geiger (1976)	Produced decreased social interaction in all subjects. Social grooming was decreased in all subjects; self-grooming and stereotypic behavior increased. Haloperidol blocked stereotypic effects (*d*-amphetamine: 1.0–4.0 mg/kg; haloperidol: 0.7–0.14 mg/kg).

d-Amphetamine	*M. arctoides*		Schlemmer et al. (1980a)	Produced decreases in social grooming, although increased overall activity.
d-Amphetamine	*M. arctoides*	3 males, 3 females	Wilson et al. (1977a)	Administered individually; produced significant decreases in social grooming, playing, and feeding. Increased frequency of sexual presentation in both males and females; frequency of mounting not affected (0.125–2.0 mg/kg).
d-Amphetamine	*M. arctoides*	3 males, 3 females	Wilson et al. (1977b)	Administered to all group members; decreases in frequency of play and feeding, while frequency of sexual presentation and vocalization increased; mounting did not increase. Dominance hierarchy affected (0.125–2.0 mg/kg).
d-Amphetamine	*M. arctoides*	3 males, 3 females	Wilson et al. (1981)	Concurrent administration to all group members for 12 days. Reduction in investigatory and fleeing behaviors and in social proximity, and elimination of social grooming. Agonistic interactions increased as duration of the study increased (1.0 mg/kg).
d-Amphetamine	*M. arctoides*	6 groups: 4–6 animals per group	Schlemmer and Davis (1981a)	Two females treated for 12 days. Treatment increased stereotyped behavior, social withdrawal, scratching, hyperactivity, checking, and initiation of submissive behaviors. Rank differences may have influenced expression. Haloperidol and pimozide antagonized increase in submissive gestures (*d*-amphetamine: 3.2 mg/kg/day; haloperidol:0.57 mg/kg; pimozide: 0.50 mg/kg).
d-Amphetamine	*M. arctoides*	1 male, 4 females	Schlemmer and Davis (1981b)	See Schlemmer and Davis (1981a).
l-Amphetamine	*C. jacchus*	6 adolescents	Scraggs and Ridley (1978)	Similar results to *d*-amphetamine (Scraggs and Ridley, 1978) (4–12 mg/kg).
Meth-amphetamine	*M. nemestrina*	30 individuals	Crowley et al. (1974)	Five males as subjects—decreased dominance-to-submission ratio; produced hyperactivity, stereotypies, and social unresponsiveness (0.0625–0.5 mg/kg).
Meth-amphetamine	*M. fuscata*	7–9 4-year-old males	Machiyama et al. (1970)	Administered to pairs of subjects. Increased behavioral activity of highest-ranking animal; decreased activity of lowest-ranking animal (1 mg/kg).
Diethyl-propion	*M. arctoides*	3 males, 3 females	Bedford et al. (1977)	See Bellarosa et al. (1980) for *d*-amphetamine.

(continued)

TABLE I. Reports of Studies of Drug Effects in Groups of Nonhuman Primates (continued)

Drug	Species	Group size	Reference	Comments
Fenfluramine	*M. arctoides*	3 males, 3 females	Bedford et al. (1977)	Produced anorexia and increase in sexual presentation; presentations were homosexual rather than heterosexual. Masturbation increased in frequency among males. Drug effects may depend on subject's status in dominance hierarchy (1–10 mg/kg).
Methyl-phenidate	*M. arctoides*	3 males, 3 females	Bedford et al. (1977)	Similar effects to that reported for *d*-amphetamine (Wilson et al., 1977a). Produced decrease in grooming and feeding, increase in frequency of sexual presentation (1.0–5.0 mg/kg).
Opiates and antagonists				
Morphine	*S. sciureus*	4 groups: 6–9 animals per group	Miczek et al. (1981)	See results for *d*-amphetamine for details. Juveniles treated with morphine increased time near mother both in and out of presence of unfamiliar male in test situation (0.5–2.0 mg/kg).
Morphine	*M. nemestrina*	30 individuals	Crowley et al. (1974)	Five males as subjects; blocked sexual behavior without impairing motor activity (0.05–0.4 mg/kg).
Morphine	*M. mulatta*		Ternes and Colon (1976)	Alpha male addicted while living in social group. Under treatment, aggression toward group members reduced; affiliative relations increased.
Naltrexone	*Miopithecus talapoin*	2 groups: 8 males, 10 females	Meller et al. (1980)	Treatment significantly reduced sexual behavior in two highest-ranking males. Grooming invitations increased for all males.
Naltrexone	*M. talapoin*	16 individuals: 8 pairs	Fabre-Nys et al. (1982)	Half of each pair drugged twice daily for seven days, the procedure reversed. Significant increase in grooming and grooming invitations (0.25–1.0 mg/kg).
Nalaxone	*M. talapoin*	16 individuals: 8 pairs	Fabre-Nys et al. (1982)	Similar to results for naltrexone (Fabre-Nys et al., 1982).
Antipsychotic agents				
Chlor-promazine	*M. mulatta*	6 juvenile males	Miller et al. (1973)	Decreased frequency of social interactions (0.25 mg/kg).
Chlor-promazine	*M. mulatta*	4 3½-year-old males	McKinney et al. (1980)	Daily administration for 113 weeks. Incidence of huddling increased; locomotory behavior, proximity, and social exploration decreased; aggression increased in initial phases (8–40 mg/kg).
Chlor-promazine	*M. cyclopis*	4 individuals	Hsi-Lin and Shih-Chie (1977)	Treatment reduced overall behavioral output, especially grooming and play (0.25 mg/kg/day).

Hallucinogens				
Δ^9-Tetrahydrocannabinol	*S. sciureus*	2 groups: 2–3 adult males, 3 adult females, 1 infant per group	Miczek (1978)	Introduced intruder animals into resident groups. Drug administration to intruder animals did not alter their reaction to defense, submission, and flight when confronted with nontreated attacking residents. Administration to resident animals reduced frequency of attacks in a dose-dependent manner (0.25–2.0 mg).
Δ^9-Tetrahydrocannabinol	*S. sciureus*	12 dyads	Jones (1976)	Observed drinking, social and competitive behaviors—found total competitive behaviors decreased in frequency when both members received 1.0 mg/kg, but increased when either the lesser member or both members of low competition dyads were treated with 0.25 mg/kg. Noncompetitive social behaviors increased when both animals were drugged (0.25–1.0 mg/kg).
Δ^9-Tetrahydrocannabinol	*S. sciureus*	14 dyads	Kaplan (1979)	Treated mothers from 2 weeks to 6 months after birth. Treated animals showed no differentiation in response to their infants from other infants (5.0 mg/kg).
Δ^9-Tetrahydrocannabinol	*M. mulatta*	2 groups: 22–24 individuals	Burgess et al. (1980)	Used two groups; 3–4 individuals administered simultaneously. Produced decreases in distance between all animals, decreases in nearest neighbor distance, and an index of clumping increased significantly (4 mg/kg).
Δ^9-Tetrahydrocannabinol	*M. mulatta*		Hooley et al. (1979)	Effects different for high- vs. low-ranking subgroups.
Δ^9-Tetrahydrocannabinol	*M. mulatta, M. fascicularis*	8 groups: 3–6 individuals per group	Sassenrath and Chapman (1975)	One subject in each group drugged. Subjects displayed less aggression toward cagemates; however, they were threatened and attacked more frequently by cagemates. Decreased frequency of grooming and play (2.4 mg/kg p.o.).
Δ^9-Tetrahydrocannabinol	*M. mulatta, M. fascicularis*	8 groups: 3–6 individuals per group	Sassenrath and Chapman (1976).	See Sassenrath and Chapman (1975).
Δ^9-Tetrahydrocannabinol	*M. mulatta, M. fascicularis*	6 groups: 3–4 individuals per group	Chapman et al. (1979)	In a long-term chronic study, relative effects predominated for the first 2–3 months. Acute effects diminished, aggressiveness increased, and low-ranking animals began to rise in dominance hierarchy (2.4 mg/kg).

(continued)

TABLE I. Reports of Studies of Drug Effects in Groups of Nonhuman Primates (continued)

Drug	Species	Group size	Reference	Comments
Δ^9-Tetrahydrocannabinol	*M. mulatta*	5 mother-infant dyads	Golub et al. (1981)	Treated mothers chronically through gestation and nursing. Maternal rejection behaviors in treated mothers were initiated earlier than in controls, while infant-initiated maternal approach increased in treated subjects (2.4 mg/kg).
5-Methoxy N,N-dimethyltryptamine	*M. arctoides*	4 individuals	Schlemmer et al. (1977)	Administered to 2 of 4 group members. Found dose-dependent induction of abnormal behaviors and attenuation of normal affiliative behavior. Induced doglike "wet shakes," involuntary limb jerks, stereotyped behavior, and hypervigilance. Dose-dependent decreases in social grooming, submissive behavior, and initiated social activity were noted (5–250 μg/kg).
5-Methoxy-N,N-dimethyltryptamine	*M. arctoides*	3 groups: 4–5 individuals per group	Schlemmer and Davis (1981a)	Administered once per day for 5 consecutive days. Observed increase in submissive behavior without increase in aggressive behavior received. Methiothepin, haloperidol, and trifluoperazine antagonized increase in submissive behavior (5-MeODMT: 0.25 mg/kg; methiothepin: 0.15 mg/kg; haloperidol: 0.2 mg/kg; trifluoperazine: 0.04 mg/kg).
5-Methoxy N,N-dimethyltryptamine and 3 serotonin antagonists (cinanserin, methiothepin, and metergoline)	*M. arctoides*	2 groups: 4–5 individuals	Schlemmer et al. (1979)	All decreased drug-induced limb jerks and body shakes to baseline level. None antagonized the decreased social grooming, and only methiothepin antagonized the increased submissive behavior (0.003–5.0 mg/kg).
N,N-dimethyltryptamine	*Pan troglodytes*	2 groups: 4 individuals per group	Brower and Siegel (1977)	Found dose-dependent increase in locomotion and decrease in social interactions. Subjects did not exhibit the high levels of bizarre behavior sometimes associated with hallucinogens (0.5–4.0 mg/kg).

Other				
Alpha-methyl-para-tyrosine	*M. arctoides*	1 adult male, 4 adult females	Redmond et al. (1971a)	Two females treated for 6 and 7 weeks, respectively. Treated animals initiated fewer social interactions, social and self-grooming decreased, and one female decreased in rank under treatment (160–250 mg/kg).
Alpha-methyl-para-tyrosine	*M. arctoides*	1 adult male, 4 adult females	Redmond et al. (1971b)	See results in Redmond et al. (1971a) above.
Phencyclidine	*M. mulatta*	6 juvenile males	Miller et al. (1973)	Decreased frequency of social interactions. Increased aggression by untreated subjects toward treated subjects (0.25 mg/kg).
Phencyclidine	*M. arctoides*	1 adult male, 4 adult females	Schlemmer et al. (1978)	Four adult females treated. Two different doses (0.025 and 0.5 mg/kg) were studied for 21 days, while a dose of 1.0 mg/kg was studied for 14 consecutive days. Stereotyped behavior was induced in all animals at all doses. Pimozide (0.1 mg/kg) was found to completely antagonize the induced stereotyped behavior.
6-Hydroxydopamine	*M. mulatta*	2 groups: 35 individuals per group	Redmond et al. (1973)	Six adult females and two adult males were used (four were treated). Subjects were treated with 30 mg/kg over 4 days and released. One treated female was found in another social group. Treated animals were attacked when they returned to their group; treated animals initiated fewer threats and attacks, and engaged in less social and self-grooming than controls. Treated male eventually became peripheral to his social group.
Parachlorophenylalanine	*C. aethiops*		Raleigh and McGuire (1980)	Social group. Chronic treatment (14 days) produced irritable, aggressive, and hypermobile animals. Treatment of alpha males resulted in significant reduction in grooming among nontreated subjects. Low-ranking males did not exhibit similar changes (80 mg/kg/day).
Tryptophan	*C. aethiops*		Raleigh and McGuire (1980)	Daily administration for 14 days in males resulted in increased approaching, grooming, resting, and eating, and decreased locomotory, solitary, vigilance, and avoidance behaviors (20 mg/kg/day).
Apomorphine	*M. arctoides*	1 male, 3 females	Schlemmer et al. (1980b)	Significant dose-dependent increases in vigilance behavior, submissive behavior, and vocalizations were found. Grooming was eliminated at all dose levels (0.05–3.0 mg/kg).

(continued)

TABLE I. Reports of Studies of Drug Effects in Groups of Nonhuman Primates (continued)

Drug	Species	Group size	Reference	Comments
Apomorphine	*M. arctoides*	1 male, 4 females	Schlemmer and Davis (1981a,b)	Results similar to *d*-amphetamine (see 1981a), except apomorphine significantly increased locomotion and significantly reduced self-grooming levels.
Piribedil	*S. sciureus*	2 groups: 8 adult males, 4 adult females	Poignant and Avril (1978)	Decreased social and solitary behaviors (5 mg/kg).
Amineptine	*S. sciureus*	2 groups: 8 adult males, 4 adult females	Poignant and Avril (1978)	Significantly increased solitary and social interactions (20 mg/kg p.o.).
Reserpine	*M. mulatta*	2 males, 4 females	McKinney et al. (1971)	One male and two females treated daily for 81 days. Frequency of abnormal posturing increased under drug treatment. Visual exploration decreased, huddling increased, locomotion decreased, and self-mouthing decreased. Dosage increased from 1 mg/kg to 4 mg/kg by 10th day and remained at 4 mg/kg/day for 10 weeks.
Imipramine	*M. mulatta*	2 males, 6 females	Suomi et al. (1978)	One male and two females treated in separation experiment. Treated subjects seemed less severely affected by separation than controls. Chronic treatment reduced passive self-directed behavior and increased exploration (10 mg/kg/day).
Amitriptyline	*S. sciureus*	2 groups: 8 adult males; 4 adult females	Poignant and Avril (1978)	Decreased social and solitary behaviors (5 mg/kg).

A group-scoring observational technique can also be used. This technique involves recording the number of individuals engaged in each of several molar classes of behavior (e.g., aggression, submission, affiliation, general social activity, play, sexual, and self-directed or solitary behavior) at 1-minute time intervals. Table III presents a detailed definition of these classes and their major constituent behaviors. This procedure does not allow the precision or detail of the focal-animal technique, but does allow the collection of group interaction profiles. The number of group members engaged in the molar classes of behavior gives an indication of the overall group interaction

TABLE II. Birthdates of Group Members

Males		Females	
Code	Birthdate	Code	Birthdate
06	1970	01	1961
10	2/04/70	02	4/29/66
13	9/16/72	03	1965
18	2/15/74	04	1965
24	8/11/75	05	1970
26	11/12/76	07	1970
28	12/24/76	08	1970
30	7/04/77	09	1970
33	3/04/78	11	6/06/72
35	8/05/78	12	8/28/72
37	1/22/79	15	1/01/73
38	6/12/80	16	1/22/73
39	7/09/80	17	6/18/73
41	9/05/80	19	9/19/74
42	12/13/80	20	2/20/75
45	4/17/82	21	3/06/75
46	6/01/82	22	3/18/75
49	11/22/82	23	7/13/75
		25	7/05/76
		27	12/16/76
		29	12/31/76
		31	9/09/77
		32	9/20/77
		34	3/22/78
		36	8/10/78
		40	8/11/80
		43	7/31/81
		44	1/20/82
		48	7/05/82

patterns. Hence, we can determine the effect of a drugged individual on other members of the group.

DRUG EFFECTS IN A GROUP

The availability of refined techniques for quantitating behavior, for administering drugs without disrupting ongoing behavior in a group, and for computer processing of data characterizing activities of members of a group has made it possible to study and describe relations between the behavioral effects of drugs and group dynamics. Using the methods described above, we have studied changes in behavior in a group as a consequence of drug administration. Typically, the drug is dissolved in sterile normal saline (0.9%) and injected intramuscularly in a volume of less than 1.0 ml; saline (0.9%) alone serves as a control (placebo) injection. On a given day, each of several adult male subjects will receive either a drug injection, a saline (placebo) injection, or no injection. However, only the experimental animal for that day will receive the drug. Those personnel responsible for data collection do not know whether saline or drug is administered. A drug may be administered 2 days per week, but a given animal is the experimental or drug subject no more frequently than once per week. In general, each dose (0.01–0.30 mg/kg) is studied two or three times in each subject. Immediately after injection in the capture unit, the subjects return to the compound and observations begin. The initial observation period encompasses the first hour post-injection (i.e., four periods of 15 minutes each), and one 15-minute period of observation is scheduled during each hour thereafter for several hours.

A general objective of our research is a detailed characterization of the way in which specific drugs can affect various naturally occurring behaviors exhibited by members of a group. Toward this objective, we have conducted studies to determine the behavioral effects of acutely administered *d*-amphetamine. In order to determine the time course of the behavioral effects of *d*-amphetamine in a group under the conditions of our research laboratory, doses of the drug were administered to two monkeys and changes in self-directed aggressive behavior (e.g., self-biting and hair pulling) were quantitated. Over a range of doses encompassing 1½ log units (0.01–0.30 mg/kg), *d*-amphetamine had dose-dependent effects on self-directed aggression and the resulting dose-effect curves were of an inverted U-shape; i.e., self-directed aggressive behavior increased at intermediate doses and then decreased at higher doses (Fig. 5). The time course of the enhancing effect of *d*-amphetamine was then determined using the dose that produced the maxi-

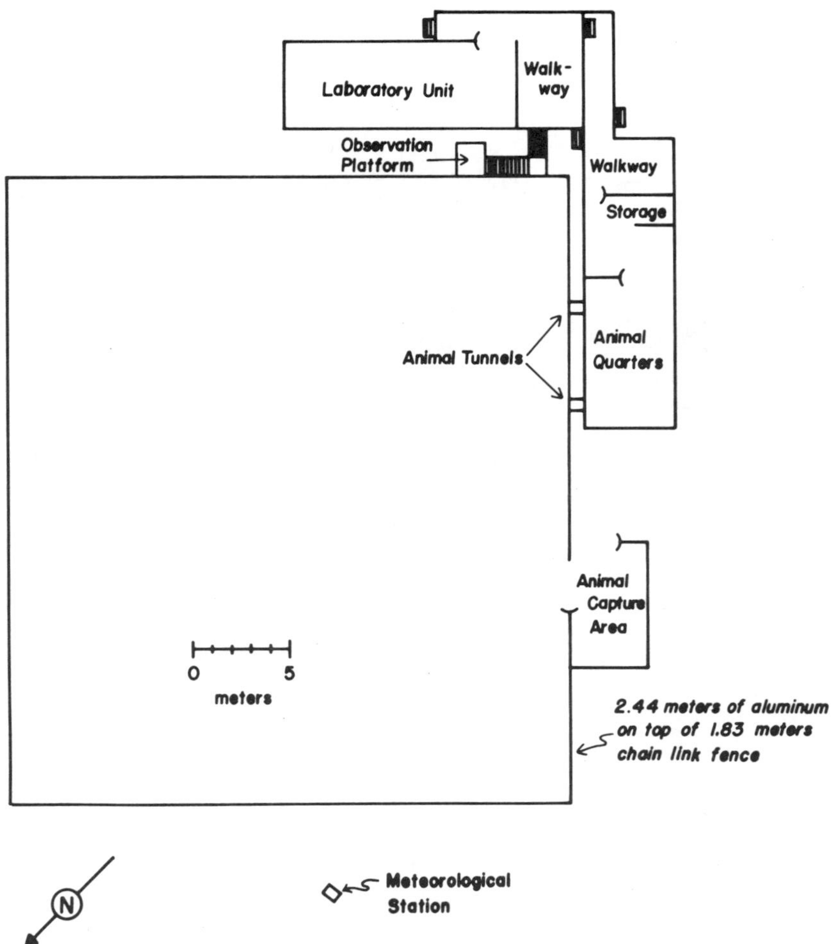

Fig. 1. Line drawing representing an aerial view of the outdoor enclosure, animal quarters, and capture/isolation unit in a group of stumptail macaques.

mum increase in self-directed aggressive behavior. After 0.1 mg/kg, self-directed aggressive behavior increased in frequency to a maximum during a period 45–105 minutes post-injection and then gradually returned to baseline levels as time since injection increased (Fig. 6). The time course of this effect was consistent with time-course data reported by others for *d*-amphetamine.

In addition to the striking effect of *d*-amphetamine in enhancing self-directed aggressive behavior, we have also obtained interesting results in experiments to study changes in affiliative and aggressive behavior as a

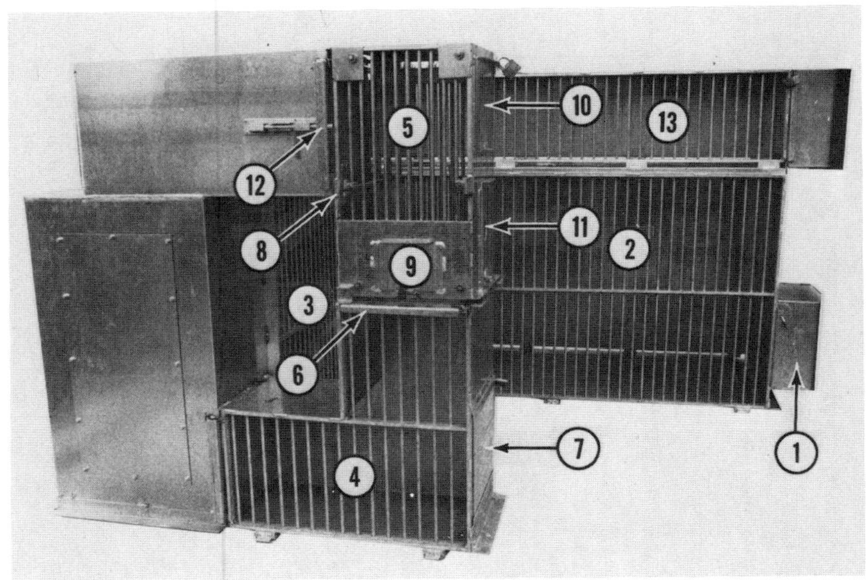

Fig. 2. Close-up view of the animal capture/isolation unit used for effecting drug administration. Specific features include (1) an entrance from the outdoor area, (2) initial holding area, (3) secondary holding area, (4) tertiary holding area, (5) isolation or restraint area, (6) removable bottom panel, (7) lower exit door, (8) restraining or squeeze accessory, (9) removable door to facilitate separation of infant from mother, (10) removable door for accessing sedated subject, (11) small opening for arm extension and drug injection, (12) sliding panel for separating the isolation/restraint area, and (13) exit tunnel to outdoor area. Reprinted by permission from Laboratory Animal Science.

consequence of *d*-amphetamine. Following the administration of a range of doses of *d*-amphetamine (0.003–0.56 mg/kg), four of five adult male subjects showed a dose-related decrease in the rate of affiliative behavior that they initiated. Doses of 0.003–0.03 mg/kg produced little effect, and higher doses (0.30–0.56 mg/kg) decreased rates in a dose-dependent manner (Fig. 7). Moreover, the initiation of affiliative behavior was affected similarly in the high-ranking and low-ranking subjects with no discernible evidence of differ-

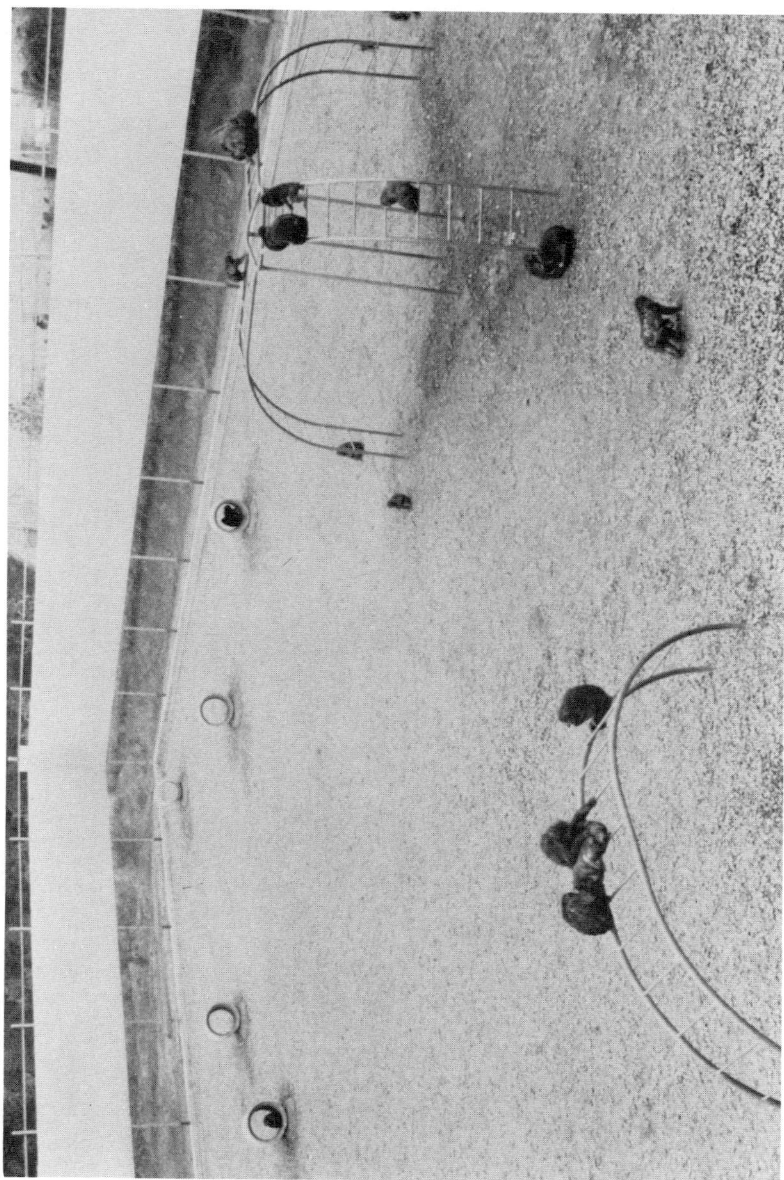

Fig. 3. View of outdoor enclosure from observation tower.

```
H1092479
H202
H31170
H4001
H50800,00000,
001*19,00021,19*030,00024,045*19,00027,040*05,00033,041*05,00036
05*052,00039,128*05,00045,05*043,00047,31*086,00051,31*137,00054
045*31,00058,101*06,00066,
H1092479
H202
H31170
H4001
H50815,00000,
001*19,00007,19*030,00012,045*19,00015,040*05,00018,041*05,00021
05*052,00023,128*05,00026,05*043,00029,31*086,00032,31*137,00036
045*31,00040,101*06,00045,
```

INITIATOR		BEHAVIOR		RECEIPIENT	TIME	DATE	OBSERVER	ENVIRONMENTAL DATA	EXPERIMENTAL CONDITIONS	FOCAL ANIMAL	START TIME	BEHAVIOR CLASS	COUNTER
01	*	001	*	19	80021	092479	02	1170	0	01	0800	1	1
19	*	030	*	01	80024	092479	02	1170	0	01	0800	3	2
01	*	045	*	19	80027	092479	02	1170	0	01	0800	3	3
01	*	040	*	05	80033	092479	02	1170	0	01	0800	3	4
01	*	041	*	05	80036	092479	02	1170	0	01	0800	3	5
05	*	052	*	01	80039	092479	02	1170	0	01	0800	4	6
01	*	128	*	05	80045	092479	02	1170	0	01	0800	2	7
05	*	043	*	01	80047	092479	02	1170	0	01	0800	3	8
31	*	086	*	01	80051	092479	02	1170	0	01	0800	5	9
31	*	137	*	01	80054	092479	02	1170	0	01	0800	2	10
01	*	045	*	31	80058	092479	02	1170	0	01	0800	3	11
01	*	101	*	06	80066	092479	02	1170	0	01	0800	6	12
01	*	001	*	19	815 7	092479	02	1170	0	01	0815	1	1
19	*	030	*	01	81512	092479	02	1170	0	01	0815	3	2
01	*	045	*	19	81515	092479	02	1170	0	01	0815	3	3
01	*	040	*	05	81518	092479	02	1170	0	01	0815	3	4
01	*	041	*	05	81521	092479	02	1170	0	01	0815	3	5
05	*	052	*	01	81523	092479	02	1170	0	01	0815	4	6
01	*	128	*	05	81526	092479	02	1170	0	01	0815	2	7
05	*	043	*	01	81529	092479	02	1170	0	01	0815	3	8
31	*	086	*	01	81532	092479	02	1170	0	01	0815	5	9
31	*	137	*	01	81536	092479	02	1170	0	01	0815	2	10
01	*	045	*	31	81540	092479	02	1170	0	01	0815	3	11
01	*	101	*	06	81545	092479	02	1170	0	01	0815	6	12

Fig. 4. Format of raw data derived during focal-animal observation (top). Data from two periods of observation are preceded by the date (line 1), observer I.D. (line 2), environmental conditions (line 3), focal-animal I.D. (line 4), and time (line 5). Lines 6–8 for each set of data are digitally encoded records of behavioral actions. The edited and formatted forms of the data as they are stored in the PDP 11/23 computer are shown in the bottom half of the figure. Reprinted by permission from Behavior Research Methods and Instrumentation.

ential effect among those monkeys. The only subject in which *d*-amphetamine did not produce a pronounced decrease in rate of affiliative behavior was monkey M-06, a mid-ranking animal. In retrospect, his data suggest that doses even moderately higher than those studied would have produced a decrease in this subject.

In contrast to the monotonically depressive effect of *d*-amphetamine on affiliative behavior initiated by the adult male subjects, the drug markedly increased the rate of aggressive behavior initiated by the same monkeys. *d*-Amphetamine increased the rate of aggressive behavior initiated by the highest- and lowest-ranking monkeys and had little or no effect in the two mid-ranking subjects (Fig. 8). The largest increase in rate was observed in monkey M-13, the highest-ranking animal in the group. Rate of aggression in that monkey increased in direct relation to increases in dose, and at the

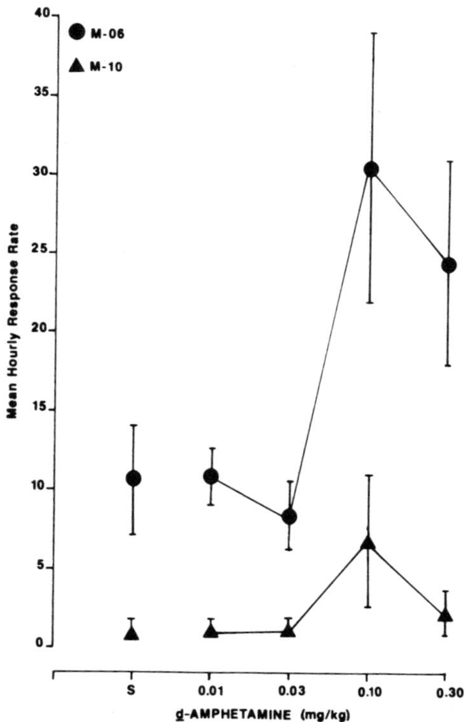

Fig. 5. Effect of *d*-amphetamine on rate of self-directed aggression in two adult male stumptail macaques. Each data point is the mean + SEM based on three administrations. Data points to the left of the dose-effect curves were obtained when saline was administered as a control.

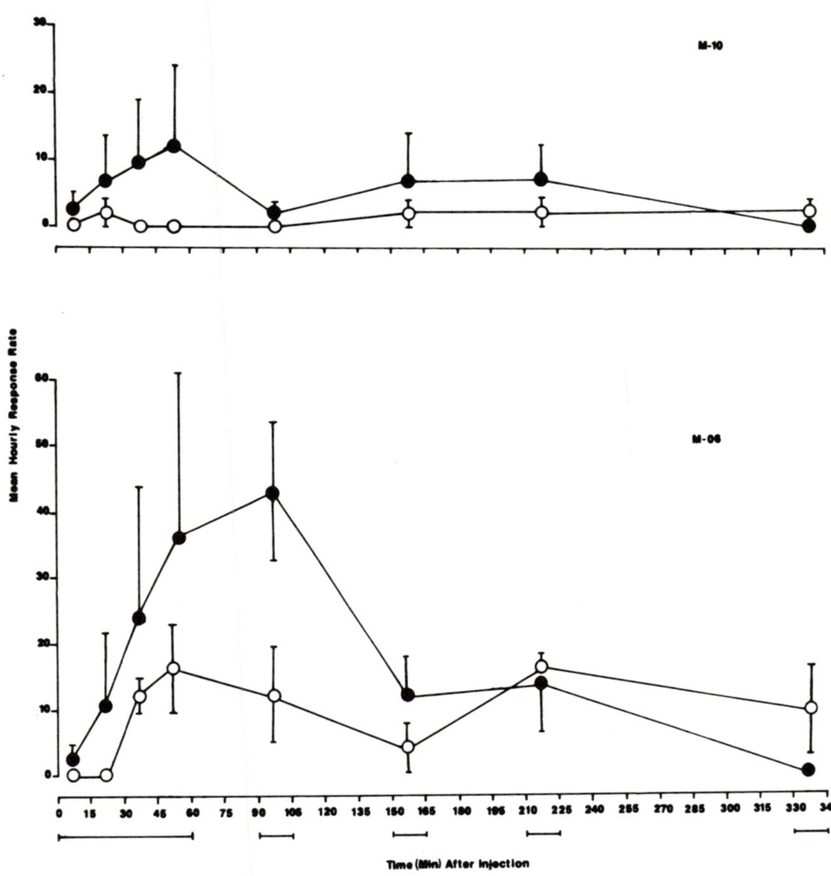

Fig. 6. Time-course effects of *d*-amphetamine (0.1 mg/kg) on self-directed aggressive behavior in monkeys M-10 (top) and M-06 (bottom). Each data point is the mean + SEM based on three administrations of the drug (solid circles) or saline (open circles).

highest dose studied (0.56 mg/kg), rate increased sixfold over the next lowest dose (0.30 mg/kg). *d*-Amphetamine also increased the rate of aggressive behavior initiated by monkeys M-18 and M-24, the two lowest-ranking adult males in the social group, with a dose of 0.003 mg/kg having no effect and a dose of 0.30 mg/kg producing decreases in rate. Intermediate doses increased rate of aggressive behavior two- to eight-fold over saline rates, and the dose-effect curves conformed to inverted U-shaped functions. There was no change in the rate of aggressive behavior over a range of doses of *d*-amphetamine (0.01–0.30 mg/kg) in monkeys M-10 and M-06, the two mid-

TABLE III. Molar Class of Behavior for Group Scan and Focal Animal Data

Molar class	Description
Aggression	Behaviors which cause actual physical injury or signal the potential for harm; also, behaviors which result in priority access to incentives.
Submission	Behaviors which are a reaction to a real or perceived possibility of bodily injury.
General social behavior	Behaviors, such as looking at another animal or moving toward or away from another, which convey no apparent specific social message and which, as a class, indicate general activity.
Affiliation	Positive association with or attempt to safeguard another.
Play	Vigorous, exaggerated but relaxed movements; structurally similar behavior seen in aggressive and submissive classes, but contact is less forceful and silent, and the roles of the interactants are frequently reversed.
Sexual behavior	Behaviors that are regularly a component of heterosexual mating; however, may be scored regardless of the reproductive potential of the participants.
Self-directed behavior	Self-maintenance behaviors, or any behavior directed to the self.

ranking subjects in the group. Their behavioral rates remained in the range of rates observed in the absence of the drug and suggested differential effects of the drug as a function of dominance position in the group.

CONCLUSIONS

The data presented here show that *d*-amphetamine can have qualitatively contrasting effects on two types of naturally occurring behavior in individual monkeys comprising part of a large, heterogeneous social group. *d*-Amphetamine decreased affiliative behavior to as little as one-third of saline control values, and the effect was dose-dependent. In contrast, comparable doses of *d*-amphetamine increased aggression in three of the subjects that exhibited marked decreases in affiliative behavior. Given the relatively uniform decrease in affiliative behavior by the subjects treated with *d*-amphetamine in the present study, it was surprising that the drug had a qualitatively dissimilar effect on aggression in the same subjects. The high- and low-ranking subjects exhibited pronounced, dose-related increases in aggressive behavior at doses that either decreased affiliation or had no effect.

These data also show that *d*-amphetamine can increase the rate of occurrence of self-directed aggressive behavior in individual monkeys living in a

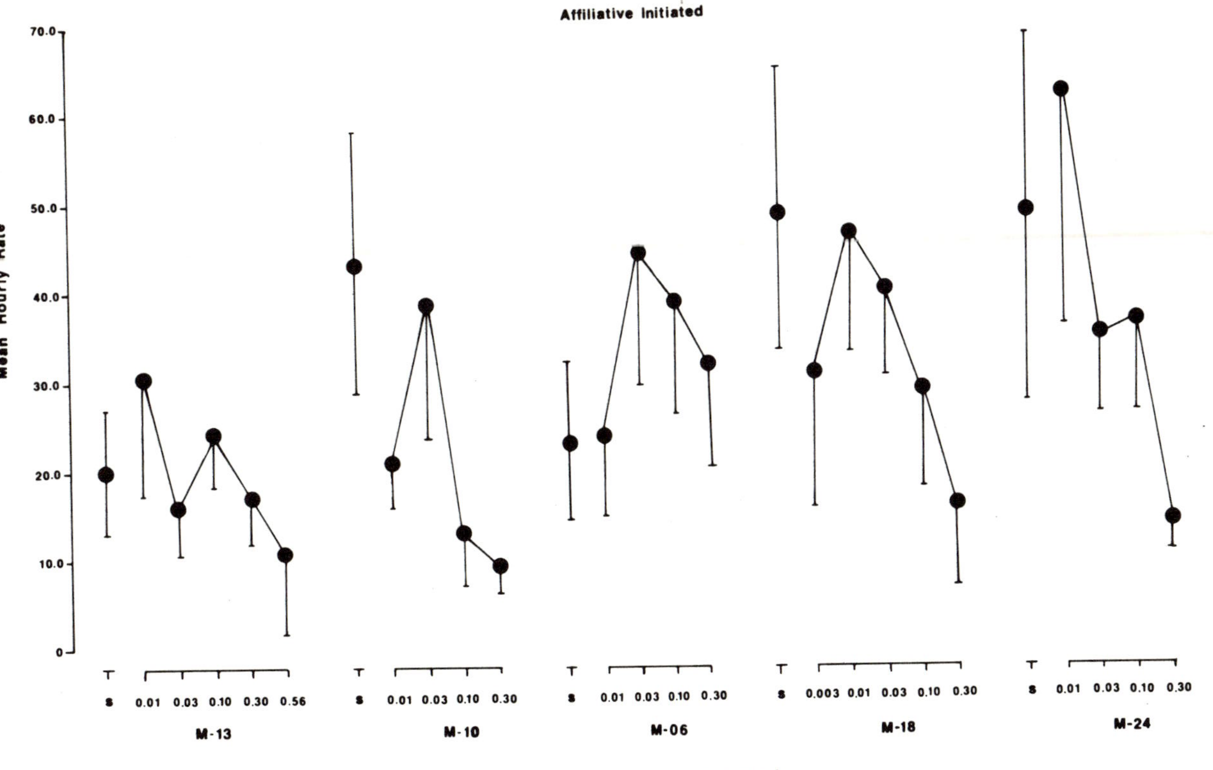

Fig. 7. Effect of *d*-amphetamine on rate of affiliative behavior initiated in five adult male stumptail macaques. Each data point is the mean + SEM based on three adminstrations (except the highest dose for monkey M-13 and the lowest dose for monkey M-18 are based on only one administration). Data ponts to the left of the dose-effect curves were obtained when saline was administered as a control.

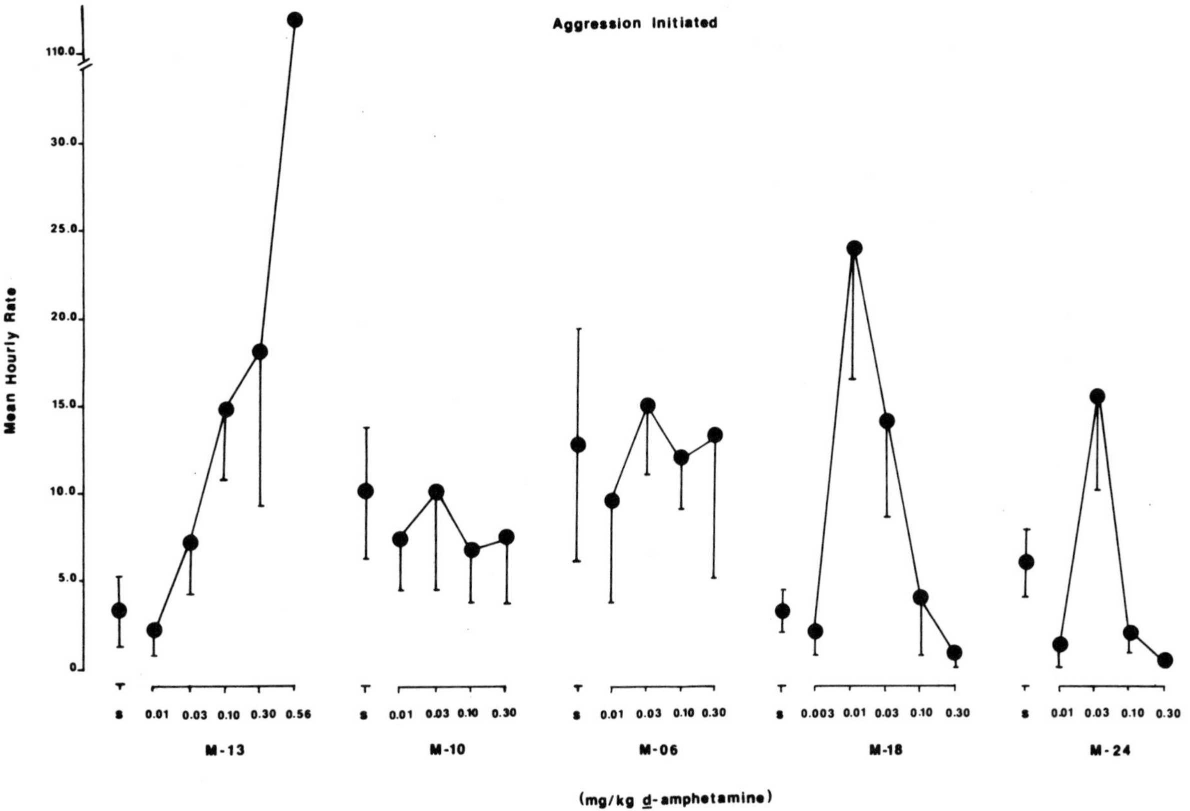

Fig. 8. Effect of *d*-amphetamine on rate of aggressive behavior initiated in five adult male stumptail macaques. Each data point is the mean + SEM based on three administrations (except the highest dose for monkey M-13 and the lowest dose for monkey M-18 are based on only one administration). Data points to the left of the dose-effect curves were obtained when saline was adminstered as a control.

large, heterogeneous social group, and that the enhancing effect is dose-dependent. The effect of *d*-amphetamine on self-directed aggression in group-living monkeys resembles the effect of *d*-amphetamine on conditioned or learned behavior in a variety of animal species. Low doses have little or no effect, higher doses result in an increase in the rate of the behavior, and still higher doses decrease or increase less the rate of the behavior (Byrd, 1973, 1981; Clark and Steele, 1966; Dews and Morse, 1958; Kelleher and Morse, 1968; McMillan, 1969). These results are also consistent with other reports of amphetamine in group-living monkeys (Bellarosa et al., 1980; Miller et al., 1973; Schlemmer, 1977; Schlemmer et al., 1980a; Scraggs and Ridley, 1978, 1979). The similarity of our results and those from laboratories in which individual animals are studied alone suggests a generality of effect of *d*-amphetamine that encompasses a wide range of behavioral conditions.

The foregoing indicates that the observation of nonhuman primates living in a group under seminatural conditions can represent a powerful paradigm for studying the behavioral effects of drugs. We have succeeded in developing a research design that allows for controlled experimentation within a stable, heterogeneous group of nonhuman primates, yet provides quantitative measures of behavior that are precise and readily amenable to a variety of analyses. More importantly, the data presented above show that a drug like *d*-amphetamine can have effects that depend qualitatively on the type of behavior under study and may depend on the social or dominance position of the subject in the group. These phenomena could not easily be studied in individual subjects removed from the group environment, and therefore these results lend credence to the value and importance of studying the behavioral effects of drugs under conditions that more closely approximate those of the human population. The research design we have described allows for closer parallels between animal experiments and the real world of human primates.

ACKNOWLEDGMENTS

This work was supported by US Public Health Service Grants DA-01161, DA-02128, RR-00165, and RR-00167 (Division of Research Resources, National Institutes of Health). P. Peffer-Smith, S. Martin, F. Haman, P. Plant, and F. Kiernan assisted in preparing the manuscript and illustrations.

REFERENCES

Altmann J (1974) Observational study of behavior: sampling methods. Behav 49:227–265

Baker HF, Ridley RM (1979) Behavioural effects of chronic amphetamine and their reversal by haloperidol in the marmoset. Brit J Pharmacol 66:117

Bedford JA, Lovell DK, Wilson MC (1977) The sociopharmacology of fenfluramine (FM), methylphenidate (MP) and diethylpropion (DP) in *Macaca arctoides*. Pharmacologist 19:227

Bellarosa A, Bedford JA, Wilson MC (1980) Sociopharmacology of *d*-amphetamine in Macaca arctoides. Pharmacol Biochem Behav 13:221–228

Bernstein IS (1980) Activity patterns in a stumptail macaque group (*Macaca arctoides*). Folia Primatologica 33:20–45

Bernstein IS, Guilloud NP (1965) Reevaluation of *Macaca speciosa* as a laboratory primate. Lab Primate Newsl 4:5–6

Bertrand M (1969) The behavioral repertoire of the stumptail macaque. A descriptive and comparative study. Bibliotheca Primatologica 11:1–123

Blurton Jones NG, Trollope J (1968) Social behaviour of stumptail macaques in captivity. Primates 9:365–394

Boelkins RC (1967) Determination of dominance hierarchies in monkeys. Psychon Sci 7:317–318

Brower KJ, Siegel RK (1977) Hallucinogen-induced behaviors of free-moving chimpanzees. Bull Psychonomic Society 9:287–290

Burgess JW, Witt PN, Phoebus E, Weisbard C (1980) The spacing of rhesus monkey troops changes when a few group members receive THC or *d*-amphetamine. Pharm Biochem Behav 13:121–124

Byrd LD (1973) Effects of *d*-amphetamine on schedule-controlled key pressing and drinking in the chimpanzee. J Pharm Exp Ther 185:633–641

Byrd LD (1977) Introduction: chimpanzees as biomedical models. In: Bourne GH (ed) Progress in Ape Research. Academic Press, New York, pp 161–165

Byrd LD (1981) Quantitation in behavioral pharmacology. In: Thompson T, Dews PB, McKim WA (eds) Advances in Behavioral Pharmacology Vol. III. Academic Press, New York, pp 75–90

Chapman LF, Sassenrath EN, Goo GP (1979) Social behavior of rhesus monkeys chronically exposed to moderate amounts of delta-9-tetrahydrocannabinol. Adv Biosci 22–23:693–712

Chevalier-Skolnikoff S (1974) The ontogeny of communication in the stumptail macaque (*Macaca arctoides*). Contributions Primatology 2:1–174

Clark FC, Steele BJ (1966) Effects of *d*-amphetamine on performance under a multiple schedule in the rat. Psychopharmacologia 9:315–335

Claus G, Kling A, Bolander K (1980) Effects of methaqualone on social behavior in monkeys (*Macaca mulatta*). Brain Behav Evol 17:391–410

Claus G, Kling A, Bolander K (1981) Effects of methaqualone on social-sexual behavior in monkeys (*M. mulatta*) II. Simultaneously dosed subjects. Brain Behav Evol 18:105–113

Cressman RJ, Cadell TE (1971) Drinking and the social behavior of rhesus monkeys. Quart J Stud Alcohol 32:764–777

Crowley TJ, Stynes AJ, Hydinger M, Kaufman IC (1974) Ethanol, methamphetamine, pentobarbital, morphine, and monkey social behavior. Arch Gen Psychiatry 31:829–838

Dews PB, Morse WH (1958) Some observations on an operant in human subjects and its modification by dextro amphetamine. J Exp Anal Behav 4:359–364

Estrada A, Estrada R (1976) Birth and breeding cyclicity in an outdoor living stumptail macaque (*Macaca arctoides*) group. Primates 17:225–231

Estrada A, Estrada R (1981) Reproductive seasonality in a free-ranging troop of stumptail macaques (*Macaca arctoides*): a five-year report. Primates 22:503–511

Evans HL (1975) Scopalamine effects on visual discrimination: Modifications related to stimulus control. J Pharm Exp Ther 195:105–113

Fabre-Nys C, Meller RE, Keverne EB (1982) Opiate antagonists stimulate affiliative behaviour in monkeys. Pharm Biochem Behav 16:653–659

Fooden J (1967) Identification of the stump-tailed monkey, *Macaca speciosa* I. Geoffrey, 1826. Folia Primatologica 5:153–164

Fooden J (1976) Provisional classification and key to living species of macaques (Primates: *Macaca*). Folia Primatologica 25:225–236

Golub MS, Sassenrath EN, Chapman LF (1981) Mother-infant interactions in rhesus monkeys treated chronically with delta-9-tetrahydrocannabinol. Child Develop 52:389–392

Gouzoules H (1975) Maternal rank and early social interactions of infant stumptail macaques, *Macaca arctoides*. Primates 16:405–418

Grove L, Wilson M, Bedford J (1977) Effects of diazepam and *d*-amphetamine on food competition in rhesus monkey. Pharmacologist 19:228

Haber SN (1979) The effects of amphetamine on social and individual behavior of rhesus macaques. PhD Diss Stanford Univ Stanford

Haber SN, Barchas PR, Barchas JD (1977) Effects of amphetamine on social behaviors of rhesus macaques: an animal model of paranoia. In: Hanin I, Usdin E (eds) Animal Models in Psychiatry and Neurology. Pergamon Press, Elmsford New York, pp 107–115

Haber SN, Berger PA, Barchas PR (1979) The effects of amphetamine on agonistic behaviors in nonhuman primates. In: Usdin E, Kopin IJ, Barchas J (eds) Catecholamines: Basic and Clinical Frontiers. Pergamon Press, Elmsford New York, pp 1702–1704.

Hooley PS, Sassenrath EN, Goo HP, Chapman LF (1979) Computer analysis of primate social behavior: acute effects of Δ^9-THC. Pharmacologist 21:189.

Hsi-Lin Y, Shih-Chie H (1977) Effects of chlorpromazine on social behavior and interaction pattern in Formosan monkey. Chung Yuan J 6:51–58

Jones BC (1976) Effects of Δ^9-tetrahydrocannabinol on squirrel monkey incentive competition behavior. Dissert Abst Intern B36:4204

Kaplan JN (1979) Maternal responsiveness in the squirrel monkey following chronic administration of Δ^9-THC. Pharm Biochem Behav 11:539–543

Kelleher RT, Morse WH (1968) Determinants of the specificity of behavioral effects of drugs. Ergebnisse Physiologie, Biologischen Chemie Experimentellen Pharmakologie 60:1–56

Kjellberg B, Randrup A (1972) Changes in social behavior in pairs of vervet monkeys (*Cercopithecus*) produced by single, low doses of amphetamine. Psychopharmacologia 26:127

Kraemer GW, Lin DH, Moran EC, McKinney WT (1981) Effects of alcohol on the despair response to peer separation in rhesus monkeys. Psychopharm 73:307–310

Lovell DK, Bedford JA, Grove L, Wilson MC (1980) Effects of *d*-amphetamine and diazepam on paired and grouped primate food competition. Pharm Biochem Behav 13:177–181

Machiyama Y, Utena H, Kikuchi M (1970) Behavioural disorders in Japanese monkeys produced by the long-term administration of methamphetamine. Proc Japan Acad 46:738–743

McGuire MT, Raleigh MJ, Brammer GL (1982) Sociopharmacology. Annual Rev Pharm Toxicol 22:643–661

McKinney WT, Eising RG, Moran EC, Suomi SJ, Harlow HF (1971) Effects of reserpine on the social behavior of rhesus monkeys. Diseases Nerv System 32:735–741

McKinney WT, Moran EC, Kraemer GW, Prange AJ Jr (1980) Long term chlorpromazine in rhesus monkeys: production of dyskinesias and changes in social behavior. Psychopharm 72:35–39

McMillan DE (1969) Effects of *d*-amphetamine on performance under several parameters of multiple fixed-ratio, fixed-interval schedules. J Pharm Exp Ther 167:26–33

Meller RE, Keverne EB, Herbert J (1980) Behavioural and endocrine effects of naltrexone in male talapoin monkeys. Pharm Biochem Behav 13:663–672

Miczek KA (1978) Δ^9-tetrahydrocannabinol: antiaggressive effects in mice, rats, and squirrel monkeys. Sci 199:1459–1461

Miczek KA, Yoshimura H (1982) Disruption of primate social behavior by *d*-amphetamine and cocaine: differential antagonism by antipsychotics. Psychopharm 76:163–171

Miczek KA, Woolley J, Schlisserman S, Yoshimura H (1981) Analysis of amphetamine effects on agonistic and affiliative behavior in squirrel monkeys (*Saimiri sciureus*). Pharm Biochem Behav 14:103–107

Miller MH (1976) Behavioral effects of amphetamine in a group of rhesus monkeys with lesions of dorsolateral frontal cortex. Psychopharmacol 47:71–74

Miller MH, Geiger E (1976) Dose effects of amphetamine on macaque social behavior: reversal by haloperidol. Res Comm Psych Psychiatr Behav 1:125–142

Miller RE, Levine JM, Mirsky TA (1973) Effects of psychoactive drugs on non-verbal communication and group social behavior of monkeys. J Per Soc Psych 28:396–405

Nail G, Bedford JA, Wilson MC (1980) The effects of *d*-amphetamine on primate food competition. Pharmacologist 22:293

Peretti PO, Lewis BR (1969) Effects of alcohol consumption on the activity patterns of individual rhesus monkeys and their behavior in a social group. Primates 10:181–188

Poignant JC, Avril A (1978) Pharmacological studies on drugs acting on the social behaviour of the squirrel monkey. Effects of amineptine, piribedil, *d*-amphetamine, and amitriptyline. Drug Res 28:267–271

Raleigh MJ, McGuire MT (1980) Biosocialpharmacology. McLean Hosp J 5:73–86

Redmond DE Jr, Hinrichs RL, Maas JW, Kling A (1973) Behavior of free-ranging macaques after intraventricular 6-hydroxydopamine. Sci 181:1256–1258

Redmond DE Jr, Maas JW, Kling A, Dekirmenjian H (1971a) Changes in primate social behavior after treatment with alpha-methyl-para-tyrosine. Psychosomatic Med 33:97–113

Redmond DE Jr, Maas JW, Kling A, Graham CW, Dekirmenjian H (1971b) Social behavior of monkeys selectively depleted of monoamines. Sci 174:423–431

Rhine RJ (1972) Changes in the social structure of two groups of stumptail macaques (*Macaca arctoides*). Primates 13:181–194.

Rhine RJ (1973) Variation and consistency in the social behavior of two groups of stumptail macaques (*Macaca arctoides*). Primates 14:21–35

Rhine RJ, Kronenwetter C (1972) Interaction patterns of two newly formed groups of stumptail macaques (*Macaca arctoides*). Primates 13:19–33

Sassenrath EN, Chapman LF (1975) Tetrahydrocannabinol-induced manifestations of the "marihuana syndrome" in group-living macaques. Fed Proc 34:1666–1670

Sassenrath EN, Chapman LF (1976) Primate social behavior as a method of analysis of drug action: studies with THC in monkeys. Fed Proc 35:2238–2244

Schiørring E (1972) Social isolation and other behavioral changes in a group of three vervet monkeys (*Cercopithecus*) produced by single, low doses of amphetamine. Psychopharmacologia 26:127

Schiørring E (1977) Changes in individual and social behavior induced by amphetamine and related compounds in monkeys and man. In: Ellinwood EH, Kilbey MM (eds) Cocaine and Other Stimulants. Plenum Press, New York, pp 481–522

Schiørring E (1979) Social isolation and other behavioral changes in groups of adult vervet monkeys (*Cercopithecus aethiops*) produced by low, nonchronic doses of *d*-amphetamine. Psychopharm 64:297–302

Schiørring E, Hecht A (1979) Behavioral effects of low, acute doses of *d*-amphetamine on the dyadic interaction between mother and infant vervet monkeys (*Cercopithecus aethiops*) during the first six postnatal months. Psychopharm 64:219–224

Schlemmer JK, Schlemmer RF Jr, Casper RC, Siemsen FK, Tichy AM, Marszynski TJ, Davis JM (1980a) Age-related differences in behavioral response to chronic *d*-amphetamine treatment in selected members of a juvenile primate social colony. Fed Proc 39:403

Schlemmer RF Jr (1977) Amphetamine-induced behavioral changes in primate social colonies. PhD Diss Univ Illinois Chicago

Schlemmer RF Jr, Davis JM (1981a) Evidence for dopamine mediation of submissive gestures in the stumptail macaque monkey. Pharm Biochem Behav 14:95–102

Schlemmer RF Jr, Davis JM (1981b) Similarities in the behavioral effects of *d*-amphetamine and apomorphine in selected members of a primate social colony. Adv Biosci 31:3–12

Schlemmer RF Jr, Jackson JJ, Preston KL, Bederka JP Jr, Garver DL, Davis JM (1978) Phencyclidine-induced stereotyped behavior in monkeys: antagonism by pimozide. Eur J Pharmacol 52:379–384

Schlemmer RF Jr, Narasimhachari N, Davis JM (1980b) Dose-dependent behavioral changes induced by apomorphine in selected members of a primate social colony. J Pharm Pharmacol 32:285–289

Schlemmer RF Jr, Narasimhachari N, Thompson VD, Davis JM (1977) The effect of a hallucinogen, 5-methoxy N,N-dimethyltryptamine, on primate social behavior. Comm Pharm 1:105–118

Schlemmer RF Jr, Tyler CB, Heinze WJ, Narasimhachari N, Davis JM (1979) The effect of serotonin antagonists on 5-methoxy N,N-dimethyltryptamine (5-MeODMT) induced behavioral changes in primate social colonies. Pharmacologist 21:152

Scraggs PR, Ridley RM (1978) Behavioral effects of amphetamine in a small primate: relative potencies of the *d*- and *l*-isomers. Psychopharm 59:243–245

Scraggs PR, Ridley RM (1979) The effect of dopamine and noradrenaline blockade on amphetamine-induced behavior in the marmoset. Psychopharm 62:41–45

Smith EO (1981) Device for capture and restraint of nonhuman primates. Lab Animal Sci 31:305–306

Smith EO, Begeman ML (1980) BORES: behavioral observation, recording, and editing system. Behav Res Meth Instrumentation 12:1–7

Suomi SJ, Seaman SF, Lewis JK, De Lizio RD, McKinney WT Jr (1978) Effects of imipramine treatment of separation-induced social disorders in rhesus monkeys. Arch Gen Psychiatry 35:321–325

Ternes JW, Colon D (1976) Morphine addiction of an alpha male acts as a leveling factor in intragroup aggression in the rhesus monkey. Bull Psychonom Soc 8:245

Thierry BH, Milhaud CL, Klein MJ (1981) The greeting behavior in nonhuman primates: a new test in pharmacology of social behavior. IRCS Med Sci Library Compendium 9:808–809

Trollope J (1978) Reproduction in a closed colony of *Macaca arctoides*. In: Chivers DJ, Lane-Petter W (eds) Recent Advances in Primatology Vol 2 Conservation. Academic Press, London, pp 243–250

Trollope J, Blurton Jones NG (1970) Breeding the stumptailed macaque, *Macaca arctoides*. Lab Animals 4:161–169

Trollope J, Blurton Jones NG (1975) Aspects of reproduction and reproductive behavior in *Macaca arctoides*. Primates 16:191–205

van Hooff JARAM (1972) An ethologist's view on organization of behaviour and behavioural pharmacology. In: van Noordwijk J (ed) Animal Behavior under the Influence of Psychoactive Drugs. Rijksinstituut voor de Volksgezondheid, Bilthoven, pp 4.1–4.11

Wilson MC, Bailey L, Bedford J (1981) Effects of subacute administration of *d*-amphetamine on nonhuman primate social behavior. Fed Proc 40:277

Wilson MC, Bellarosa A, Bedford J (1977a) Sociopharmacology of *d*-amphetamine (DA) in *Macaca arctoides*. Fed Proc 36:1039

Wilson MC, Bellarosa A, Bedford J (1977b) Sociopharmacology of *d*-amphetamine in *Macaca arctoides* II. Pharmacologist 19:227

Ethopharmacology: Primate Models of Neuropsychiatric Disorders,
pages 33–78

A Comparison of Three Psychotomimetic-Induced Models of Psychosis in Nonhuman Primate Social Colonies

R. Francis Schlemmer and John M. Davis

Department of Research, Illinois State Psychiatric Institute, Chicago, Illinois 60612

INTRODUCTION

One of the more fruitful approaches used to study psychosis in animals has been the study of behavioral changes induced in animals by psychotomimetic drugs. Although a number of drugs under appropriate conditions have been reported to induce psychosis in normal individuals (cf. Snyder, 1972), psychotic behavior induced by three classes of these substances most closely resembles symptoms of endogenous psychosis: (1) the psychomotor stimulants which include the amphetamines and cocaine, (2) the arycyclohexylamines, including phencyclidine (PCP or Angel Dust) and ketamine, and (3) the hallucinogens or psychedelics such as LSD and mescaline. It is also these drugs which have been studied most extensively in animals in regard to psychosis.

Over the past 10 years, we have studied the behavioral effects of representative drugs from each of the three classes of psychotomimetics in selected members of adult stumptail macaques social colonies. With each drug, we have attempted to replicate in monkeys the same conditions which have been known to induce psychosis in humans. In this chapter, the effects of d-amphetamine, phencyclidine (PCP), and several hallucinogens on nonhuman primate social and solitary behavior will be compared and evaluated as animal models of psychosis. Only significant behavioral changes which may have relevance to human psychosis will be discussed; however, more detailed reports of these experiments have been published elsewhere as noted throughout the text.

GENERAL METHODS

The subjects in all experiments were adult stumptail macaques *(Macaca arctoides)*. This species was selected because of the highly affiliative nature of stumptail macaques and the relative ease at which they could be handled when necessary. *Macaca arctoides* is native to Southeast Asia. They are particularly noted for their rich variety of social interaction in their natural habitat and in the laboratory setting (Bertrand, 1969; Chevalier-Skolnikoff, 1974). Jolly (1972) has noted that in the wild, stumptail macaques are among the most affiliative nonhuman primates, spending a large percentage of their waking hours engaged in social interaction. Stumptails typically travel in troops and form a rather stable, well-defined hierarchy which appears to carry over to laboratory-formed groups as well. Together, these characteristics of the stumptail macaque provide a particularly good species for studies in which drug-induced alterations of social behavior are of primary interest.

The animals were continuously housed in colonies of 4–6 members in large group cages (1.5 × 2.5 × 3.5 m or 1.75 × 3.0 × 5.25 m) throughout an experiment. Prior to the initiation of any experiment, each colony was allowed sufficient time to stabilize, usually 4–6 months. During an experiment, individual monkeys were only briefly removed from their home cages for weekly weighings, when drug administration required nasogastric intubation, or when the animal's safety was considered in jeopardy owing to physical injury or illness. In the latter instance, the experiment was either canceled and restarted or temporarily discontinued. Throughout the study, each group received a generous supply of food (Purina Monkey Chow) supplemented with fruits and vegetables, and had access to water continuously. The status of the monkeys during the experiments was monitored at all times by licensed veterinarians who were experienced in treating nonhuman primates and who had the right to intervene or discontinue an experiment when they believed it was necessary.

Each experiment began with observation of undrugged or normal behavior which was used to determine baseline behavior. This ranged from 4 to 50 days, but typically was 2 weeks. During this time, normal saline or drug vehicle (acidified saline) was injected or tap water administered nasogastrically at a specified time prior to behavioral observation to control for the drug administration process. The drug administration which followed varied with each experiment and therefore will be discussed in relation to each drug class.

In general, the behavioral observation technique was similar for each experiment with the exception of the PCP experiments. A 1-hour behavioral observation was conducted on specified days (usually 5–7 days per week) by the same experienced "blind" observer throughout an individual experiment. During that time, the observer quantified and recorded the behavior of each monkey in the colony from a checklist (Table I) which was originally 28, but later expanded to 48 social, solitary, and abnormal behaviors for this species using the focal sampling technique. Each monkey was observed in rotation for 30 seconds every 5 minutes for 60 minutes. Scores from the twelve 30-second intervals were summed for each behavior for the individual animals, which represented the daily score for each monkey. In addition, the total number of body shakes that occurred for each animal during the entire observation period was recorded. The PCP experiments, which were completed early in our series of studies, were conducted with the group sampling technique. Each of the 20 behaviors was scored by frequency or duration. The latter was recorded using a clock where one unit equaled 20 seconds.

All data are presented as the daily score or the mean daily score for each behavior unless otherwise noted. Data for each behavior were analyzed using a two-way or three-way (partially crossed) analysis of variance. Means within the analysis were compared using the least significant difference method.

TABLE I. Behavioral Checklist

I. General assessment

A. Active or passive: each 30-second interval marked active when social and/or solitary activity occurred excluding the non-active behaviors of huddling, contact, staring, vigilance or vocalization.

B. Distancing: during each 30-second scoring period for an individual monkey, the observer notes whether the closest animal was at a distance *greater than or less than three feet* away from the animal being scored for most of the 30 seconds. For each scoring period, the monkey received one score for *either* greater than or less than three feet from the nearest animal and the *total* of the distance categories always equalled 12. To avoid repetition, distancing scores for each monkey are only reported for *distance greater than three feet*.

II. Social behavior

A. Affiliative

1. Social groom: discrete picking or spreading of the hair of another animal.
2. Approach: when one monkey walks or runs toward another animal from a distant point to within an arm's length distance so that one animal could touch the other animal.
3. Social present: presentation of a body part to another monkey for the purpose of grooming.
4. Social explore: oral or manual examination of a body part of another animal, usually the genital area.
5. Body jerk: quick, voluntary jerks of the body while the animal is looking directly at another monkey who is in close proximity.
6. Huddle: when two animals are sitting together where at least one monkey's arm is embracing the other animal.
7. Contact: when the body of one animal is touching the body of another animal, but no social interaction or huddling takes place.

(continued)

TABLE I. Behavioral Checklist (Continued)

B. Aggressive
1. Threat: eye-brows up, ears back, mouth open, stare at another animal sometimes accompanied by a specific, low-pitched vocalization.
2. Chase: pursuit of another animal for purpose of attack.
3. Attack: vigorous, hostile biting and/or hair pulling of another monkey.
4. Limb bite: non-vigorous bite of an outstretched arm or leg of another animal.

C. Submissive
1. Lipsmack: a submissive gesture made by smacking the lips and/or teeth together rapidly.
2. Submissive present: presentation of genitalia with the tail erect to another animal as a submissive gesture.
3. Yield: movement away from a location in the cage so that a more dominant monkey may assume that location. Reciprocal of displace.
4. Grimace: smile-like face in response to threatening situation.
5. Limb present: presentation of an arm (usually) or leg to another animal for a limb bite. A limb bite does not necessarily follow.

D. Sexual
1. Mount: one monkey climbing atop another animal where all appendages of the mounting monkey are off the floor or perch and the animal is totally supported by the mounted monkey.
2. Intromission: insertion of a penis into a vagina.
3. Ejaculation: scored by noting a series of vocalizations from the male during copulation and evidence of ejaculate on the penis after the dismount.

III. Solitary behavior

A. Food forage
1. Handle food: manipulation of food with the hands.
2. Chew food: mastication of food.
3. Drink: drinking water from water spout.

B. Active
1.* Locomotion: the number of ambulations by the observed monkey from one point to a distant point.
2. Self groom: discrete picking or spreading of monkey's own hair.
3.* Scratch: scratching of a single specific location (for example, scratching of the leg followed by scratching of the arm would be scored as two distinct scratches).
4.* Checking (vigilance): the number of observed changes of visual field determined by head and eye movements.
5.* Yawn: involuntary opening of mouth wide for intake of air.
6.* Vocalization: the number of clearly audible sounds emanating from the observed animal.
7. Vomit: emesis into pouches or out of mouth.
8. Pick genitalia: manipulation or grooming of genitals excluding masturbation.
9. Masturbation: self-initiated manipulation of genitalia other than discrete grooming of the area.

(continued)

TABLE I. Behavioral Checklist (Continued)

C. Inactive

1. Stare: fixation of eyes on no apparent object with a blank, expressionless face for greater than 15 seconds.
2. Lying down: assumes horizontal position on cage floor or perch.
3. Resting with eyes open: maintaining a relaxed posture initiating no active behaviors for 30 seconds while eyelids remain open for more than half of the 30 seconds.
4. Resting with eyes closed: maintaining a relaxed posture initiating no active behaviors for 30 seconds where the eyelids are shut for more than half of the 30 seconds.

IV. Abnormal behavior

A. Social

1. Inappropriate response: any situation where an animal initiates or acknowledges a social cue from another animal improperly. For example, a dominant animal responds to a submissive present from a subordinate animal with a submissive present.

B. Social or solitary

1. Stereotyped behavior: repetitive, often rhythmic fragments of behavior performed continuously over a period of time that interrupt normal behavior. Each form of stereotypy is counted separately.
2. Rocking: moving back and forth in a swaying movement. May or may not be associated with a series of threats.

C. Solitary

1.* Limb jerks: involuntary myoclonic spasm of an extremity, usually the leg.

2.* Body shake (wet shake): a specific response similar to that of a dog after emerging from water.

3. Posturing: a cataleptiform posture where the animal maintains an unnatural stance for more than 15 seconds.
4. Dyskinesia: abnormal, repetitive localized movements of specific muscle groups usually involving the mouth.
5. Self bite: biting of own arm or body.
6. Ataxia: irregular, uncoordinated or staggering movement when walking, running or standing is attempted.
7. Other: space is provided for any other abnormal behaviors noted by the observer (e.g., ptosis, play by adult animals).

*Scored by the frequency of occurrence during each 30 second observation interval. All other behaviors scored by presence (1) or absence (0) during the 30-second observation interval.

d-AMPHETAMINE EXPERIMENTS

Chronic administration of large doses of amphetamines to normal individuals often leads to the induction of amphetamine psychosis. Many clinicians believe that amphetamine psychosis is very similar to, if not virtually indistinguishable from, paranoid schizophrenia (Connell, 1958; Snyder, 1972; Angrist et al., 1974). The hallmark characteristics of this disorder are paranoid ideation, autistic behavior or withdrawal, hyperactivity, and assorted stereotypies which all occur in a setting of clear consciousness and correct orientation (Connell, 1958; Snyder, 1972; Davis and Schlemmer, 1980). Visual, auditory, and tactile hallucinations have been reported in a number of individuals. In addition, schizophrenic patients are particularly sensitive to the psychotogenic effects of amphetamines. When low doses of either amphetamine isomer or methylphenidate (Ritalin) were administered to schizophrenic patients, their psychosis was markedly worsened within minutes (Janowsky and Davis, 1974). Moreover, the patients believed that the change was an actual deterioration of their behavioral status rather than a distinct drug-induced phenomenon.

One of the key aspects of amphetamine psychosis is that this syndrome has been most frequently reported in individuals who had been on an "amphetamine binge"; that is, amphetamine users who had administered relatively large doses frequently over a period of several days. We attempted to replicate the amphetamine binge in monkeys by administering a sustained release preparation of d-amphetamine to provide around-the-clock blood levels of the drug for 12 days.

Methods

In the amphetamine experiments, two females from each of six social colonies received amphetamine treatment. d-Amphetamine sulfate in time-release form (Dexedrine Spansules, Smith, Kline, French, Philadelphia, PA), 1.6 mg(base)/kg, was administered nasogastrically every 12 hours (6 AM and 6 PM) for 12 consecutive days. The same two monkeys received tap water nasogastrically at 6:00 AM during the baseline period which preceded each treatment period. Behavioral observation was conducted at the same time each day for individual experiments once daily for 12 consecutive days during treatment and on specified days during baseline.

Upon completion of five of the amphetamine experiments, a second experiment followed where an antipsychotic or other relevant psychotropic drug was tested alone then concomitantly with d-amphetamine in the same two monkeys that had previously received amphetamine treatment. Following a drug "wash-out" period from amphetamine of no less than 3 weeks, the antipsychotics haloperidol, chlorpromazine, pimozide, or clozapine, or the nonantipsychotics diazepam or promethazine, were administered alone for 4–21 days followed immediately by concomitant treatment with the antipsychotic or nonantipsychotic plus d-amphetamine. Haloperidol (McNeil, Ft. Washington, PA), 0.57 mg(base)/kg, was administered once daily for 21 days followed by 12 days of haloperidol plus d-amphetamine. Chlorpromazine (Smith, Kline, French), 11.25 mg(base)/kg, and pimozide (Mc-

Neil),0.50 mg(base)/kg, were each given once daily for 14 days followed by each drug plus d-amphetamine for 12 days. Clozapine (Sandoz, Hanover, NJ), 7.0 mg(base)/kg, was given in two equally divided doses daily for 14 days followed by concomitant treatment with d-amphetamine for 12 days. Diazepam (Roche, Nutley, NJ), 0.50 mg(base)/kg, was administered in two divided doses daily for 5 days followed by concomitant treatment with d-amphetamine for 5 days. Promethazine (Wyeth, Philadelphia, PA), 11.25 mg(base)/kg, was given in two divided doses for 4 days followed by concomitant treatment with d-amphetamine for 4 days. All drugs were administered nasogastrically.

In the final amphetamine experiment, a cross-over study was conducted. Initially, two females from a colony of five monkeys received the 12-day d-amphetamine treatment. Six weeks later, the other two females from the colony received identical amphetamine treatment. The dominant male remained untreated. Following a 1-year drug wash-out period, the experiment was repeated substituting the direct dopamine receptor agonist apomorphine for d-amphetamine. Apomorphine (Lilly, Indianapolis, IN), 0.5 mg(base)/kg, was administered intramuscularly at 10:30 AM (15 minutes prior to observation) and at 2:30 PM for 12 consecutive days using the same crossover technique used in the first part of the experiment.

Results

Chronic d-amphetamine administration induced hyperactivity, abnormal behaviors, and general disruption of baseline interactions with other members of the colony in all treated monkeys. Throughout the amphetamine study, though, we were particularly impressed by the large individual variation in response to d-amphetamine. This has also been noted in other monkey studies (Machiyama et al., 1970; Schiorring, 1977) and with amphetamine psychosis in humans as well (Davis and Schlemmer, 1980). Therefore, although several amphetamine-treated monkeys often displayed a particular behavioral change, others did not or may have even had a change in the opposite direction. To illustrate this point, the behavioral response of four amphetamine-treated monkeys is shown for each behavioral change represented in Figs. 1–3 and 5–7. The graphs depict three monkeys that displayed a response to amphetamine typical of most treated monkeys and a fourth (lower right) that had an "atypical response."

The major change noted in social behavior was progressive social withdrawal, reflected best by the grooming and distancing scores. d-Amphetamine reduced or eliminated social grooming (heterogroom) in 12 of 13 monkeys while it increased self-grooming (autogroom) in 11 monkeys (Fig.

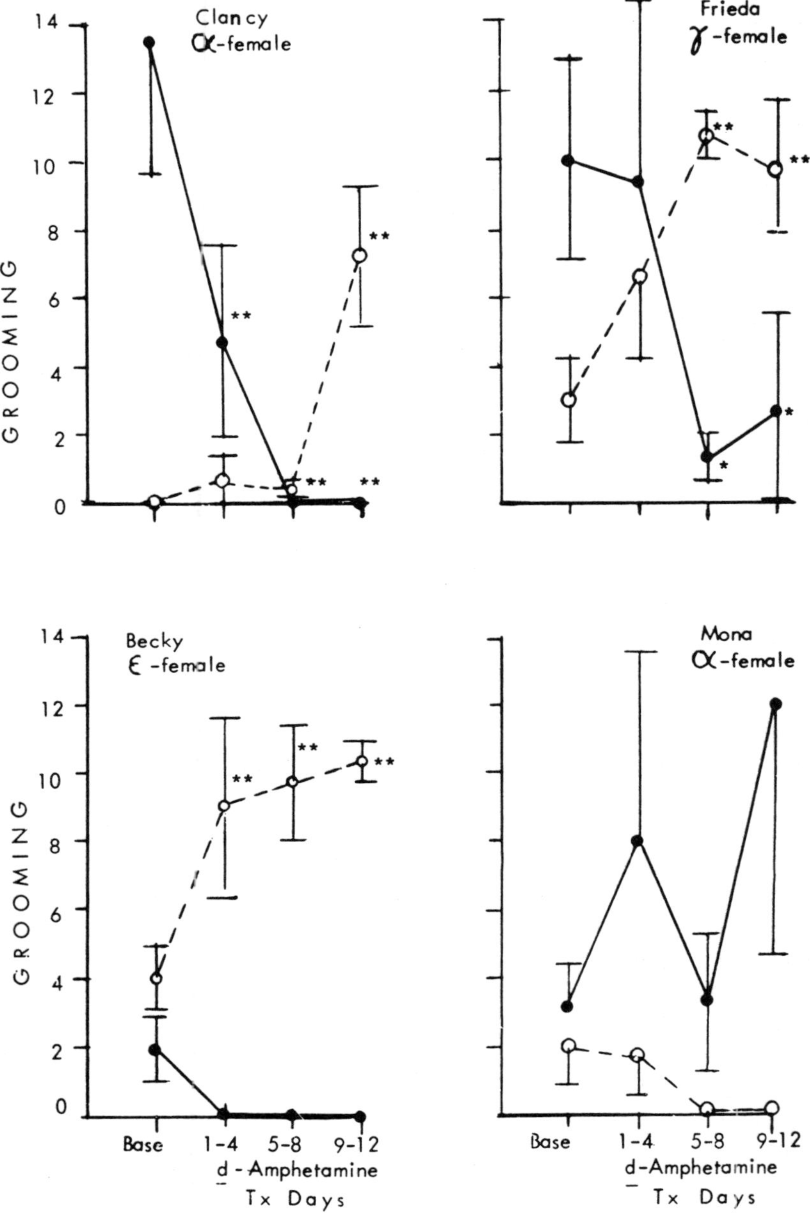

Fig. 1. The effect of chronic d-amphetamine treatment on initiated grooming scores by four treated monkeys. Each point represents the mean ± SEM for baseline (base), early (days 1–4), mid (days 5–8), and late (days 9–12) d-amphetamine treatment. Each animal's hierarchical rank within her respective colony is noted under each name. The solid line represents social groom and the dotted line represents self-groom. Statistical significance is denoted by * — $p < 0.05$ or ** — $p < 0.01$ when compared to the respective baseline.

1). The self-groom seen during amphetamine treatment was almost always stereotyped. Distancing scores reflect the number of observation intervals in which the closest monkey was more than 3 feet (an arm's length for this species) from the treated monkey. Thus, the highest isolation score would be 12. d-Amphetamine increased distancing scores, often dramatically, in 12 of 13 treated monkeys (Fig. 2). Lower-ranking monkeys tended to become isolated earlier in treatment that higher-ranking monkeys. The exception was the alpha female, Mona, who had reduced distancing scores. During amphetamine treatment, Mona displayed an interesting shadowing behavior where she continually followed control monkeys around the cage, resulting in decreased distancing scores. Note that Mona also had an atypical grooming response during amphetamine administration (Fig. 1).

Another significant behavioral change induced by chronic d-amphetamine was an increase in the number of submissive gestures given by several (9/13) treated animals (Fig. 3). In most cases, this change was not accompanied by a significant increase in the number of aggressive gestures received by these animals, suggesting that the increase in submissive responses was not elicited by aggression directed toward the treated monkeys by control animals. Interestingly, higher-ranking females were more affected than lower-ranking females (Fig. 4).

The most consistent changes in solitary behavior induced by amphetamine included the induction of stereotyped behavior and a large increase in checking behavior or vigilance. A behavior was considered to be stereotyped when it became a repetitive (often rhythmical) fragment of behavior which occurred in the virtual absence of other behaviors. "Checking" is the number of obvious changes in visual field as determined by head and eye movement. All amphetamine-treated animals developed intense stereotyped behavior (Fig. 5). Most stereotypies involved solitary forms of behavior (self-grooming, scratching, licking), but occasionally social behavior also became stereotyped (stereotyped threatening, submissive presents, social grooming). Higher-ranking monkeys developed more social stereotypies than lower-ranking animals. In total, more than 20 distinct behaviors became stereotyped throughout the amphetamine experiments. Checking increased significantly for all treated monkeys at least during one treatment period during chronic amphetamine administration (Fig. 6). Tolerance developed to d-amphetamine-induced checking within the 12-day treatment in all but one animal (Cheryl). However, tolerance did develop in the latter case by day 17 when treatment was continued. One other relevant change in solitary behavior was the intense scratching seen in nine amphetamine-treated monkeys (Fig. 7). Occasionally scratching became so intense that scarring occurred.

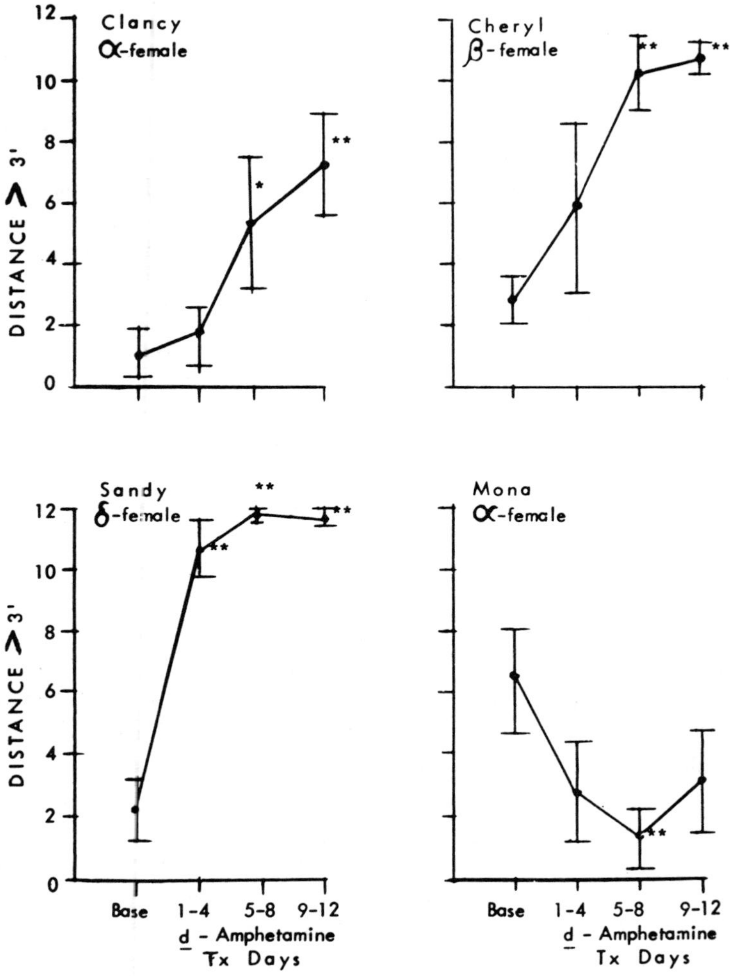

Fig. 2. The effect of chronic d-amphetamine treatment on distancing scores for four treated monkeys. Each point represents the mean ± SEM for baseline (base), early (days 1–4), mid (days 5–8), and late (days 9–12) d-amphetamine treatment. Each animal's hierarchical rank within her respective colony is noted under each name. Statistical significance is denoted by * — $p < 0.05$ or ** — $p < 0.01$ when compared to baseline.

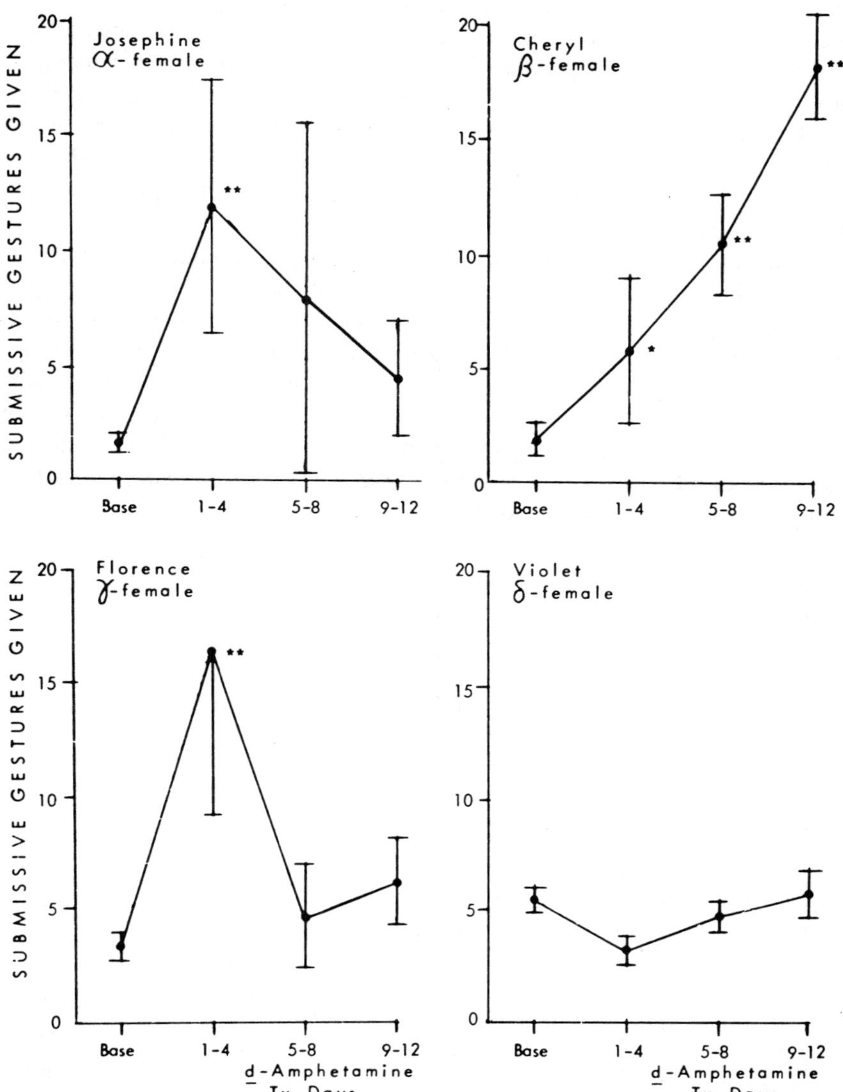

Fig. 3. The effect of chronic d-amphetamine treatment on submissive gestures given by four treated monkeys. Each point represents the mean ± SEM for baseline (base), early (days 1–4), mid (days 5–8), and late (days 9–12) d-amphetamine treatment. Each animal's hierachical rank with her respective colony is noted under each name. Statistical significance is denoted by * — $p < 0.05$ or ** — $p < 0.01$ when compared to baseline. (From Schlemmer and Davis, 1981b.)

Although significant changes in other behaviors in some monkeys were noted, these changes were seen only with one to three monkeys. Some monkeys occasionally displayed bizarre behaviors which were not recorded but may be relevant. These included eye tracking then reaching and grabbing into the air at apparently imaginary objects by three monkeys, repeatedly peering under the cage when nothing was there by two monkeys, shadowing behavior by two monkeys, and submissive presents simultaneously to each other by two sets of two treated monkeys.

When antipsychotic agents were administered in combination with d-amphetamine, amphetamine-induced hyperactivity was greatly reduced. Antipsychotic agents had the most profound effect on amphetamine-induced abnormal behaviors such as stereotypy (Fig. 8) and increased checking. Note, however, that clozapine was not as effective as the other antipsychotics, similar to reports in rodents (Burki et al., 1975). The antipsychotics were less consistently effective in restoring the disruption of social interaction to baseline levels. However, the reduction in initiated social groom induced by d-amphetamine was returned to or in the direction of baseline by the anti-

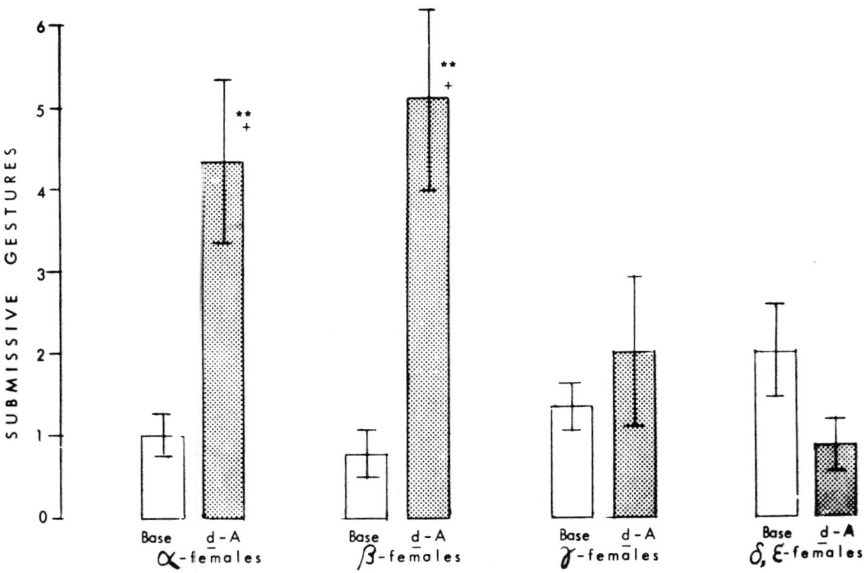

Fig. 4. The effect of hierarchical rank on submissive gestures given by d-amphetamine-treated monkeys. Each bar represents the mean ± SEM score for two to four monkeys for baseline and treatment. Statistical significance is denoted by: ** — $p < 0.01$ when compared with respective baseline or + — $p < 0.05$ when compared with d-amphetamine treatment of delta and epsilon females. (From Schlemmer and Davis, 1981b.)

psychotics in most animals (Fig. 8). Similarly, elevated distancing scores approached baseline levels with concomitant antipsychotic treatment in most treated monkeys (Fig. 8). However, two nonantipsychotic agents tested failed to significantly antagonize amphetamine-induced behavior as seen with stereotyped behavior (Fig. 9). Neither promethazine, a phenothiazine antihistamine, nor the anxiolytic diazepam antagonized amphetamine-induced stereotypy in two monkeys.

When the effects of chronic d-amphetamine were compared with those seen with chronic apomorphine, it was evident that apomorphine not only induced hyperactivity comparable to d-amphetamine, but also induced a behavioral syndrome which in general was strikingly similar to the amphetamine syndrome. Both drugs significantly reduced initiated social grooming and increased distancing scores (Fig. 10). Both apomorphine and d-amphetamine significantly increased the number of submissive gestures given by treated monkeys approximately threefold during the early days of treatment (Fig. 10). Both drugs induced stereotyped behavior, but at the apomorphine dose selected (0.5 mg/kg), there was significantly less stereotypy with apomorphine than d-amphetamine (Fig. 10). However, other studies from our laboratory have demonstrated that larger doses of apomorphine (3 mg/kg) induced more intense stereotypy comparable to the levels seen with d-amphetamine in this experiment (Schlemmer et al., 1980). Apomorphine and d-amphetamine also induced comparable responses in hyperactivity and increased checking, but not locomotion and self-grooming (Schlemmer and Davis, 1981a).

Discussion

When evaluating the amphetamine syndrome in monkeys as an animal model of psychosis, one must consider that this paradigm should better model amphetamine psychosis than schizophrenia. Therefore, any comparisons between the behavioral changes in monkeys and schizophrenia symptomatology are highly dependent on the similarities between amphetamine psychosis and schizophrenia. Fortunately, many investigators believe there are many commonalities between the drug-induced and endogenous psychopathologies (Connell, 1958; Griffith et al., 1972; Snyder, 1972; Angrist et al., 1974; Davis and Schlemmer, 1980). Similar inducing conditions were used to elicit the behavioral changes seen in monkeys in these experiments as those which frequently induce amphetamine psychosis in humans—i.e., large, repeated doses of amphetamine.

Some of the significant symptoms of amphetamine psychosis involve disturbances of thought processes and are difficult to detect in animals with

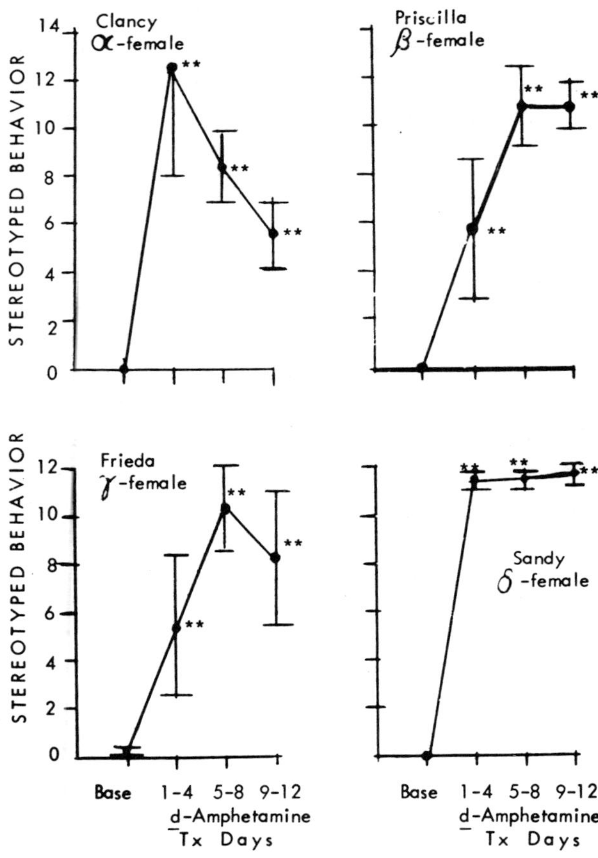

Fig. 5. The effect of chronic d-amphetamine treatment on stereotyped behavior in four treated monkeys. Each point represents the mean ± SEM for baseline (base), early (days 1–4), mid (days 5–8), and late (days 9–12) d-amphetamine treatment. Each animal's hierarchical rank within her respective colony is noted under each name. Statistical significance is denoted by ** — $p < 0.01$ when compared with baseline.

no spoken language; however, some do not. It is the latter changes in which we are particularly interested. In our experiments, at least four behavioral changes induced in monkeys by chronic administration of d-amphetamine bear direct resemblance to behavior reported in individuals with amphetamine psychosis. These include stereotyped behavior, progressive social withdrawal, excessive scratching, and general hyperactivity. As reported with amphetamine psychosis, monkey stereotypies varied considerably between individuals (Rylander, 1972; Schiorring, 1977; Davis and Schlemmer, 1980).

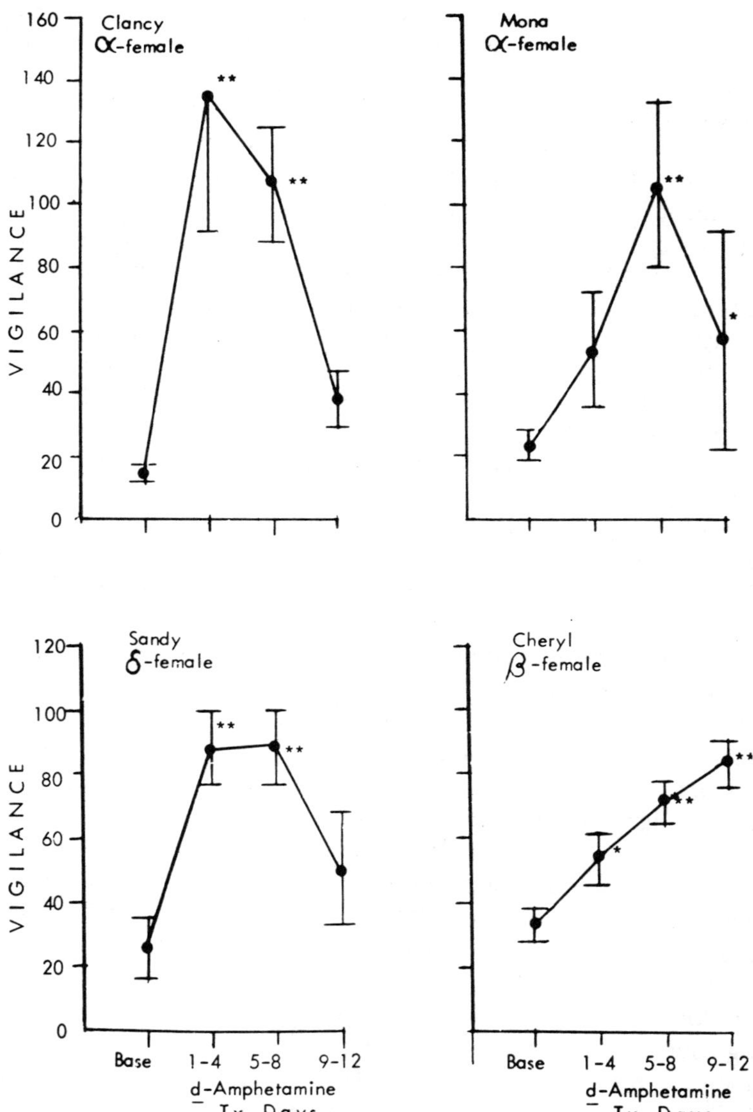

Fig. 6. The effect of chronic d-amphetamine treatment on checking or vigilance by four treated monkeys. Each point represents the mean ± SEM for baseline (base), early (days 1–4), mid (5–8), and late (days 9–12) d-amphetamine treatment. Each animal's hierarchical rank within her respective colony is noted under each name. Statistical significance is denoted by * — $p < 0.05$ or ** — $p < 0.01$ when compared to baseline.

In our view, the large increase in checking behavior induced by d-amphetamine does not necessarily constitute a stereotypy. This is based on several significant inconsistencies between increased checking and clearly distinguishable stereotypies such as stereotyped self-grooming. In our paradigm, tolerance always develops to d-amphetamine-induced increased checking during chronic treatment, whereas tolerance rarely develops to amphetamine-induced stereotypies during the same period. Two potent dopamine antagonists, haloperidol and pimozide, fail to return the increased checking induced by d-amphetamine back to baseline levels, yet completely antagonize amphetamine-induced stereotypies in the same monkeys (Garver et al., 1975). Checking may be significantly increased from baseline levels by amphetamine and other drugs without any other behaviors becoming stereotyped. In subsequent experiments, it was found that hallucinogen-induced increased checking could be antagonized by serotonin antagonists and pentobarbital, drugs which fail to antagonize rodent stereotypy (Randrup and Munkvad, 1970; Wallach 1974).

Social withdrawal is a response which has been consistently reported in adult amphetamine-treated monkeys studied in a social setting (Machiyama et al., 1970; Kjellberg and Randrup, 1971, 1973; Crowley et al., 1974; Garver et al., 1975; Schiorring, 1977; Schlemmer and Davis, 1981a; Miczek and Yoshimura, 1982). Social groom is a major affiliative behavior in this species undoubtedly serving an important role in providing cohesion between members of the colony. The elimination or large reduction in initiated social grooming in amphetamine-treated monkeys demonstrates a significant disruption in interaction between the subject and other colony members. The increase in distancing scores reveals a spatial isolation between treated and control animals. It might be argued that the reduction in initiated social grooming is a result of nonspecific effects of the drug or is simply replaced by other amphetamine-induced behavior such as stereotypy. This is not likely since self-grooming, a behavior requiring the same motor skills but in a nonsocial context, was frequently increased while social grooming was reduced. Moreover, both social and self-grooming often became sterotyped during amphetamine treatment. Although subtle, social withdrawal is also a common feature of amphetamine psychosis (Griffith et al., 1972; Rylander, 1972; Schiorring, 1977). Amphetamine users frequently feel as if they are "in a world of their own," confining themselves to a room or off in a corner.

Increased checking or looking around is also a commonly reported behavioral change in monkeys treated with amphetamines (Garver et al., 1975; Ridley et al., 1980; Schlemmer and Davis, 1981a; Nielsen et al., 1982; Miczek and Yoshimura, 1982); however, it is not specifically induced by

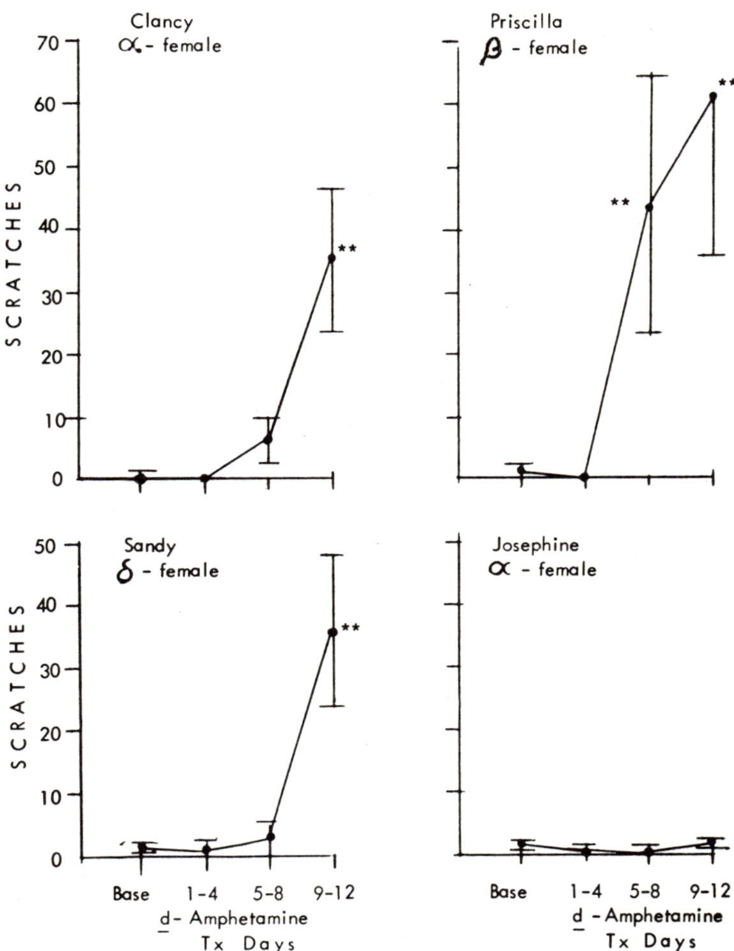

Fig. 7. The effect of chronic d-amphetamine treatment on scratching by four treated monkeys. Each point represents the mean ± SEM for baseline (base), early (days 1–4), mid (days 5–8), and late (days 9–12) d-amphetamine treatment. Each animal's hierarchical rank within her respective colony is noted under each name. Statistical significance is denoted by ** — $p < 0.01$ when compared to baseline.

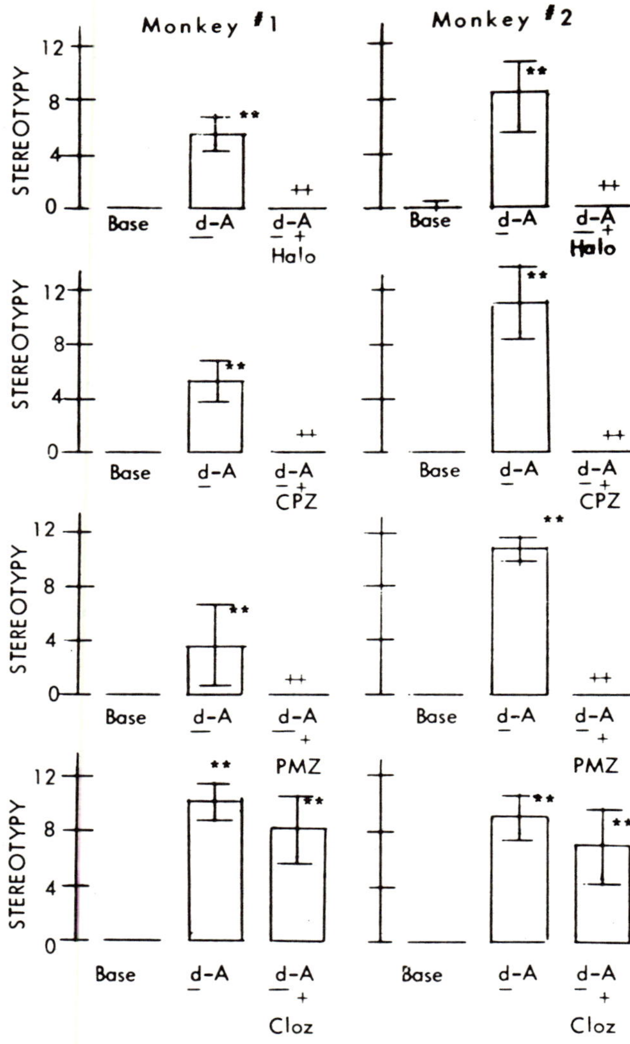

Fig. 8. The effect of four antipsychotic agents on d-amphetamine-induced changes in stereotyped behavior (A), initiated social grooming (B), and distancing (C) in monkeys. Each bar represents the mean ± SEM score per treatment period. The antipsychotics tested included haloperidol (Halo), chlorpromazine (CPZ), pimozide (PMZ), and clozapine (Cloz). No monkey received more than one antipsychotic drug in this experiment. Statistical significance is denoted by * — $p < 0.05$ or ** — $p < 0.01$ when compared to baseline (base), or + — $p < 0.05$ or ++ — $p < 0.01$ when compared to d-amphetamine (d-A) treatment period.

Monkey #1
Monkey #2
SOCIAL GROOM
20
15
10
5
0
Base
d-A
d-A + Halo
d-A + CPZ
d-A + PMZ
d-A + Cloz
**
++
*
+

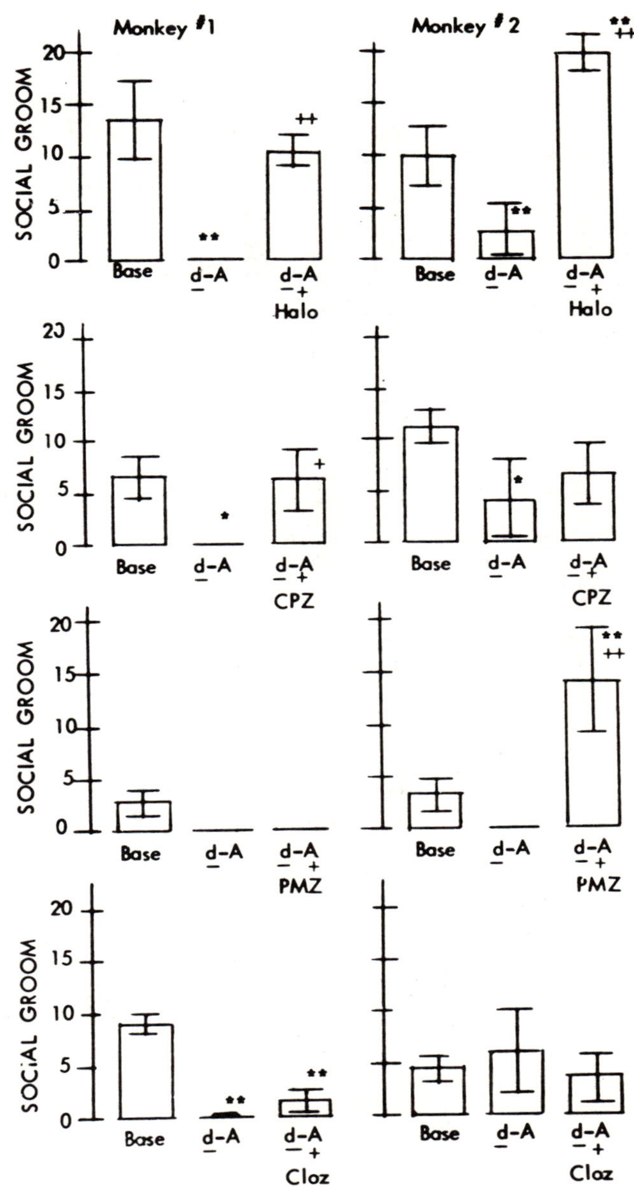

Figure 8B.

Monkey #1
Monkey #2
DISTANCE >3'
12
8
4
0
Base
d-A
d-A + Halo
d-A + CPZ
d-A + PMZ
d-A + Cloz

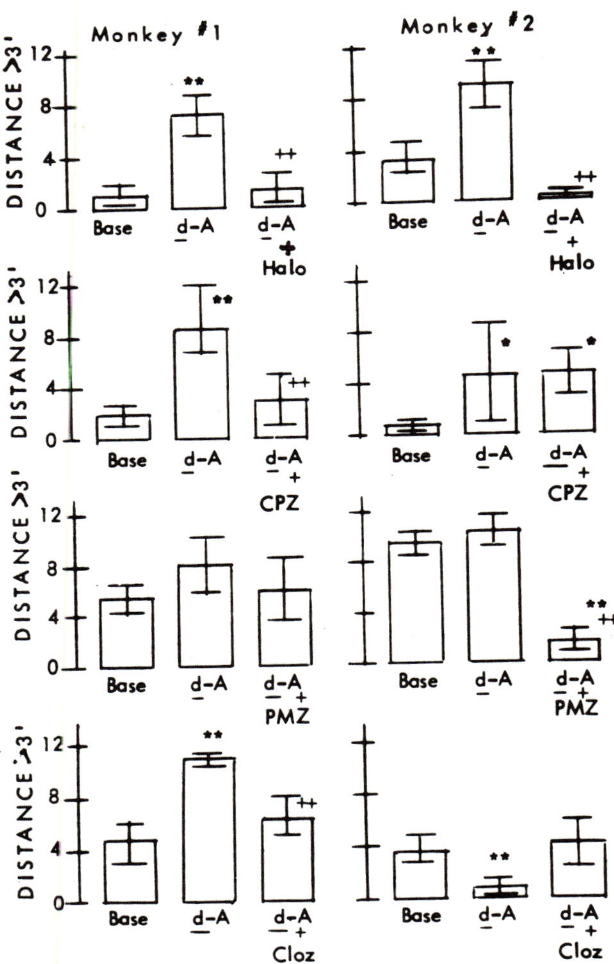

Figure 8C.

psychomotor stimulants. Many amphetamine psychotics are described as hypervigilant with increased visual scanning (Snyder, 1972).

Other behavioral changes seen in monkeys during chronic d-amphetamine treatment may have relevance to amphetamine psychosis but must be considered speculative in nature. For example, we have argued that the large increase in submissive gestures given by treated monkeys without an increase in aggressive gestures received by these animals may have relevance to human paranoia (Schlemmer and Davis, 1981b). That is, the treated monkey is apparently perceiving a nonthreatening situation as being threatening. Excessive scratching by amphetamine abusers has been related to the presence of tactile hallucinations or paresthesias (Griffith et al., 1972), leading to the speculation that a similar phenomenon may be occurring in monkeys. The eye-tracking accompanied by grabbing of nonexistent objects in the air in three monkeys in our experiments and several vervet monkeys in the studies of Nielsen and co-workers (this volume) makes it tempting to postulate that these animals are experiencing visual hallucinations. However, this speculation must be viewed with caution since administration of several potent visual hallucinogens including LSD and mescaline failed to elicit this behavior in stumptail macaques throughout numerous trials in our laboratory. Other isolated incidents with amphetamine-treated monkeys suggest a possible disturbance of thought processes such as the shadowing behavior seen with the monkey Mona, repetitive or stereotyped threatening behavior of a

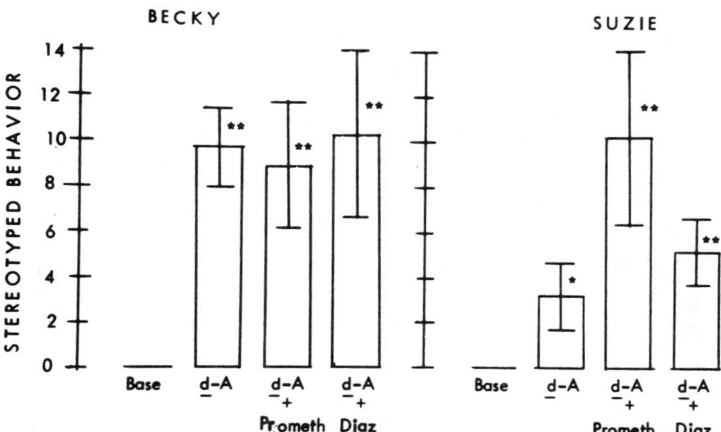

Fig. 9. The effect of two nonantipsychotic drugs on d-amphetamine (d-A)-induced stereotyped behavior in two monkeys. Each bar represents the mean ± SEM per treatment period. The nonantipsychotics tested were promethazine (Prometh) and diazepam (Diaz). Statistical significance is denoted by * — $p < 0.05$ or ** — $p < 0.01$ when compared with baseline (base).

dominant treated animal toward a subordinant without any subsequent attack, and consistent inappropriate elicitation of or response to social cues.

Antipsychotic agents are effective in suppressing many schizophrenic symptoms (Appleton and Davis, 1980) as well as amphetamine psychosis (Bell 1973; Angrist et al., 1974). To be a valid model of psychosis, antipsychotics should at least partially antagonize amphetamine-induced behavioral changes in monkeys. The results of our experiments demonstrate that antipsychotics are clearly potent in antagonizing the abnormal behavior induced by d-amphetamine such as stereotyped behavior and increased checking. The four antipsychotic agents tested were less consistent in returning disrupted social behavior to baseline levels. Yet, in many instances, they were clearly effective in this regard. This finding may be in better agreement with clinical response to antipsychotic drugs than first appears. It is commonly recognized that not all schizophrenic patients respond favorably to antipsychotic treatment or to a particular antipsychotic agent (Appleton and Davis, 1980). Furthermore, antipsychotic drugs rarely totally restore "normal" behavior, but instead suppress psychotic behavior to the extent that a patient can hopefully lead a more productive life. Interestingly, clozapine, an antipsychotic which rarely induces extrapyramidal side effects (EPS), failed to antagonize amphetamine-induced stereotypy, but returned distancing scores to baseline levels. Since social withdrawal is a more fundamental symptom of schizophrenia than stereotypy, and since stereotypy, like EPS, is presumably mediated through the nigrostriatal dopamine system (Randrup and Munkvad, 1970; Wallach, 1974), the "normalization" of distancing without antagonism of stereotypy may detect potential antipsychotic drugs with low incidence of EPS. Likewise, psychoactive drugs lacking antipsychotic activity should not antagonize the amphetamine effect in this paradigm. Promethazine, a phenothiazine without antipsychotic action but a potent histamine-1 receptor antagonist, and diazepam, an anxiolytic, failed to return amphetamine-induced behavior to baseline levels. It is also important to note that, as with the four antipsychotics, both nonantipsychotics tested possess potent sedative properties, suggesting that the antagonism of amphetamine effects by the antipsychotic agents can not be attributed to a general sedative effect.

Two of the antipsychotic agents which were particularly effective in antagonizing the behavioral changes induced by amphetamine were haloperidol and pimozide. Coincidentally, these neuroleptics are two of the more selective dopamine receptor antagonists (Anden et al., 1970; Peroutka and Snyder, 1980), suggesting that dopamine systems may be involved in the mediation of this syndrome. To test this hypothesis, we administered the direct dopamine receptor agonist apomorphine to monkeys to compare its

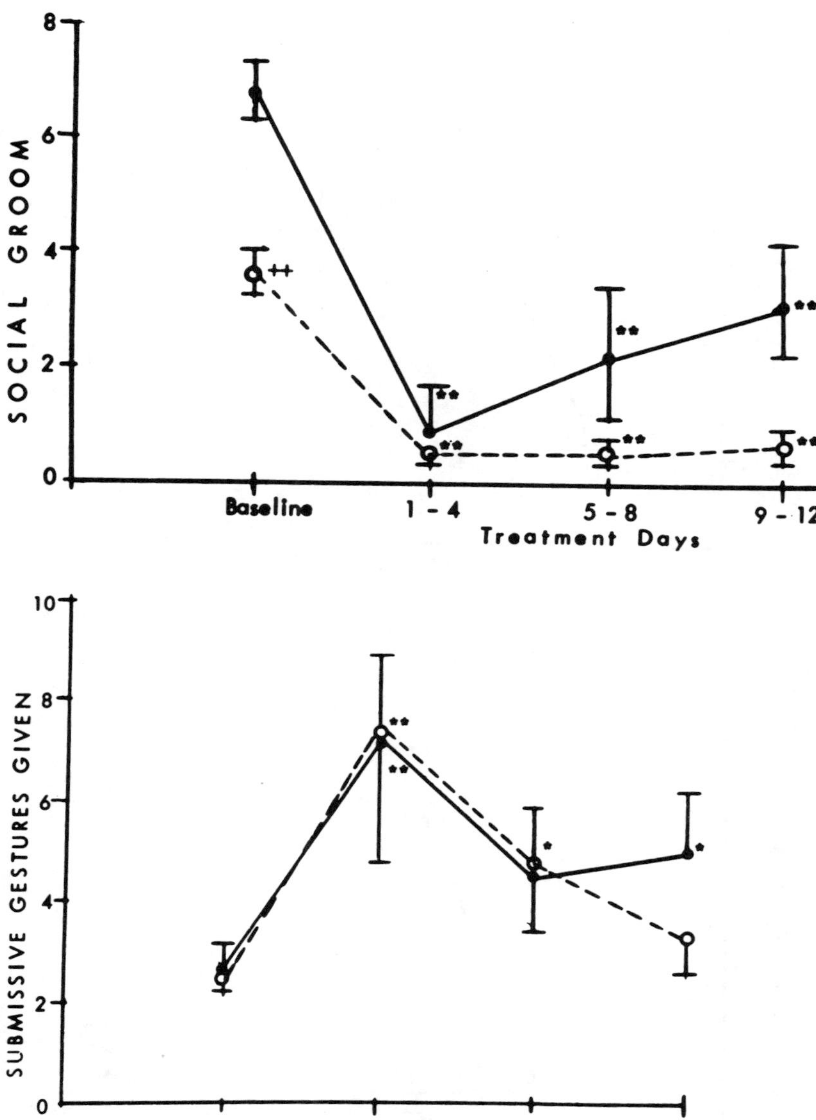

Fig. 10. The comparative effects of chronic d-amphetamine and chronic apomorphine treatment on four behaviors in four monkeys. d-Amphetamine is represented by the solid line and apomorphine by the dotted line. Each point represents the mean ± SEM for four monkeys for each treatment period. Statistical significance is denoted by * − $p < 0.05$ or ** − $p < 0.01$ when compared to respective baseline, or + − $p < 0.05$ or + + − < 0.01 when compared to d-amphetamine during the same period. (From Schlemmer and Davis, 1981a.)

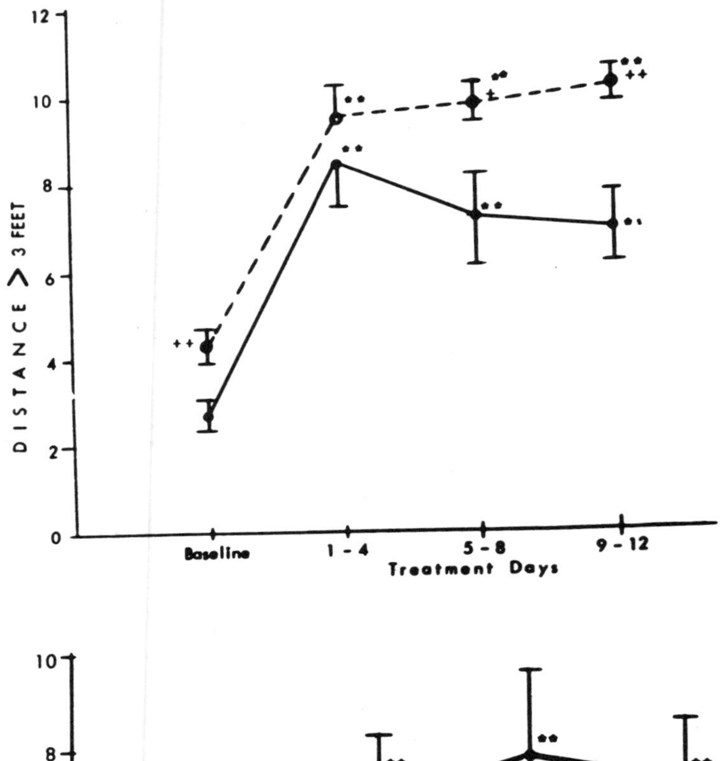

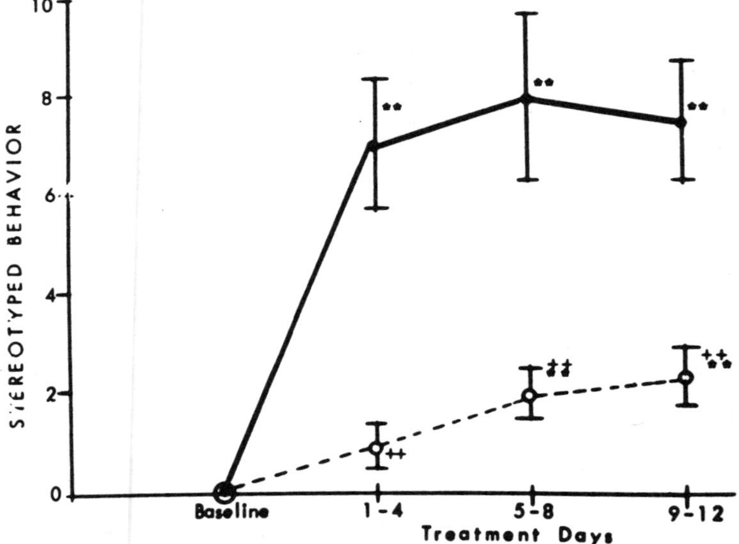

Figure 10 (continued).

effect to d-amphetamine. Importantly, large doses of apomorphine do not induce emesis in most nonhuman primate species (Brizzie et al., 1955; Peng and Wang, 1962; Schlemmer et al., 1980) as is seen in humans. The results reveal a striking similarity in response to chronic apomorphine and d-amphetamine in the same monkeys with the major behavioral changes of the syndrome. The data strongly implicate dopamine systems in the mediation of amphetamine-induced social withdrawal, increased submissiveness, increased checking, stereotypy, and hyperactivity. Since some of these changes are also reported with schizophrenia as well as amphetamine psychosis, this experiment provides additional support for the dopamine theory of psychosis.

PHENCYCLIDINE EXPERIMENTS

Some clinicians believe that phencyclidine (PCP) intoxication mimics endogenous psychosis better than amphetamine (Allen and Young, 1978). The major characteristics of PCP intoxication include paranoid ideation, body-image disturbances, depersonalization, visual and auditory hallucinations, repetitive purposeless movements, autistic behavior, and unpredictable violent behavior (Luby et al., 1962; Davies and Beech, 1960; Burns and Lerner, 1976; Fauman et al., 1976; Petersen and Stillman, 1978). However, PCP users are almost always disoriented and have severe clouding of consciousness while intoxicated. Note that there are some similar characteristics of PCP intoxication and amphetamine psychosis, but that a major difference is the disorientation seen with PCP. A full-blown schizophreniform psychosis occurs in a small percentage of PCP users (Luisada and Brown, 1976; Luisada, 1978). PCP psychosis may occur after acute or chronic intoxication with a wide range of PCP doses, and may persist for weeks after the last exposure to PCP (Luisada and Brown, 1976). PCP psychosis responds well to antipsychotic therapy (Luisada and Brown, 1976). The persistent PCP psychosis bears even greater resemblance to endogenous psychosis than PCP intoxication.

We have studied the effects of acute and chronic administration of several doses of PCP on the behavior of group-housed monkeys and the effect of the antipsychotic pimozide on PCP-induced behavior.

Methods

In the first experiment, two females from a colony of five stumptail macaques received five acute doses of PCP ranging from 0.01 to 0.50 mg(base)/kg to ascertain the dose-dependent behavioral changes induced by PCP. At least 3 days separated each drug administration.

In the next three experiments, three doses of PCP were administered daily for 2–3 weeks. Four monkeys from a colony of five animals received PCP, 0.025 mg/kg, once daily for 21 consecutive days in a crossover design. In the next two experiments, two monkeys from the same group received PCP once daily 0.05 mg/kg for 21 consecutive days and 0.10 mg/kg for 14 consecutive days. A drug wash-out period of at least 3 weeks separated each experiment.

In the final experiment, pimozide, 0.10 mg(base)/kg, was administered once daily alone for the first 7 days followed by combined pimozide and PCP, 0.025 mg/kg, treatment for the next 14 days. The four monkeys that had previously received the 0.025 mg/kg dose of PCP also received drug treatment in this experiment using the same crossover design.

Phencyclidine HCl (Sernalyn, Bio-Ceutics Laboratories, St. Joseph, MO) was administered intramuscularly 15 minutes prior to observation throughout the experiments. Pimozide (McNeil), was administered nasogastrically at 6:00 AM daily.

Results

In general, PCP suppressed most active forms of behavior at doses of 0.025 mg/kg and greater (Fig. 11). PCP decreased both social and self-grooming in a dose-dependent manner. Many changes in social behavior seen with amphetamine were not seen with PCP such as no change in the number of submissive gestures given by PCP-treated monkeys (Fig. 11). The major effect of acute PCP administration appeared to be sedation seen primarily as an increase in resting with eyes open (Fig. 11). At no time was a significant increase in any aggressive behavior noted in PCP-treated monkeys. In fact, at higher doses, PCP-treated monkeys were attacked by control animals, but were essentially unresponsive to either facial threats or biting and hair pulling.

The effects of chronic administration of PCP were similar to those induced by acute doses of the drug with the exception of stereotyped behavior. Although stereotypy was rarely seen upon acute PCP administration, it appeared in all treated animals within the first 4 days of treatment and became more prevalent with continued daily administration (Fig. 12; see also Schlemmer et al., 1978). The most common stereotypies induced by PCP were oral stereotypies (licking, chewing, tongue protrusion) and self-grooming. PCP stereotypies were performed at a much slower rate than those seen with d-amphetamine, but both were repetitive and continuous. When the same monkeys later received a test treatment with chronic d-amphetamine, a different pattern of stereotyped behavior developed from that seen with PCP.

Pimozide significantly antagonized PCP-induced stereotypy, leaving only a small amount of residual stereotypy (Fig. 12). However, pimozide failed

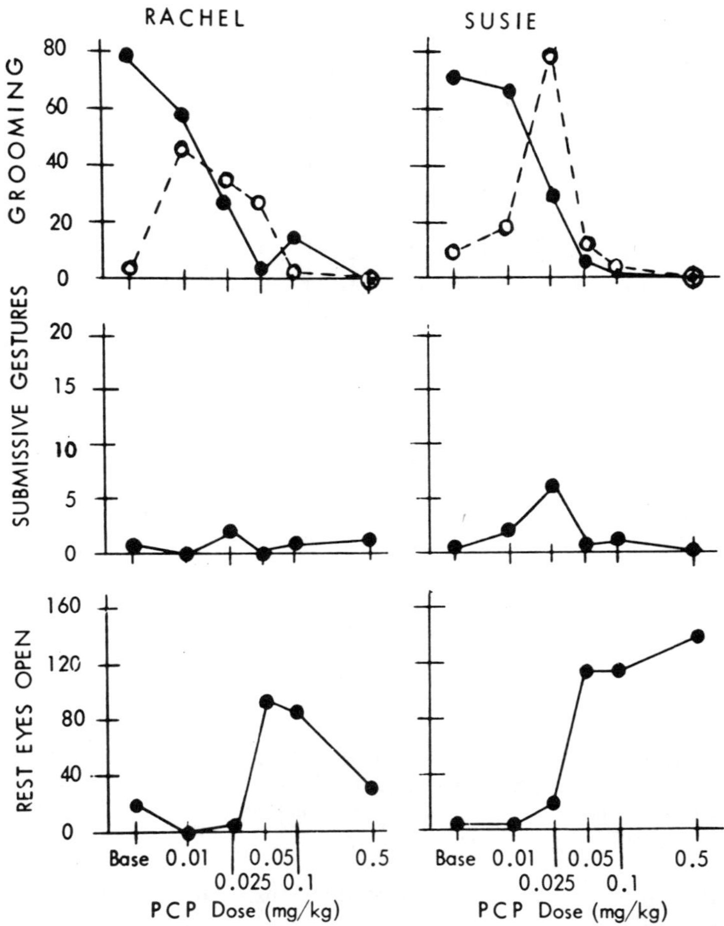

Fig. 11. The dose-dependent effects of acute phencyclidine (PCP) administration on three behaviors in two monkeys. In the top graphs, initiated social grooming is represented by the solid line and self-grooming by the dotted line.

to improve other significant behavioral changes induced by PCP, and in some cases, such as initiated social grooming, actually worsened the effect (Fig. 12).

Discussion

The behavioral effects of PCP in monkeys were considerably less dramatic than those seen with amphetamine. However, the behavioral changes seen

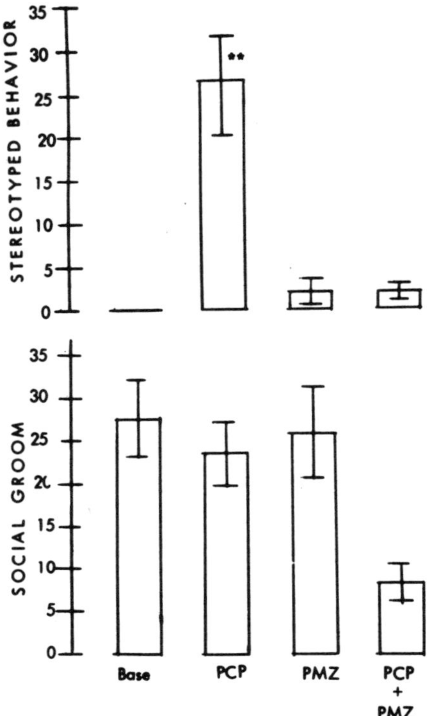

Fig. 12. The effect of the antipsychotic pimozide (PMZ) on two behavioral changes induced by chronic phencyclidine (PCP) treatment in monkeys. Each bar represents the mean ± SEM for each treatment period. Statistical significance is denoted by ** — $p < 0.01$ when compared to baseline (base).

with PCP in this study were essentially consistent with those reported for rhesus monkeys *(M. mulatta)* treated with PCP (Miller et al., 1973).

Some similarities were noted between PCP-induced behavior in monkeys and human PCP intoxication and PCP psychosis. Both monkeys and humans appear sedated during PCP intoxication whereas rodents are hyperactive when treated with PCP (Chen et al., 1965; Kanner et al., 1975a). Ataxia may be present in all three species as well (Lerner and Burns, 1978; Sturgeon et al., 1982). Perhaps the most significant behavioral change seen with PCP was the induction of stereotyped behavior which may be related to the repetitive, purposeless movements described in some individuals with PCP intoxication or PCP psychosis (Lerner and Burns, 1978). More recently, PCP-induced stereotypy has also been reported in rodents (Smith et al., 1978; Sturgeon et al., 1982). Even more intriguing is the finding that PCP stereotypy becomes more persistent over time in monkeys (Schlemmer et al., 1978) and rats (Smith et al., 1978), suggesting that reverse tolerance to PCP may develop at least with regard to stereotypy.

Other behaviors seen during human PCP intoxication which would presumably be detected in monkeys were not noted. The most conspicuous was the absence of any increase in aggression in PCP-treated monkeys whereas unpredictable, violent behavior is frequently reported in humans (Burns and Lerner, 1976; Fauman et al., 1976).

The antipsychotic, pimozide, was not effective in antagonizing the effects of PCP with the exception of stereotyped behavior. This could be due in part to additive sedative properties of the two drugs and is not inconsistent with reports of the effect of neuroleptic drugs on individuals with PCP intoxication (Luisada, 1978). However, antagonism of PCP-induced stereotyped behavior by pimozide, a preferential dopamine receptor antagonist, suggests that PCP acts, at least in part, through dopamine systems to induce abnormal behavior in monkeys. This finding is consistent with biochemical (Garey and Heath, 1976; Smith et al., 1977) and other behavioral studies (Kanner et al., 1975b; Tyler and Miczek, 1982) which suggest indirect dopamine agonist properties.

HALLUCINOGEN EXPERIMENTS

Hallucinogens or psychedelics are one of the oldest group of drugs to be studied for their psychotomimetic properties. The immediate effect of hallucinogens is, of course, hallucinations which are predominantly visual although auditory and tactile hallucinations are occasionally reported (Hoffer and Osmond, 1967; Sankar, 1975). However, other significant but less heralded behavioral changes occur during or after the hallucinatory experience. These include frank paranoia, body-image disturbances, depersonalization, and multiple changes in affect or mood (Hoffer and Osmond, 1967; Sankar, 1975). In contrast to amphetamines and PCP, hallucinogens induce their effects upon acute administration, usually in small doses, with a rapid partial tolerance developing upon repeated administration.

Several objections have been raised against the use of hallucinogen intoxication as a model psychosis. 1) Hallucinogen-induced hallucinations are primarily visual whereas schizophrenic hallucinations are primarily auditory (Aggernaes, 1972). 2) Hallucinations are the predominant effect of hallucinogens, yet hallucinations are considered a secondary, not a primary symptom of schizophrenia (Bleuler, 1961). 3) A rapid partial tolerance develops to repeated administration of most hallucinogens whereas psychosis is typically more prolonged. Nevertheless, there is continued interest in the study of hallucinogens and their relationship to psychosis since at least two potent hallucinogens, N,N-dimethyltryptamine (DMT) and 5-methoxydimethyltryptamine (5-MeODMT), to which tolerance apparently does not develop, may be formed endogenously through aberrant tryptamine metabolism and may serve as endogenous psychotogens (cf. Gillin et al., 1978).

We have tested ten known hallucinogens and several structurally related nonhallucinogen congeners in stumptail macaques.

Methods

The hallucinogens tested, dose most frequently used, and time administered before observation in the experiments were: the ergot derivative d-lysergic acid diethylamide (d-LSD, NIDA, Bethesda, MD), 0.01 mg/kg, 15 min; the phenylethylamine derivatives mescaline (Sigma, St. Louis, MO), 17 mg/kg, 60 min; 3,4,5-trimethoxyamphetamine (TMA), 8 mg/kg, 45 min; 4-methyl 2,5-dimethoxyamphetamine (DOM, NIDA), 0.17 mg/kg, 30 min; 3,4-methylenedioxyamphetamine (MDA, NIDA), 3 mg/kg 15 min; and the tryptamine derivatives N,N-dimethyltryptamine (DMT, Sigma), 2 mg/kg, 5 min; 5-methoxy N,N-dimethyltryptamine (5-MeODMT, Sigma), 0.25 mg/kg, 5 min; N,N-diethyltryptamine (DET, Sigma), 2 mg/kg, 5 min; psilocin and psilocybin (NIDA), 0.4 mg/kg, 15 min. Relevant nonhallucinogens tested included the LSD congeners 2-brom LSD (BOL, NIDA), 0.1 mg/kg, 15 min, and lisuride (Schering AG, Berlin, Germany), 0.05 mg/kg, 15 min; the phenylethylamine 3,4-dimethoxyphenethylamine (DMPEA, Sigma), 17 mg/kg, 60 min; and tryptamine (Sigma), 10 mg/kg, 15 min. All drug doses are expressed as mg(base)/kg. All drugs were administered intramuscularly.

The hallucinogens were tested in either two female dyad groups or social colonies of 4–5 monkeys each. In both situations, the drug was given in a crossover design with all members of the group receiving drug by the completion of the experiment. Those members of the group not receiving drug treatment on a particular day received an injection of normal saline at the time of drug administration. All drugs were tested for acute effects and most hallucinogens were also given once daily for 5–12 days to test for chronic effects. In addition, the effect of five doses of d-LSD were examined to determine if the behavioral changes seen with this hallucinogen were dose-dependent. In this experiment, a colony of five monkeys (one male, four females) received five doses of d-LSD ranging from 0.0003 to 0.03 mg(base)/kg in a Latin-square design. Only one monkey received drug treatment on a given day, and at least 14 days elapsed before that monkey received another LSD injection. Those monkeys not receiving a drug received an injection of normal saline at the same time the treated monkey received LSD, 15 min prior to observation.

The effects of two antipsychotic agents and several selected nonantipsychotics on the behavioral effects of the hallucinogen 5-MeODMT were also tested. Following baseline, 5-MeODMT, 0.25 mg/kg, was administered i.m. once daily 5 minutes prior to observation for 5 consecutive days to members of a social colony of 4–5 animals in a crossover fashion. Then the antipsychotic or nonantipsychotic was administered i.m. for 14 consecutive days. During the last 5 days of treatment, 5-MeODMT, 0.25 mg/kg, was given concomitantly. The drugs, dose, and time of administration prior to observation included: the antipsychotics haloperidol (McNeil), 0.1 mg(base)/kg, twice daily, the last 2.5 hr prior to observation, trifluoperazine HCl (Smith, Kline, French), 0.02 mg(salt)/kg, twice daily, 2.5 hr; the serotonin antagonists cinanserin HCl (Squibb; Princeton, NJ), 5 mg(salt)/kg, 2.5 hr; metergoline (Farmitalia; Milan, Italy), 0.30 mg(base)/kg, 2 hr; methysergide maleate (Sandoz; Hanover, NJ), 1.0 mg(salt)/kg, 2 hr; cyproheptadine HCl (Merck, Sharp, Dohme, West Point, PA), 1.0 mg(salt)/kg, 2 hr; and methiothepin maleate (gift from Dr. M. Protiva, Prague, Czechoslovakia), 0.15 mg(salt)/kg, 22 hr; and the phenothiazine antihistamine promethazine HCl (Wyeth), 2.0 mg(salt)/kg, twice daily 2.5 hr; the anxiolytic diazepam (Roche), 1.0 mg(base)/kg, 2.5 hr. The hypnotic pentobarbital Na (Abbott, North Chicago, IL), 10 mg(salt)/kg, was given acutely 30 min prior to observation, 1 day alone and 1 week later concomitantly with 5-MeODMT.

Results

Some behavioral changes induced by individual hallucinogens were common to several hallucinogens. In general, hallucinogen-treated monkeys appeared sedated with the exception of those receiving DMT and 5-MeODMT. Most hallucinogens induced a dose-dependent reduction in both social and self-grooming as seen with LSD (Fig. 13). There was typically a significant increase in distancing scores, although not to the extent seen with amphetamine (Fig. 13). Interestingly, though, treated monkeys were at the same time approached more frequently by control animals while receiving certain hallucinogens such as LSD (Fig. 13). Control monkeys would occasionally approach treated animals, but would not stay and interact with the animal. This unusual phenomenon has not been noted with other drugs. Most hallucinogens induced an increase in the number of submissive gestures given by the treated monkeys. In the case of 5-MeODMT, this was not accompanied with an increase in aggressive gestures received by these monkeys (Fig. 14). Hallucinogens also induced significant changes in several individual behaviors including increased checking, ptosis, increased lying down, and some stereotypy. However, the most reliable changes in solitary behavior induced

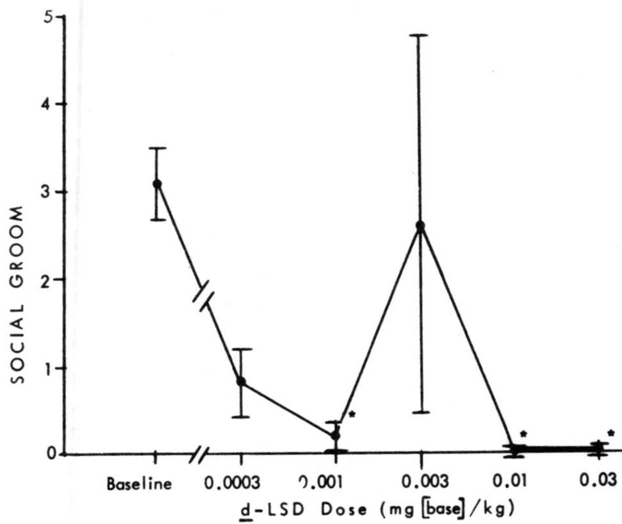

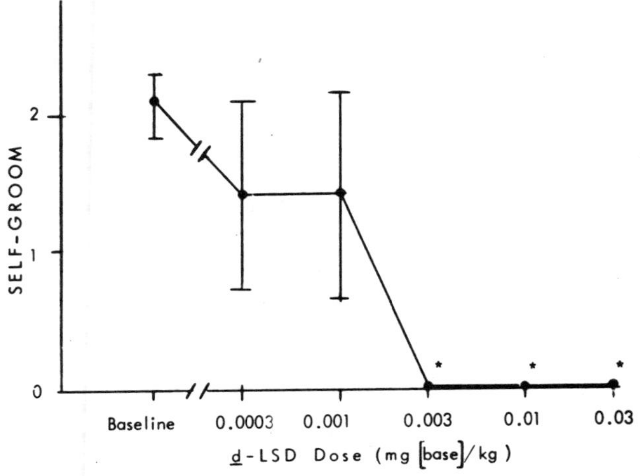

Fig. 13. The dose-dependent effects of acute d-LSD on four behaviors in monkeys. Each point represents the mean ± SEM per dose for five monkeys. Statistical significance is denoted by * — $p < 0.05$ or ** — $p < 0.01$ when compared to baseline.

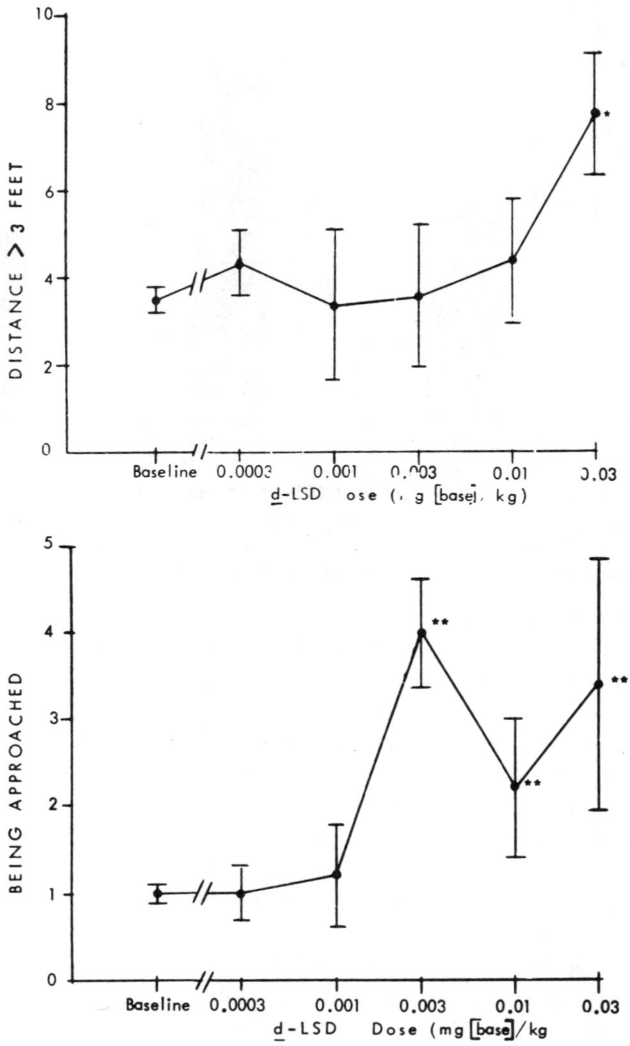

Figure 13 (continued).

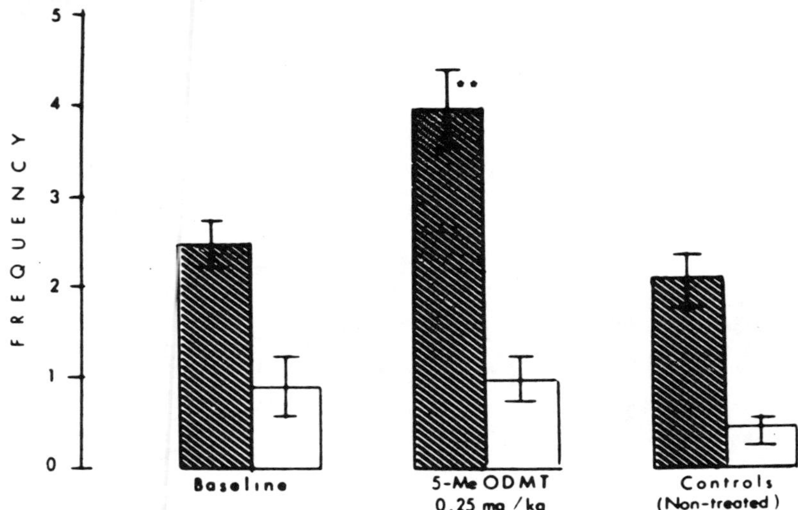

Fig. 14. The effect of chronic 5-MeODMT treatment on submissive gestures given (hatched bars) and aggressive gestures received (open bars) by treated monkeys. Each bar represents the mean ± SEM per treatment period. Statistical significance is denoted by ** — $p < 0.01$ when compared with baseline. (From Schlemmer and Davis, 1981b.)

by hallucinogens were two emergent behaviors, limb jerks (i.e., a myoclonic-like spasm of an extremity) and body shakes, resembling a wet-dog shake. These behaviors had a similar dose-dependent response effect with each hallucinogen with limb jerks having a dose-dependent linear increase with increasing drug dose while there was a biphasic, "inverted U" dose-response curve for body shakes (Fig. 15). Note also that neither behavioral change was significantly induced by the structurally related ergot lisuride (Fig. 15).

Limb jerks and body shakes appear to be behaviors specifically induced by hallucinogens in this species. Ten hallucinogens have been tested in adult stumptail macaques in our laboratory. Upon acute administration, all hallucinogens induced a significant number of limb jerks (Fig. 16). All but three hallucinogens (psilocin, psilocybin and DET) induced a significant number of body shakes (Fig. 16). Conversely, the nonhallucinogens BOL, DMPEA, lisuride, and tryptamine did not induce a significant number of limb jerks or body shakes (Fig. 16). Over 40 other psychoactive drugs not considered hallucinogenic upon acute administration which were tested in this species also failed to induce a significant level of limb jerks or body shakes. Morever, there is a highly significant correlation ($r = 0.991$) between the log of the dose of the hallucinogen necessary to induce limb jerks in monkeys and the log of the human hallucinogenic dose (Fig. 17).

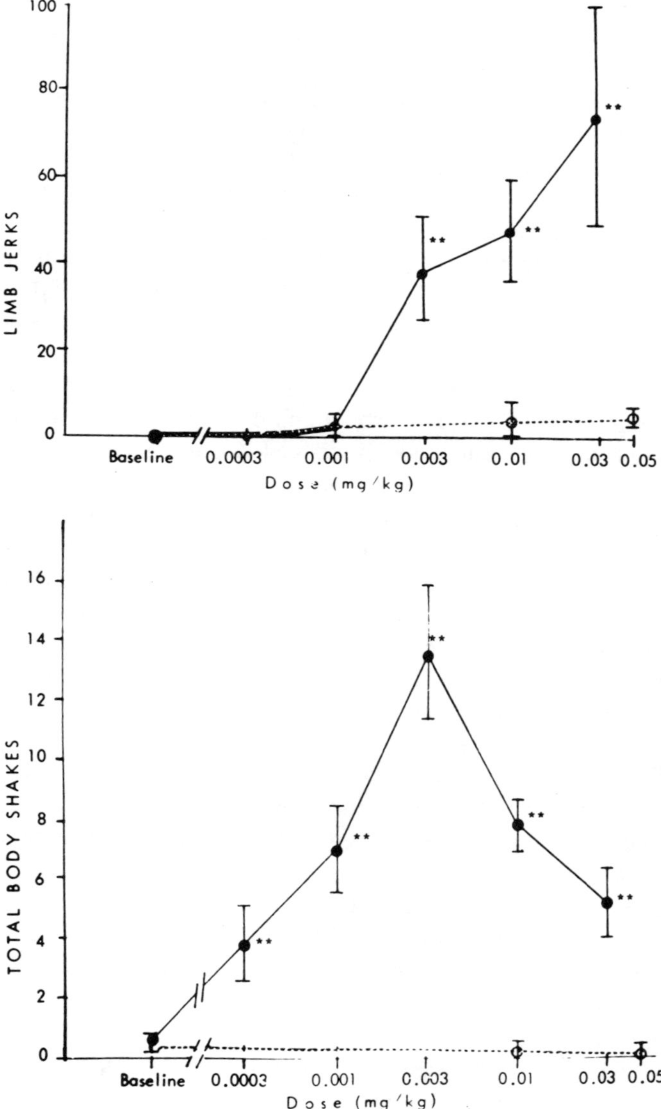

Fig. 15. The dose-dependent effect of d-LSD (solid line) and lisuride (dotted line) on the induction of two emergent behaviors in monkeys. Each point represents the mean ± SEM per dose for the same five monkeys. Statistical significance is denoted by ** — $p < 0.01$ when compared to respective baseline.

The best antagonists of hallucinogen-induced behavior in monkeys were serotonin antagonists and antipsychotic agents. Still, the effectiveness of these agents varied considerably between behaviors. Most antagonism experiments were conducted with 5-MeODMT (Table II). Serotonin antagonists were most effective in significantly antagonizing the emergent behaviors, limb jerks and body shakes, induced by 5-MeODMT as seen with cinanserin (Table II). Metergoline, methysergide, methiothepin, and cyproheptadine were approximately equieffective. The antipsychotics haloperidol and trifluoperazine also significantly antagonized 5-MeODMT-induced limb jerks and body shakes, but not to the extent as the serotonin antagonists did (Table II). Similar results have been obtained for LSD-induced limb jerks and body shakes with cinanserin and haloperidol. Promethazine, a nonantipsychotic, failed to antagonize either 5-MeODMT-induced emergent behavior to near baseline levels (Table II). Pentobarbital and diazepam were also ineffective. As with amphetamine, hallucinogen-induced disruption of normal behavior was more difficult to antagonize than abnormal emergent behavior. No antagonist tested restored the reduced scores for initiated social grooming to baseline levels (Table II). Distancing scores which were increased by 5-MeODMT were only partially reduced by cinanserin (Table II). Interestingly, though, the antipsychotics were clearly the most effective agents in reducing elevated scores for submissive gestures given (Table II). Cinanserin as well as all other nonantipsychotic serotonin antagonists increased initiated submissive gestures even further (Schlemmer and Davis, 1981b).

Discussion

Despite the infrequent use of hallucinogens to induce a model psychosis, certain aspects of hallucinogen-induced behavior in monkeys might be useful in the study of psychotic processes, particularly when the less sedative hallucinogens DMT and 5-MeODMT are used. Some of these behavioral changes were identical to those seen with chronic d-amphetamine treatment. Therefore, arguments used for similarities between these behavioral changes induced by amphetamine and psychotic behavior could be applied here as well. These hallucinogen-induced behavioral changes include: the social withdrawal noted by increased distancing scores and decreased initiated social grooming; increased submissive gestures given by treated monkeys; increased checking; and several instances of inappropriate responses to social cues from control monkeys. However, these changes were usually of a lower magnitude than those seen with chronic amphetamine.

The behavioral effects induced by most hallucinogens in monkeys (e.g., d-LSD) were not unlike the reactions seen with human hallucinogen intoxi-

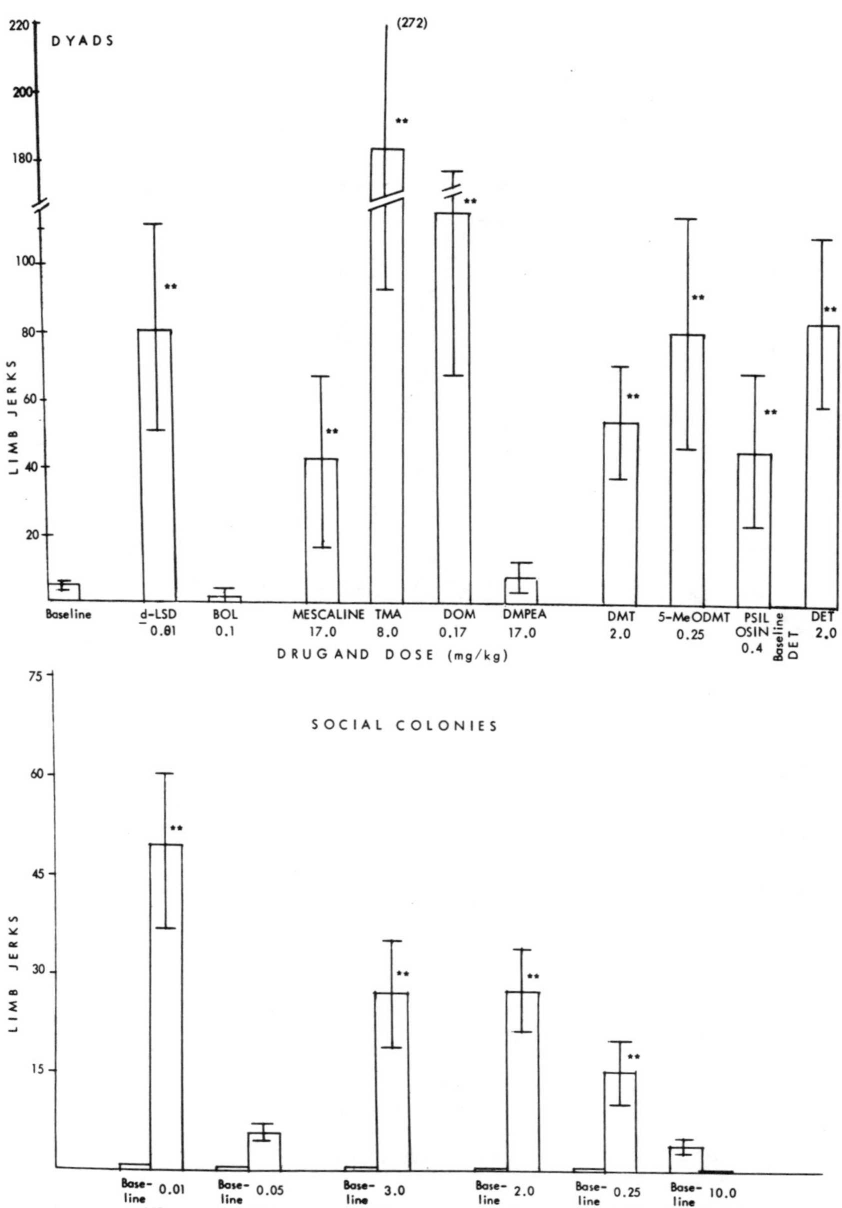

Fig. 16. The effect of nine hallucinogens and four related nonhallucinogens on the emergent behaviors limb jerks and body shakes. Each bar represents the mean ± SEM for an acute drug dose for four monkeys in the dyads and four to five monkeys in the social colonies. Statistical significance is denoted by ** – $p < 0.01$ when compared to respective baseline.

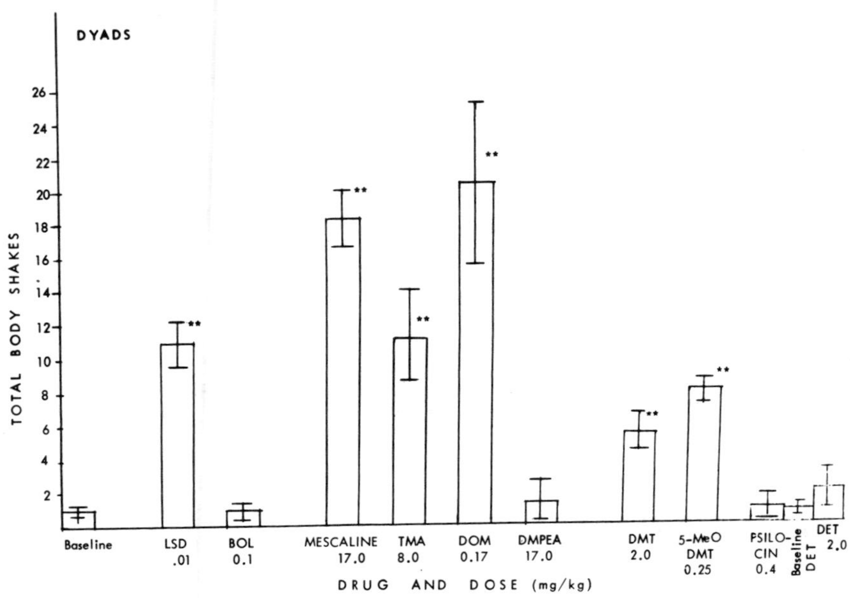

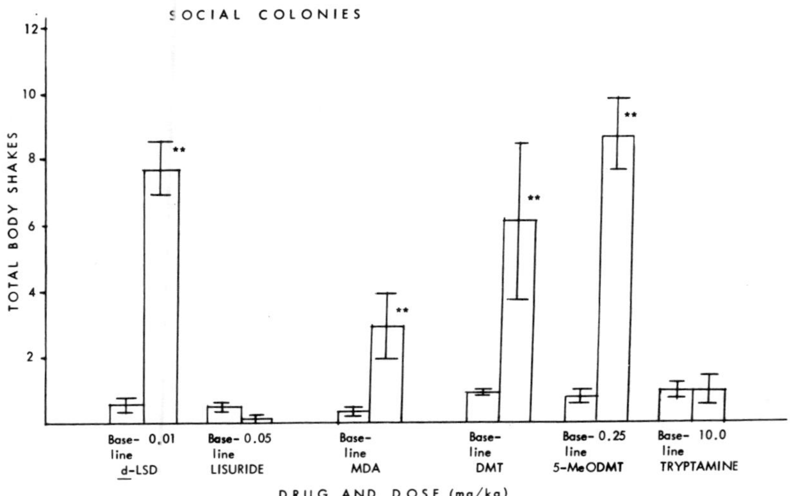

Figure 16 (continued).

cation. It is somewhat unremarkable, sedative effects including ptosis can be noted, and the individual initiates interaction with others infrequently.

Aside from viewing the effects of hallucinogens in monkeys as an animal model of psychosis, the experiments suggest that the emergent behaviors induced by hallucinogens, particularly limb jerks, may serve as a model for hallucinogenic activity of drugs. Specificity has been demonstrated since all hallucinogens tested induced limb jerks whereas closely related nonhallucinogens did not. Importantly, lisuride, a nonhallucinogenic ergot which has given false-positives in cat tests for hallucinogens (White et al., 1981; Marini, 1981), failed to elicit a positive response in stumptail macaques. Moreover, the dose necessary to elicit limb jerks in monkeys correlates well with the human hallucinogenic dose of these substances. Also, of the hallucinogens tested chronically, rapid partial tolerance developed to limb jerks induced by d-LSD, mescaline, DOM, and psilocin, but not to DMT, which agrees precisely with the hallucinogenic effects of these drugs in humans. This aspect of hallucinogen-induced behavior in monkeys may prove useful in further delineating the mechanism(s) of action of hallucinogens and in detecting potential hallucinogenic activity of new drugs prior to clinical testing.

The lack of a consistent antagonism by antipsychotic drugs across all behaviors was not totally surprising since previous reports of patients with hallucinogen intoxication who were tested with neuroleptics suggested that the response was variable (Schwarz, 1967). It does appear, however, that antipsychotics are particularly effective in antagonizing the increase in submissive gestures given by treated monkeys and somewhat less effective in attenuating limb jerks and body shakes induced by hallucinogens. The antagonist experiments do suggest that both serotonin and dopamine systems are involved in the mediation of hallucinogen-induced behavior in primates.

CONCLUSIONS

Each of the three classes of psychotomimetics studied induced behavioral changes in monkeys which may prove useful in the study of psychotic processes. Therefore, there is merit in the continued investigation of each substance.

To evaluate which is the best animal model of psychosis, we have compared the three paradigms using the criteria for an ideal animal model of a mental disorder suggested by McKinney (1977) (Table III). To meet the criteria, four conditions must be satisfied: 1) similarity of inducing conditions, 2) similarity to the behavioral state in humans, 3) similar underlying biological mechanism, and 4) reversal by clinically effective drugs, but not

TABLE II. The Effect of Selected Antagonists on 5-MeODMT-Induced Behavioral Changes in Stumptail Macaques

Treatment period	Limb jerks	Total body shakes	Social groom	Distance > 3 ft.	Submissive gestures given
Baseline	0.08 ± 0.08	0.52 ± 0.14	5.84 ± 0.98	4.04 ± 0.48	2.72 ± 0.32
5-MeODMT (0.25)	11.96 ± 1.95	8.44 ± 0.59**	1.00 ± 0.32**	8.56 ± 0.49	3.92 ± 0.60
Antipsychotics:					
Haloperidol (0.2)	0.00 ± 0.00††	0.12 ± 0.08††	0.08 ± 0.08**	7.24 ± 0.65*	0.84 ± 0.27**††
Haloperidol + 5-MeODMT	4.08 ± 0.74**††	2.52 ± 0.37*†	0.00 ± 0.00**	7.56 ± 0.63*	0.64 ± 0.28**††
Trifluoperazine (0.04)	0.00 ± 0.00††	0.04 ± 0.04††	0.08 ± 0.08**	7.48 ± 0.56*	1.16 ± 0.31**††
Trifluoperazine + 5-MeODMT	3.64 ± 0.96*††	3.77 ± 0.66**††	0.00 ± 0.00**	9.09 ± 0.42**	0.84 ± 0.28**††
Serotonin antagonists:					
Cinanserin (5.0)	0.16 ± 0.16††	0.00 ± 0.00††	4.76 ± 1.06††	4.92 ± 0.67††	1.20 ± 0.23
Cinanserin + 5-MeODMT	0.28 ± 0.15††	1.88 ± 0.38††	1.68 ± 0.38**	6.00 ± 0.47†	4.92 ± 0.98*
Non-antipsychotic:					
Promethazine (2.0)	0.05 ± 0.05††	0.00 ± 0.00	1.76 ± 0.52*	6.39 ± 0.56	1.84 ± 0.39
Promethazine + 5-MeODMT	8.32 ± 1.61**†	6.64 ± 0.54**†	0.20 ± 0.12**	8.04 ± 0.53**	6.40 ± 1.95**††

Each value represents the mean ± SEM for 5 monkeys for each respective treatment period. The daily dose in mg/kg is shown in parentheses next to the drug. Statistical significance is shown as:

*$p < 0.05$ when compared with baseline
**$p < 0.01$ when compared with baseline
†$p < 0.05$ when compared with 5-MeODMT alone
††$p < 0.01$ when compared with 5-MeODMT alone

TABLE III. Comparison of Three Psychotomimetic-Induced Models of Psychosis in Monkeys

Similarity to human condition	d-Amphetamine	PCP	Hallucinogens
Inducing conditions	Yes	Yes	Yes
Behavioral state	Certain aspects	No	Certain aspects
Underlying mechanism	Dopamine Norepinephrine(?)	Dopamine Other NTs(?)	Serotonin Dopamine
Reversal by clinically effective drugs	Partial	Only stereotypy	Partial
Not reversed by clinically ineffective drugs	Yes	Not tested	No

by ineffective drugs. All three models are induced by drugs which under the right conditions can induce psychotic behavior in normal individuals (Davis and Schlemmer, 1980; Burns and Lerner, 1976; Hoffer and Osmond, 1967). Certain aspects of the hallucinogen-induced and particularly the amphetamine-induced behavior in monkeys may be comparable to schizophrenic symptoms. Although the behavioral changes induced by PCP may resemble some PCP behavior in humans, PCP-induced behavior was the least like that seen in endogenous psychoses. The third criterion cannot be met since the etiology of schizophrenia is unknown. However, dopamine systems have been most frequently implicated in the mediation of psychosis (Meltzer and Stahl, 1976). The results of these experiments provide evidence that some behavioral changes from each of the three models are mediated by dopamine. Finally, our laboratory and other laboratories (Kjellberg and Randrup, 1971; Miczek and Yoshimura, 1982) have been unable to find an agent which antagonizes any of these syndromes in monkeys such that normal baseline activity and interaction are completely restored. Yet the same statement can likely be made for antipsychotics and schizophrenia. Antipsychotic drugs may suppress certain psychotic behavior in individual schizophrenic patients while other symptoms remain untouched (Klein and Davis, 1969; Appleton and Davis, 1980). Antipsychotic agents were at least partially effective in restoring several important behavioral changes induced by chronic d-amphetamine and a few changes induced by hallucinogens. Conversely, nonantipsychotic agents were ineffective in antagonizing amphetamine-induced behavior. However, the nonantipsychotic serotonin antagonists partially antagonized hallucinogen-induced behavior in monkeys although other nonantipsychotics did not.

Therefore, we conclude that the behavioral syndrome induced by chronic d-amphetamine treatment is the best model of psychosis of the three tested in

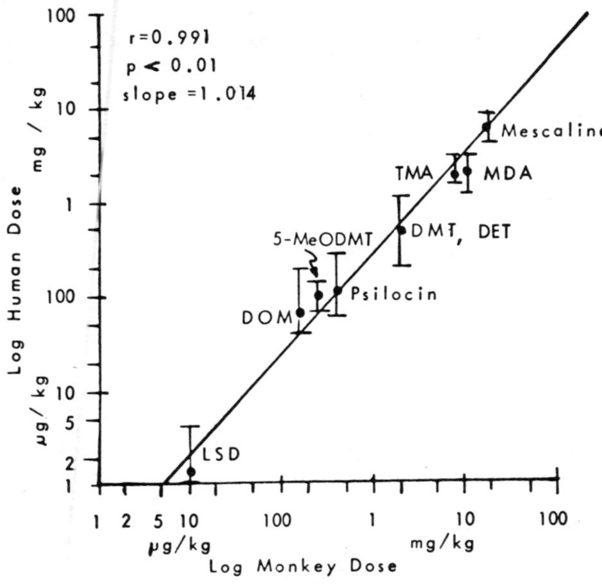

Fig. 17. The correlation between the hallucinogen dose used to induce limb jerks in monkeys and the reported human hallucinogenic dose. The vertical brackets represent the reported human hallucinogenic dose range for each drug.

stumptail macaques. In addition to at least partially satisfying all the criteria of an ideal animal model of psychosis, the amphetamine model had the most behavioral changes suggestive of human psychotic behavior and was best antagonized by the antipsychotic agents. However, the hallucinogen model may be a reasonable alternative because it partially fulfills the criteria and because of the similarity of a number of behavioral changes induced by the nonsedative hallucinogens (DMT and 5-MeODMT) and d-amphetamine.

ACKNOWLEDGMENTS

Most of the experiments were conducted at the University of Illinois Biological Resources Laboratory, Chicago, The authors thank Jane Ann Retallack, Corinne Tyler, Wonnie Jones, Reuben Johnson, James Edwards, Larry Monroe, Dr. Kenzie Preston, Dr. Alan Jackson, Carol Nawara, Lilly Beluhan, and Dr. Frank Beluhan for their excellent technical expertise throughout the experiments, and Drs. D.L. Garver, W.J. Heinze, N. Narasimhachari, J.W. Maas, and J.P. Bederka Jr. for their helpful comments and contributions during the experiments. Drugs used in the study were generously provided by McNeil Laboratories, Ft. Washington, PA (pimozide); the

Squibb Institute for Medical Research, Princeton, NJ (cinanserin HCl); Sandoz Pharmaceuticals, Hanover, NJ, (clozapine and methysergide maleate); Merck, Sharp, and Dohme Research Laboratories, West Point, PA (cyproheptadine HCl); Farmatalia Laboratories, Milan, Italy (metergoline); Schering AG, Berlin, Germany (lisuride hydrogen maleate); Dr. M. Protiva, Prague, Czechoslovakia (methiothepin maleate); and the National Institute on Drug Abuse, Rockville, MD (d-LSD, MDA, DOM, psilocin, psilocybin, and BOL).

REFERENCES

Aggernaes A (1972) The difference between the experienced reality of hallucinations in young drug abusers and schizophrenic patients. Acta Psychiatr Scand 48: 287–299

Allen RM, Young SJ (1978) Phencyclidine-induced psychosis. Am J Psychiatr 135: 1081–1084

Anden NE, Butcher SG, Corrodi H, Fuxe K, Ungerstedt U (1970) Receptor activity and turnover of dopamine and noradrenaline after neuroleptics. Eur J Pharmacol 11: 303–314

Angrist BM, Sathananthan G, Wilk S, Gershon S (1974) Amphetamine psychosis: Behavioral and biochemical aspects. J Psychiatr Res 11: 13–23

Appleton WS, Davis JM (1980) Practical Clinical Psychopharmacology. Baltimore Williams and Wilkins

Bell DS (1973) The experimental reproduction of amphetamine psychosis. Arch Gen Psychiatr 29: 35–40

Bertrand M (1969) The Behavioral Repertoire of the Stumptail Macaque: A Descriptive and Comparative Study. Basel Karger

Bleuler E (1961) Dementia Praecox or the Group of Schizophrenias. Translated by Zinkin J New York International Universities Press

Brizzie KR, Neal LM, Williams PM (1955) The chemoreceptor trigger zone for emesis in the monkeys. Am J Physiol 180: 659–662

Burki HR, Eichenberger E, Sayers AC (1975) Clozapine and the dopamine hypothesis of schizophrenia: A critical appraisal. Pharmakopsychitr Neuropsychopharmakol 8: 115–121

Burns RS, Lerner SE (1976) Perspectives: Acute phenyclidine intoxication. Clin Toxicol 9: 451–477

Chen G, Ensor CR, Bohner B (1965) An investigation of the sympathomimetic properties of phencyclidine by comparison with cocaine and desoxyephedrine. J Pharmacol Exp Ther 49: 71–78

Chevalier-Skolnikoff S (1974) The Ontogeny of Communication in the Stumptail Macaque *(Macaca arctoides)*. Basel Karger

Connell PH (1958) Amphetamine Psychosis. Maudsley Monographs No 5, London Oxford Univ

Crowley TJ, Stynes AJ, Hydinger M, Kaufman IC (1974) Ethanol, methamphetamine, pentobarbital, morphine, and monkey social behavior. Arch Gen Psychiatr 31: 829–838

Davies BM, Beech HR (1960) The effect of l-arylcyclohexylamine (Sernyl) on twelve normal volunteers. J Ment Sci 106: 912–924

Davis JM, Schlemmer RF Jr (1980) The amphetamine psychosis. In: Caldwell J (ed) Amphetamines and Related Stimulants: Chemical, Biological, Clinical, and Sociological Aspects. Boca Raton, CRC Press, pp 161–173

Fauman B, Aldinger G, Fauman M, Rosen P (1976) Psychiatric sequelae of phencyclidine abuse. Clin Toxicol 9: 529–538

Garver DL, Schlemmer RF Jr, Maas JW, Davis JM (1975) A schizophreniform behavioral psychosis mediated by dopamine. Am J Psychiatr 132: 33–38

Garey RE, Heath RG (1976) The effects of phencyclidine on the uptake of H-catecholamines by rat striatal and hypothalamic synaptosomes. Life Sci 18: 1105–1110

Gillin JC, Stoff DM, Wyatt RJ (1978) Transmethylation hypothesis: A review. In: Lipton MA, DiMascio A, Killam KF (eds) Psychopharmacology: A Generation of Progress. Raven Press, New York, pp 1097–1112

Griffith JD, Cavanaugh J, Held J, Oates JA (1972) Dextroamphetamine-evaluation of psychomimetic properties in man. Arch Gen Psychiatr 26: 97–100

Hoffer A, Osmond H (1967) The Hallucinogens. Academic Press, New York

Janowsky D, Davis JM (1974) Dopamine, psychomotor stimulants, and schizophrenia: Effects of methylphenidate and the stereoisomers of amphetamine in schizophrenia. In: Usdin E (ed) Neuropsychopharmacology of Monoamines and Their Regulatory Enzymes. Raven Press, New York, pp 317–323

Jolly A (1972) The Evolution of Primate Behavior. Macmillan Press, New York

Kanner M, Meltzer HY, Davis JM (1975a) Pharmacologic aspects of the locomotor stimulation produced by phencyclidine in the rat. Neurosci Abst 1: 366

Kanner M, Finnegan K, Meltzer HY (1975b) Dopaminergic effects of phenyclidine in rats with nigrostriatal lesions. Psychopharmacol Comm 1: 393–401

Kjellberg B, Randrup A (1971) The effects of amphetamine and pimozide, a neuroleptic, on the social behavior of vervet monkeys *(Cercopithecus)*. In: Vinar O, Votava Z, Bradley P (eds) Advances in Neuro-Psychopharmacology. North Holland Publ. Amsterdam, pp 305–310

Kjellberg B, Randrup A (1973) Disruption of social behavior of vervet monkeys *(Cercopithecus)* by low doses of amphetamine. Pharmakopsychiatr Neuropsychopharmacol 6: 287–293

Klein DF, Davis JM (1969) Diagnosis and Drug Treatment of Psychiatric Disorders. Baltimore Williams and Wilkins

Lerner SE, Burns RS (1978) Phencyclidine use among youth: History, epidemiology,and acute and chronic intoxication. In: Petersen RC, Stillman RC (eds) Phencyclidine (PCP) Abuse: An Appraisal. NIDA Research Monograph 21 Rockville, NIDA, pp 66–118

Luby ED, Gottlieb JS, Cohen BD, Rosenbaum G, Domino EF (1962) Model psychoses and schizophrenia. Am J Psychiatr 119: 61–67

Luisada PV (1978) The phencyclidine psychosis: Phenomenology and treatment. In: Petersen RC, Stillman RC (eds) Phencyclidine (PCP) Abuse: An Appraisal. NIDA Research Monograph 21 Rockville, NIDA, pp 241–253

Luisada PV, Brown BI (1976) Clinical management of the phencyclidine psychosis. Clin Toxicol 9: 539–545

Machiyama Y, Utena H, Kituchi M (1970) Behavioral disorders in Japanese monkeys produced by the long-term administration of methamphetamine. Proc Japan Acad 46: 738–743

Marini JL (1981) Pilocarpine, a non-hallucinogenic cholinergic agonist, elicits limb flicking in cats. Pharm Biochem Behav 15: 865–869

McKinney WT Jr (1977) Biobehavioral models of depression in monkeys. In: Hanin I, Usdin E (eds) Animal Models in Psychiatry and Neurology. Pergamon Press, Oxford, pp 117–126.

Meltzer HY, Stahl SM (1976) The dopamine hypothesis of schizophrenia. Schizophrenia Bull 2:19–77.

Miczek KA, Yoshimura H (1982) Disruption of primate social behavior by d-amphetamine and cocaine: Differential antagonism by antipsychotics. Psychopharmacol 76: 163–171

Miller RE, Levine JM, Mirsky IA (1973) Effects of psychoactive drugs on nonverbal communication and group social behavior of monkeys. J Pers Soc Psychol 28: 396–405

Nielsen EB, Lyon M (1982) Behavioral alterations during prolonged low level continuous amphetamine administration in a monkey family group *(Cercopithecus aethiops)* Biol Psychiatr 17: 423–435

Peng MT, Wang SC (1962) Emetic response of monkeys to apomorphine, hydergine, deslanoside, and protoveratrine. Proc Soc Exp Biol Med 110: 211–215

Peroutka SJ, Snyder SH (1980) Relationship of neuroleptic drug effects at brain dopamine, serotonin, alpha-adrenergic, and histamine receptors to clinical potency. Am J Psychiatr 137: 1518–1522

Randrup A, Munkvad I (1970) Biochemical, anatomical, and physiological investigations of stereotyped behavior induced by amphetamines. In: Costa E, Garattini S (eds) Amphetamines and Related Compounds. Raven Press, New York, pp 695–713

Ridley RM, Baker HF, Crow TJ (1980) Behavioral effects of amphetamines and related stimulants: The importance of species differences as demonstrated by a study in the marmoset. In: Caldwell J (ed) Amphetamines and Related Stimulants: Chemical, Biological, Clinical and Sociological Aspects. CRC Press, Boca Raton, pp 97–116

Rylander G (1972) Psychoses and the punding and choreiform syndrome in addiction to central stimulant drugs. Psychiatr Neurol Neurochir 75: 203–212

Sankar DVS (1975) LSD—A Total Study. Westbury PJD Publications

Schiorring E (1977) Changes in individual and social behavior induced by amphetamine and related compounds in monkeys and man. In: Ellinwood EH Jr, Kilbey MM (eds) Cocaine and Other Stimulants. Plenum Press, New York, pp 481–522

Schlemmer RF Jr, Davis JM (1981a) Similarities in the behavioral effects of d-amphetamine and apomorphine in selected members of a primate social colony. In: Angrist B, Burrows GD, Lader M, Lingjaerde O, Sedvall G, Wheatley D (eds) Recent Advances in Neuropsychopharmacology, Advances in the Biosciences, Vol. 31. Pergamon Press, Oxford, pp 3–12

Schlemmer RF Jr, Davis JM (1981b) Evidence for dopamine mediation of submissive gestures in the Stumptail macaque monkey. Pharmacol Biochem Behav 14(Suppl. 1): 95–102

Schlemmer RF Jr, Jackson JA, Preston KL, Bederka JP Jr, Garver DL, Davis JM (1978) Phencyclidine-induced stereotyped behavior in monkeys: Antagonism by pimozide. Eur J Pharmacol 52: 379–384

Schlemmer RF Jr, Narasimhachari N, Davis JM (1980) Dose-dependent behavioral changes induced by apomorphine in selected members of a primate social colony. J Pharm Pharmacol 32: 285–289

Schwarz CJ (1967) Paradoxical response to chlorpromazine after LSD. Psychosomatics 8: 210–211

Smith RC, Biggs CA, Leelavathi DE, Altshuler HL (1978) Behavioral effects of acute and chronic phencyclidine in the rat. Neurosci Abst 4: 503

Smith RC, Meltzer HY, Arora RC, Davis JM (1977) Effects of phencyclidine on (^{3}H) catecholamine and (^{3}H) serotonin uptake in synaptosomal preparations from rat brain. Biochem Pharmacol 26: 1435–1439

Snyder SH (1972) Catecholamines in the brain as mediators of amphetamine psychosis. Arch Gen Psychiatr 27: 169–179

Sturgeon RD, Fessler RG, London SF, Meltzer HY (1982) Behavioral effects of chronic phencyclidine administration in rats. Psychopharmacol 76: 52–56

Tyler C, Miczek KA (1982) Effects of phencyclidine on aggressive behavior in mice. Pharmacol Biochem Behav 17: pp 503–510

Wallach MB (1974) Drug-induced stereotyped behavior: Similarities and differences. In: Usdin E (ed) Neuropsychopharmacology of Monoamines and Their Regulatory Enzymes. Raven Press, New York, pp 241–260

White FJ, Holohean AM, Appel JB (1981) Lack of specificity of an animal behavior model for hallucinogenic drug action. Pharmacol Biochem Behav 14: 339–343

Ethopharmacology: Primate Models of Neuropsychiatric Disorders,
pages 79–100

Hallucinatory Behaviors in Primates Produced by Around-the-Clock Amphetamine Treatment for Several Days via Implanted Capsules

Erik B. Nielsen, Michael S. Eison, Melvin Lyon, and Susan D. Iversen

Psychopharmacological Research Laboratory, Sct. Hans Mental Hospital DK-4000 Roskilde, Denmark (E.B.N., M.L.), and Department of Experimental Psychology, University of Cambridge, Cambridge, England (M.S.E., S.D.I.)

THE PSYCHOPHARMACOLOGY OF AMPHETAMINE PSYCHOSIS AND RELEVANCE TO SCHIZOPHRENIA

The behavioral and biochemical effects of central stimulants, such as the amphetamines, have for several decades been associated with the symptoms of schizophrenia (for recent reviews see Snyder et al., 1974; Segal and Janowsky, 1978; Nausieda, 1979). Although several of these symptoms can individually be seen following intake of drugs such as hallucinogens, anticholinergics, opiates, phencyclidine and steroids, it has generally been acknowledged that only central stimulants can produce the spectrum of psychiatric symptoms that sometimes is difficult to distinguish from genuine schizophrenia (ibid.). These symptoms include paranoid delusions, auditory and visual hallucinations, thought disturbances as well as the more variable symptoms of withdrawal or extreme agitation.

In addition to the clinical similarity between amphetamine psychosis and schizophrenia, several other lines of evidence have implicated the actions of amphetamines in the psychopharmacology of schizophrenia; most important is the well-established fact that the clinical efficacy of antipsychotic drugs (i.e., neuroleptics) closely parallels their ability to block brain dopamine (DA) receptors (see review by Seeman, 1981), which in turn are critically involved in the expression of many of the behavioral effects of amphetamines (Scheel-Krüger, 1971). Most recently, evidence is accumulating that the number of DA receptors is increased in the postmortem schizophrenic brain, and this increase is apparently unrelated to prior neuroleptic drug treatment (Lee and Seeman, 1980; Reisine et al., 1980).

An important task in delineating the critical mechanism of action of amphetamines with respect to their psychotomimetic properties is the identification of the relevant dosage and intake patterns that in humans lead to the induction of amphetamine psychosis. With respect to intake patterns, however, it was established early that amphetamine psychosis was commonly observed in addicts taking high doses for an extended period of time, i.e., during "runs" of continuous intake often lasting for several days (see for example, Kramer et al., 1967). The importance of a chronic exposure to the drug in eliciting psychosis was later indicated in studies of human volunteers who were given amphetamine in controlled settings. In the first of these experiments, Griffith et al. (1970) administered low oral doses of amphetamine every few hours around the clock to prior amphetamine addicts and the expression of paranoid psychosis followed during 2–5 days of generally identifiable stages of behavioral effects. Thus, initial mild euphoric symptoms were replaced by dysphoric or depressive symptoms after which psychosis erupted. These findings were later confirmed by Angrist and Gershon (1970) when higher doses of amphetamine were given, and accordingly a more rapid onset of psychosis was observed. However, the importance of an extended, continued presence of the drug was later questioned by Bell (1973), who collected data from cases where hospitalized addicts had been given a single, or few, intravenous dose(s) of amphetamine; here, psychotic symptoms developed as rapidly as 30 min following the injection. However, it should be noted that the patients in whom psychosis developed were heavily addicted to amphetamine (one patient is listed with a daily intake of 1 g for 18 years) and some were even diagnosed schizophrenics. Furthermore, in the same study, the only two patients who failed to develop psychosis did not have a prior history of drug addiction.

Based on both clinical evidence (see for example, Snyder, 1973) and the above experimental studies, it appears that, in most cases, amphetamine psychosis develops as a result of the acute presence of the drug in the organism with a background of prior chronic exposure. Furthermore, it has generally been established that once psychosis has been experienced under the drug, the individual has a heightened sensitivity to the psychotomimetic effects of the drug (see discussion in Segal and Janowsky, 1978). Whether this increased sensitivity reflects "state-dependent learning" or a permanent, physiological effect of the drug is at present unknown, and on the whole, the pharmacodynamics of amphetamine psychosis has not been fully explored. It has been established, however, that in acute amphetamine psychosis, the decline of circulating amphetamine corresponds quite well with the clearance of psychotic symptoms (see for example, Änggard et al., 1973). Less clear, however, is the contribution of the prior chronicity of drug intake with respect to dosage or duration to the development of psychosis.

The experimental analysis of the psychopharmacology of amphetamine psychosis has been hampered by the fact that there is as yet no clear analogue of amphetamine psychosis in animals, nor has any actual neurochemical mechanism been identified for the expression of amphetamine psychosis. Part of the difficulty of establishing a model, with face validity, of amphetamine psychosis in animals is probably due to the fact that many of the symptoms associated with psychosis in humans are identified via cognitive and social features (i.e., thought disturbances, hallucinations, etc.), that are not easily recognizable in animal behavior. Thus, while "stereotyped" behavior patterns following amphetamine administration in animals undoubtedly mimic certain basic processes involved in amphetamine psychosis, these behaviors may not per se model psychotic symptoms, since in animals, stereotyped behaviors are elicited after low acute doses within minutes after an injection, while in humans, psychosis often develops after chronic high-dose intake of the drug. However, since the antagonism of acute amphetamine "stereotypies" in animals can reliably predict antipsychotic efficacy of most drugs (Janssen et al., 1967), it would seem that any model for human amphetamine psychosis and schizophrenia would include the concept of stereotypy.

On the basis of the pharmacological antagonism by neuroleptics of the acute effects of amphetamine, stereotyped behaviors have been utilized for decades as a (drug) model for schizophrenia and amphetamine psychosis (see for example, Janssen et al., 1967; Angrist et al., 1974). In a recent elaboration on this model, it was suggested that the increase in behavioral response following repeated administration of amphetamine (sensitization or "reverse tolerance") may represent an analogue of the increase in psychotomimetic effect of central stimulants when chronically taken by humans (Segal et al., 1980). However, it remains to be established that this drug regimen of repeated, but not continuous, administration is relevant to the intake patterns that characterize the development of amphetamine psychosis in humans. In experiments on humans given moderate daily doses of amphetamine, tolerance typically develops to the acute effects of the drug (i.e., subjectively experienced euphoria) (see for example, Rosenberg et al., 1962). Furthermore, in animal experiments using continuous administration of amphetamine via implanted capsules (Nielsen, 1981) sensitization does not develop, but rather, tolerance is seen to the drug-induced stereotyped behaviors. This finding as well as other evidence (Post et al., 1981) has indicated that the sensitization effect depends on contextual variables (environment/conditioning) which are absent, for example, with implanted reservoirs of the drug, and which may indicate that the sensitization effect is not directly related to the expression of the psychotomimetic properties of central stimulants.

It is worth noting that relatively few attempts have been made to model the intake patterns that, at least in controlled studies (above), reliably elicit psychosis—that is, the continuous around-the-clock administration of amphetamine for periods of up to several days. Thus, for example, in experiments on primates, the daily repeated-injection paradigm has commonly been utilized (see for example, Ellinwood, 1971). However, the massive acute doses (up to 20 mg/kg/injection, ibid.), used in many of these experiments may have confounded the expression of the chronic, delayed drug effects which perhaps would occur with continuous drug exposure regimens with moderate doses. Although many bizarre behavioral effects have been documented with such heroic doses, these behaviors have been commonly associated with the acute "stereotypy" effects of the drug.

For these reasons we became interested in studying the continuous drug regimen in primates with the intent of characterizing behavioral abnormalities that possibly could reflect the unique "human" features of psychosis, i.e., paranoia and hallucinations.

THE IMPLANTED CAPSULE TECHNIQUE FOR ACHIEVING AROUND-THE-CLOCK AMPHETAMINE INTOXICATION FOR SEVERAL DAYS

The continuous drug regimen can easily be achieved in animals by subcutaneously implanted silicone capsules as described by Huberman et al., (1977). The design of the capsule, modified for use in primates, is shown in Fig. 1. An inner reservoir is formed by two pieces of propylene tubing leaving a center gap through which the drug diffuses through the outer wall

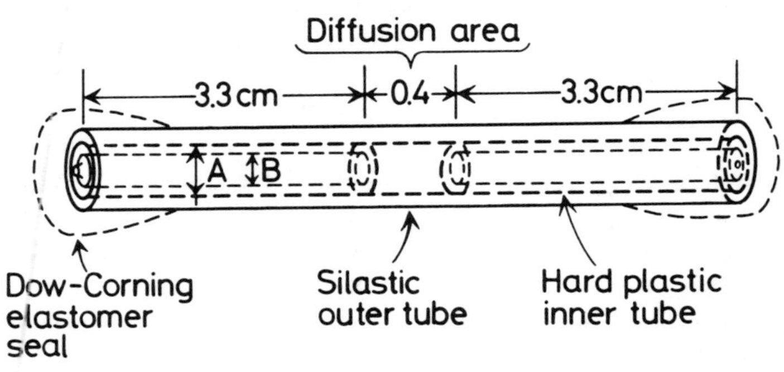

Fig. 1. The design of the silicone capsule. (Reproduced by permission of Pergamon Press, Ltd., from Ellison et al., 1981.)

of silicone plastic. The capsule is capped at the ends with Silastic Elastomer. The release rate of the capsule is shown in Fig. 2. It can be seen that the rate of release is not linear, which is a technical drawback, but in some experiments we have used the ALZET osmotic minipump to assess the role of the nonlinearity of the release rate of the silicone capsule. Minipumps filled with amphetamine base (as is also used in the silicone capsule) have a close to linear release rate (Nielsen, 1981).

The capsules used in the present experiments were surgically implanted under the skin at the level of the shoulder blades on the back of the animal. The capsules were removed using similar procedures upon completion of the drug treatment phase. At no time has infection or tissue damage been observed, even after extended implant time (up to several months).

General Experimental Procedures

In experiments on drug-induced changes in individual behaviors, primates of the following species were used: baboon (*Papio papio*, N=2); cynomologous (*Macaca fascicularis*, N=2); rhesus (*Macaca mulatta*, N=7); and African green vervet (*Cercopithecus aethiops*, N=8). Behavior was recorded using low-level light-sensitive video cameras placed in front of the animals'

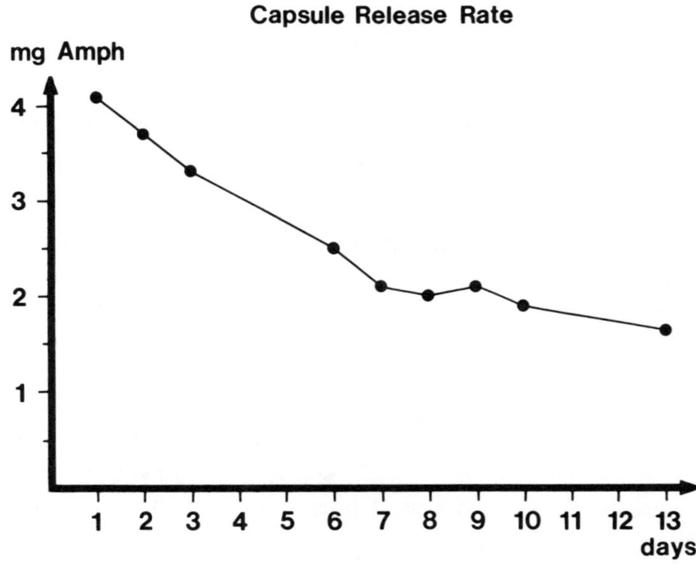

Fig. 2. Rate of release of the silicone capsule filled with amphetamine at a concentration of ca. 31 mg/kg (for a 5-kg subject). The standard error of the mean is less than the size of the symbols.

home cages which, during drug treatment, were located in a special experimental room, adjacent to the general colony room. During nights, dim red lights illuminated the experimental room. The animals were filmed every 30 min around the clock for at least 1 min, and the tapes were later scored into predefined behavioral categories using stopwatches or a computer-controlled scoring keyboard. Recordings were taken for 2–3 days prior to, during, and 2–3 days following the capsule treatment.

Socially housed primates consisted of family groups of vervet monkeys; each group was formed by the father, mother and a laboratory-born infant. During the day, the animals were released into a large arena that featured ropes, swings and concrete platforms; during the night they stayed in a smaller adjacent compartment. Owing to the size of the arena and the complexity of the social situation, a direct behavioral observation procedure was used. Twice daily, an observer sitting in an adjacent room was presented with a tone (not audible to the animals), 5 sec in duration, during which the animals were observed in a fixed sequence (i.e., mother, father, infant). Following the tone period, the observer simply indicated on a checklist which behaviors had occurred during the tone period. The animals were observed for approximately 40 min daily (representing a total of 40 individual tone/observation periods). During nights, a video camera was used to record the animals' behavior for 1 min every hour. These recordings were later scored for the presence of sleep posture and gross motor behaviors.

BEHAVIORAL EFFECTS OF AMPHETAMINE CAPSULES IN INDIVIDUALLY-HOUSED MONKEYS

Following recovery from the anesthesia used during implantation of the capsules, all monkeys exhibited strong but typical acute amphetamine behaviors such as prolonged staring or various repetitive behaviors such as biting or grooming at one particular spot on the body, biting the cage walls or bars, or "fingering" with the cage (i.e., manipulating the doors or walls). Representative examples of these behavioral changes are shown in individual animals in Fig. 3. Species differences during the acute drug phase were apparent; thus, cynomologous monkeys showed primarily prolonged staring behavior, while the baboons typically showed cage fingering. Mixed staring and/or stereotyped behaviors were present in both rhesus and vervet monkeys. These apparent species differences may also reflect actual differences in the dose of drug: although the animals received an implanted dose of amphetamine that was based on mg per kg, it has not been established if the release of drug from the capsule is a simple linear function of concentration.

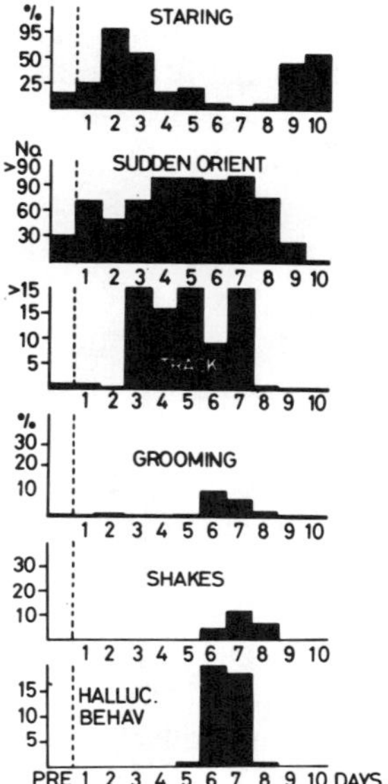

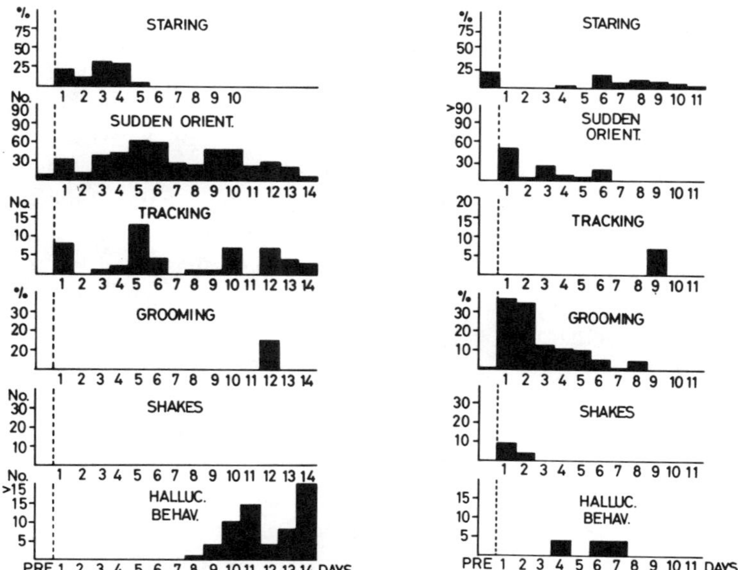

Fig. 3. Behavioral alterations in three individual vervet monkeys during several days of continuous amphetamine. Staring was defined as focused, uninterrupted staring maintained for periods longer than five seconds. Sudden orienting was defined as brief visual orienting with or without identifiable stimulus. Tracking denotes a visual orienting sequence as if a fly caught the animal's attention. See text for other details. Ordinate is behavior as a percentage of observation time per day or total number of daily observations.

One vervet monkey showed little apparent drug effect. Another vervet monkey was behaviorally unusual in that it faced the back wall of its cage while staring intensively at the same spot. However, these drug-induced behavioral changes were continuously present throughout the day/night cycle for the next 3–6 days, and at no time was sleep observed, except in the one vervet monkey that was relatively unaffected by the drug. Normal grooming (excluding stereotyped grooming), as well as drinking and eating behavior, was severely depressed. However, when a human observer entered the experimental room, the animals ceased their stereotyped activities (with the exception of staring, which, however, is a normal displacement behavior) and showed quite normal responses (such as aggressive displays) to strong stimuli such as sudden threat by the observer or being gently prodded with a wooden stick. The stereotyped behaviors were, however, resumed immediately when the observer left the room, as could be seen on the closed-circuit TV monitor.

The acute amphetamine behaviors gradually declined; however, more complex reactions evolved during the "late" phase of the drug treatment (i.e., days 6–14). An increase in sudden orienting reactions was often the first change in the animals' behavior. Over time the sudden orienting behavior became more evolved and the animals began to show striking and vivid episodes of sequences of behaviors that we termed "hallucinatory" since no eliciting stimuli could be determined. These behaviors were: (1) Flight hallucinations: Starting with a sudden orienting behavior and visual tracking, followed by a startle reaction and rapid flight from the point where the animal's initial attention was focused and finally looking back over the shoulder. This was often accompanied by emotional reactions such as fearful grimacing, vocalization and tail erection. (2) Attack hallucinations: The animal, after visual orienting behavior, pounced with great force at a point in midair or the cage wall, followed by various coordinated visual tracking behaviors and emotional reactions as noted above. (3) Eating hallucinations: This type of hallucinatory behavior was the most difficult to score, since monkeys under normal circumstances often pick up small pieces of food stuff from the bottom of their cage. However, an eating hallucination was scored if the animal slowly grasped "something" from midair, while visually following it with coordinated hand/eye movements. Often the animal, while engaged in this behavior, held the caught "object" out between the empty hands, while appearing to stretch it out, looking from hand to hand, and biting the imaginary object, as if the animal were trying to manipulate curled strings or pieces of spaghetti. This behavior could go on for several minutes at a time. (4) Other hallucinatory behaviors: These included variations of the above, such as sudden threat gestures while picking at the cage wall, and head moving slowly back and forth as if oriented to a particular "object" when none was observable to us.

On numerous occasions, the hallucinatory "objects" appeared to be at close proximity to the animal, but we were not able (on close inspection, see later) to determine any eliciting stimuli for these behaviors, such as drops of water on the shelves, bugs, sounds, reflections on metal shelves, etc. We are of course aware of the danger in inferring perceptual processes from the animals' overt behavior. However, the hallucinatory behaviors were of a great complexity, and furthermore occurred as elements of the animals' normal behavior (i.e., when threatened or in fighting). This suggests that these behaviors could not, for example, be explained as fragmentation of stereotyped behavior occurring under strong amphetamine effects.

In contrast to the early phase, the monkeys were very unresponsive in this late phase of the drug treatment. Thus, they did not show any apparent reaction to the presence of a human observer, or even to strong stimuli such as sudden threat or gentle prodding (although the animals regained normal responsivity following capsule removal).

In addition to the hallucinatory behaviors, several other abnormal behaviors were observed in the late phase of the drug treatment. These included holding a limb in a frozen position in space for an unusual amount of time. Often, a particular limb assumed an almost autonomous character: the animal would orient to a frozen-limb-in-space, and with the other hand or foot try to bring the frozen limb back to a normal position; this was usually not successful since the limb would immediately resume its unusual position. This behavior was predominantly observed in the rhesus monkeys. Another motor disturbance observed during this drug phase was vigorous shaking behavior (similar to "wet-dog" shakes), particularly in those animals exhibiting strong hallucinatory behaviors. In addition, spasms, tremor, recurrent lip smacking, jerk-like movements, facial grimacing and oral dyskinesias were noted in many animals.

Abnormal grooming behaviors were present in several animals in the late phase. However, unlike the quiet, narrowly focused grooming observed during the initial stereotypy phase of the drug treatment, the late-phase grooming was directed toward many parts of the body. Often, it appeared as if the animal were frantically trying to catch bugs in its fur; sometimes, strong emotional reactions accompanied this grooming, such as sudden startle reactions, grimacing or dance-like movements as if the animal were trying to kill insects under its feet. At times, the apparent bug-catching behavior was directed to imaginary "bugs" in the immediate visual field of the animal. We were, however, never able to find any signs of actual infestation of the animals or their quarters.

In a few vervet monkeys, intense and prolonged barking-like vocalizations were heard, lasting for up to 16 hours continuously, while the animals were intensively watching a spot outside their cage. Normal eating and drinking resumed in this late phase of the drug treatment, but total sleeplessness lasted throughout this period, with the one exception mentioned above.

Upon removal of the capsules, marked behavioral depression was observed for the next few days, during which the animals often yawned and frequently slept. None of the hallucinatory or other abnormal behaviors were observed, but some visual tracking behavior continued for several weeks. Following the initial behavioral depression, the animals were thereafter more active and showed increased "reactivity," and animals that had achieved some degree of tameness prior to the capsule treatment had now lost it.

BEHAVIORAL PROCESSES INVOLVED IN THE LATE-PHASE AMPHETAMINE STATE: CLINICAL IMPLICATIONS

The present series of experiments parallels the cited controlled studies of amphetamine psychosis in humans methodologically. Thus, the development of apparent hallucinatory behaviors in monkeys during this type of drug schedule may represent an animal analogue of the delayed appearance of psychosis in humans undergoing a similar drug regimen. This contention is supported by the observation that many of the behaviors here termed hallucinatory are also present following typical hallucinogenic drugs such as LSD and mescaline in monkeys (Siegel and Jarvik, 1975; own unpublished data). Furthermore, some of the motor symptoms observed in the late amphetamine phase, such as wet-dog shakes, are commonly elicited by hallucinogens (Schlemmer et al., 1979) and may indicate a common pharmacological mechanism (see Nielsen et al., 1980a, 1980b; Trulson and Jacobs, 1979). Finally, the observation that the animals were very unresponsive to external stimulation in this phase suggests an internal basis for the hallucinatory behaviors.

Although many similarities exist between the present findings in animals and the human experimental situation (above), some important differences can also be pointed out. Thus, if indeed the hallucinatory behaviors in the monkeys represent a correlate to human amphetamine psychosis, their development at a later time point (6–10 days following implantation) than in humans undergoing a similar drug treatment (2–5 days following the beginning of the drug treatment) requires comment. Although this can be due to many factors (such as sleep deprivation in the monkeys, see below), it is possible that sensitization had developed in the human subjects given their prior history of addiction; it is noteworthy that in Bell's study (1973), the two subjects that failed to develop amphetamine psychosis had no such history of prior drug abuse. For this reason, some monkeys in the present experiments were reimplanted with amphetamine capsules, from 2 to 8 months following the initial capsule treatment, in order to assess possible changes in drug sensitivity. In general, sensitization was found to have developed to the hallucinatory behaviors, since they appeared sooner during the reimplantation, although generally not with increased frequency. Furthermore, the duration and intensity of stereotyped behavior during the first few days following reimplantation was generally decreased compared to the first implantation, possibly indicating tolerance development to this aspect of the drug effect. It should, however, be kept in mind that an increased sensitivity to these effects may also have been present, since the apparent decrease of motor sterotypies may have been replaced by other behaviors, less identifiable as obviously stereotyped (see below).

Sleep deprivation is a potentially important variable in the present experiment since it has been established that in humans, 4–5 days of sleep deprivation produces psychotic symptoms, including paranoia and hallucinations (West et al., 1962). However, the finding of a rapid development of hallucinatory behaviors (1–2 days following capsule reimplantation), in some animals, suggests that sleep deprivation does not play an important role in drug-experienced subjects in the evolution of hallucinatory behaviors. A similar reasoning applies to amphetamine psychosis in humans, since this has been documented long before sleep deprivation could play a major role (i.e., Angrist et al., 1974; Bell, 1973). In some experiments, we attempted to sleep-deprive two rhesus for 7 days prior to implantation of amphetamine capsules. This was accomplished by a loud buzzer which frequently, at irregular intervals, would awake the animals. However, no noticeable effect on the subsequent drug-induced behavors could be established.

With the present capsule technique, release rate is not constant over time, and therefore changes in behavior over time might reflect this phenomenon. However, when some animals (of all species) were implanted with ALZET osmotic minipumps releasing a relatively constant amount of amphetamine for one week, a generally similar progression of behavioral effects was found. This indicates that release rate changes over time with the silicone capsule probably do not play a major role in the expression of phasic drug effects.

In summary, the present results suggest that a behavioral syndrome can be identified in primates which parallels amphetamine psychosis in humans with respect to drug dosage, temporal development, and the nature of the behavioral state. This syndrome is characterized by hallucinatory behaviors of a complex and highly evolved nature, motor disturbances, and decreased responsivity to the external environment.

THE EFFECTS OF IMPLANTED AMPHETAMINE CAPSULES IN FAMILY GROUPS OF PRIMATES

Since important symptoms of schizophrenia involve bizarre social responses (such as autism and inappropriate affect), it was of interest to determine the effects of the amphetamine capsule treatment in social colonies of primates. For this reason, we have conducted experiments using both the previously described high-dose amphetamine capsule (as used in individually housed animals), as well as a modified capsule designed to release its contents at a much lower rate, but for a prolonged period of time (Nielsen and Lyon, 1982). The intent with the slow-release capsule was to establish a continuous amphetamine regimen that would not produce strong acute behavioral changes, but allow for many types of social interactions, thereby perhaps providing a way to determine the specificity of the amphetamine-induced behavioral changes. Many, if not all, drugs in high enough doses can probably eliminate all social interactions of the drugged animal. The design of the slow-release capsule is similar to that of the high-dose capsule, but the window in the inner reservoir is a small hole (2 mm), through which the drug diffuses. Again, release rate is not constant (Fig. 4), but declines very gradually over a period of approximately 8–10 weeks.

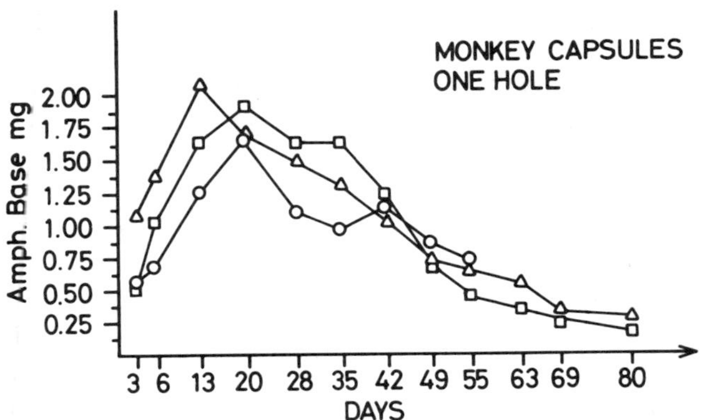

Fig. 4. Rate of release of the slow-release amphetamine capsule. Reproduced by permission of Plenum Press Corp., from Nielsen and Lyon, 1982.

It was established in preliminary experiments, that the high-dose capsule in socially housed monkeys produced a pattern of behavioral effects similar to that seen in individually housed animals, that is, an initial period of strong, stereotyped behaviors, followed by a late phase of hallucinatory and other abnormal behaviors as previously described. With respect to the changes in social behavior induced by this drug regimen, it was clear that the drug-treated animal engaged in few, if any, social interactions (such as normal social grooming, etc), but was often seen "avoiding" the other animals. These data should be regarded as preliminary, however, as they have not yet been fully analyzed.

In subsequent experiments with naive animals, the slow-release capsule was studied in one family group of vervet monkeys. The infant was born in the laboratory and the family had stayed together for 4 months prior to the beginning of the experiments. After several weeks of behavioral observations, the two adult monkeys were implanted with the slow-release capsule and the family was observed for the next 12 weeks of drug treatment. The major behavioral effects are summarized in Figs. 5–7. While gross locomotor activity was relatively unaffected in the two adult monkeys, marked increases in staring behavior developed and were maximally expressed during 6–8 weeks following implantation. Of particular interest was the lack of any of the hallucinatory behaviors that were observed with the stronger capsule, although approximately double the total amount of amphetamine was administered with the slow-release capsule. It may well be, however, that the increased staring behavior observed in the present experiment represented a first stage in the development of the later hallucinatory behaviors, as seen with the high-dose capsule. The changes in individual behaviors, seen in the present experiment, were associated with a decrease in sleep during nights, so that once sleep had recovered to preimplantation levels, most of the changes in individual behaviors had also recovered.

With the exception of infant/female contact, which gradually increased, social proximity behaviors were decreased very early with the slow-release capsule and remained depressed even after capsule removal. Although it is possible that some of these changes were developmental in nature (i.e., would have occurred anyway over time), they may reflect social-learning phenomena. This possibility is substantiated by the fact that the infant's locomotor activity was depressed for several weeks following implantation of the adult monkeys, although the infant did not receive any drug treatment. One may speculate that the increased amount of infant/female contact could be due to an increased seeking of contact by the infant, possibly related to decreased interest or attention by the mother or to other drug-induced changes

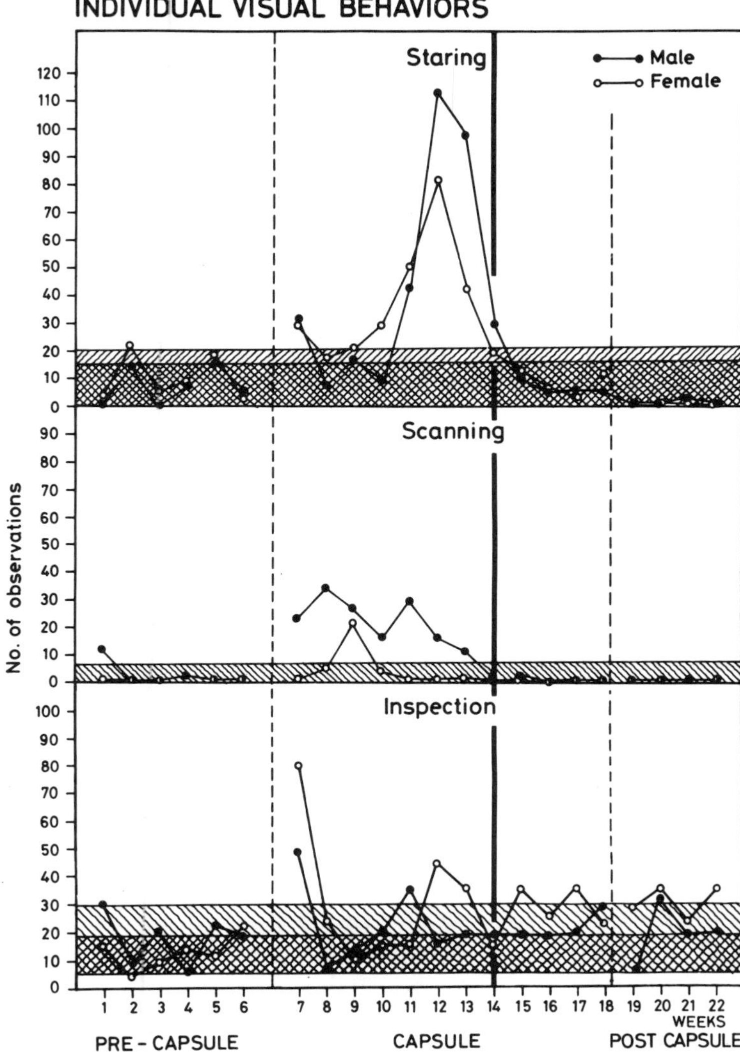

Fig. 5. Changes in individual behaviors during several weeks of treatment with the slow-release amphetamine capsule. Staring was defined as uninterrupted, focused staring throughout an individual 5-sec observation period. Ordinate is the total no of weekly observations. Scanning was defined as unfocused orienting throughout an individual 5-sec observation period. Inspection denotes all instances of orienting toward own body, with or without grooming. The shaded area indicates a confidence interval based on the precapsule baseline. Points outside this interval are statistically significant with $p < .0027$. Reproduced from Nielsen and Lyon (1982) with permission of Plenum Publishing Corp. The solid line indicates return of normal sleep. See also Fig. 7.

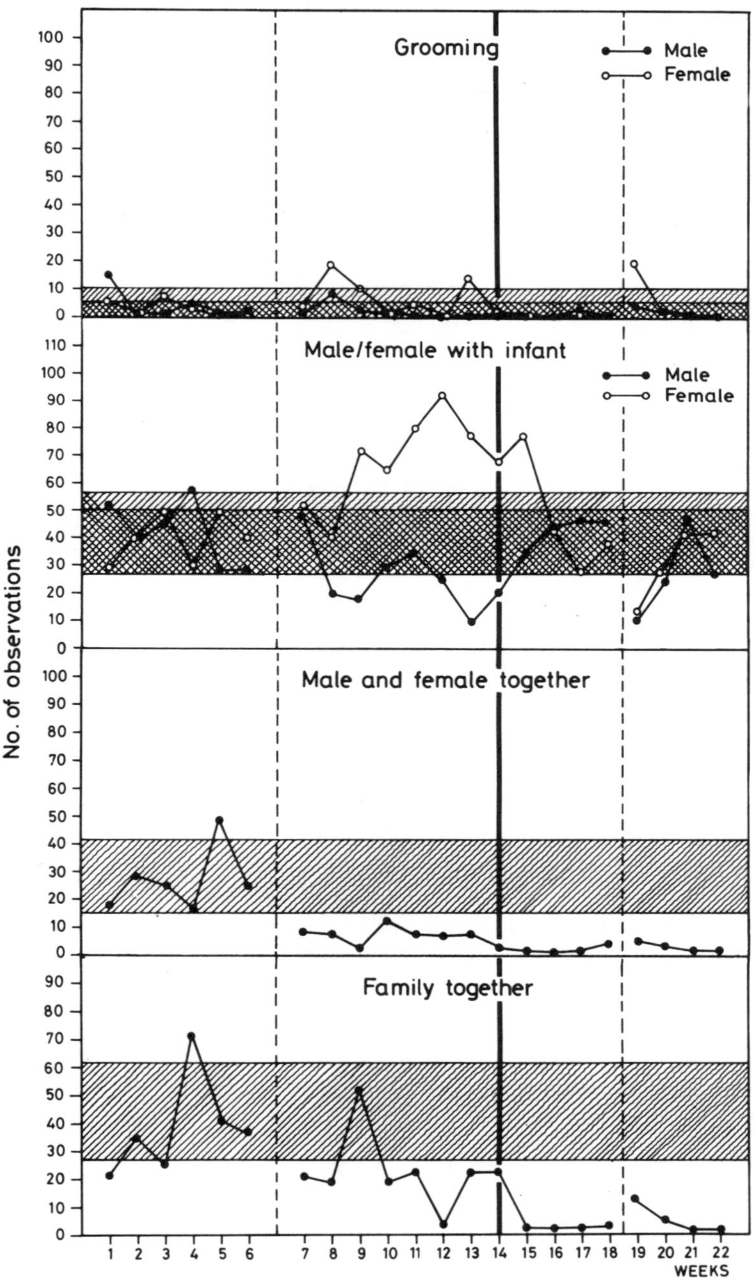

Fig. 6. Changes in social behavior during several weeks of treatment with the slow-release amphetamine capsule. The contact measures are based on physical proximity to the extent that the animals could reach each other. See legend to Fig. 5 for other details. Reproduced by permission.

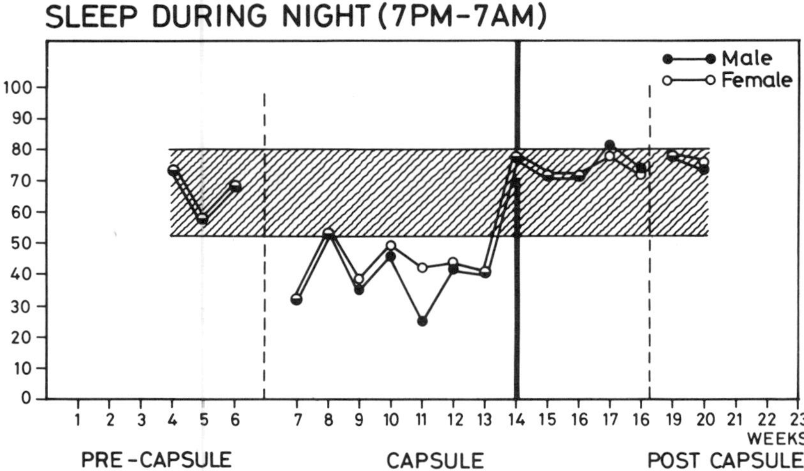

Fig. 7. Sleep during nights during the slow-release amphetamine capsule treatment based on presence of typical sleep posture (the infant was not observed). Reproduced by permission.

in the parents' behavior. Furthermore, the apparent lack of behavioral recovery was mainly present in the social behavors where a greater role of social learning factors presumably would occur. The general decrease in social contact behaviors reported with acute amphetamine treatment (Schiorring, 1977; Schiorring and Hecht, 1979) is confirmed in the present data which furthermore indicated that no tolerance develops to this effect.

In order to further assess tolerance phenomena with respect to the slow-release capsule, this capsule was implanted in one single-caged vervet monkey previously treated with the high-dose capsule. In this animal, very gradual behavioral changes occurred during the first few weeks. However, by the fourth week following implantation, pronounced hallucinatory behaviors had developed characterized by "parasitotic-like" grooming, rapid visual tracking, and grasping in midair after invisible objects. Following a period of intense barking lasting for many hours, these abnormal behaviors were rapidly terminated by an injection of the neuroleptic drug flupenthixol. Although the experiment was only performed in one animal, the result again indicates that following the high-dose capsule treatment, sensitization develops to the hallucinatory behaviors since they did not develop in naive animals. Furthermore, once sensitization has developed, the occurrence of apparent hallucinatory behaviors probably does not require high circulating levels of amphetamine. However, actual plasma or brain levels of amphetamine need to be determined to assess accurately the role of circulating drug levels in these experiments.

The finding of gradually developing alterations in social and individual behavior represents an interesting parallel to the type of change that conceivably would appear with endogenous psychotomimetic substances; thus, tolerance does not develop, evidence of accumulating behavioral changes is present, and their gradual development over time may be an analogue of gradually developing schizophrenic symptoms characterized by decreased social contact and increased time spent on idiosyncratic behaviors. It is of interest in this connection that endogenous amphetamine-like substances, such as phenylethylamine (PEA), have been implicated in schizophrenia (Wyatt, 1978).

It is also of interest that many of the behavioral changes in the present experiment quite closely paralleled the decrease and recovery of normal sleep. Sleep disturbances have been reported during the initial phases of the development of schizophrenia (i.e., Kupfer et al., 1970), although findings of sleep disturbances in chronic schizophrenia have been infrequent (see, however, Zarcone et al., 1975).

THE ROLE OF STEREOTYPED BEHAVIORS IN THE DEVELOPMENT OF THE LATE-PHASE HALLUCINATORY BEHAVIORS AND IN PSYCHOSIS IN HUMANS

A fundamental aspect of how central stimulants alter behavior in many experimental situations involves the concept of stereotyped behavior. Thus, according to the theory of Lyon and Robbins (1975), many of the behavioral effects of amphetamines can be seen as due to increased repetition rate of the ongoing behavior. Furthermore, with increasing doses, the increasing repetition rate decreases the number of observable behavioral categories. Thus, at very high doses, few behaviors may be seen, such as in the rat, for example, only biting and licking. In monkeys, the same high doses may almost "immobilize" the animal such that only staring is present, eventually interrupted by brief eye and head movements. Other important behavioral effects of amphetamines are their strong reinforcing effects (Yokel and Wise, 1975) and their strong discriminative stimulus properties (Schechter and Cook, 1975). The modulation of these reinforcing and discriminable drug effects during various chronic drug regimens has been relatively little studied with respect to the psychotomimetic properties of amphetamines. The significance of the various behavioral tolerance and sensitization effects observed during chronic drug intake has been difficult to evaluate considering parallels between human and animal data. Thus, while humans may rapidly become "tolerant" to the subjectively experienced euphoric effects of amphetamines (Rosenberg et al., 1962), comparable low doses in animals cause apparent behavioral sensitization (Segal et al., 1980). In the present experiments, examples of both tolerance and sensitization phenomena can be found. Thus, the initially strong stereotyped behaviors following implantation of the high-dose amphetamine capsule had generally declined after the first 3–6 days, an effect which was also observed with the steady-release osmotic minipump and confirmed in other experiments in rats (Nielsen, 1981). However, with the slow-release capsule, some of the acute effects of the drug (i.e., staring behavior) were increasing over time, even when drug output was steady or declining. Furthermore, upon reimplantation of amphetamine capsules, sensitization had developed to the hallucinatory effects of the drug. However, since stereotyped behaviors, such as staring or repetitive motor acts, always preceded the later hallucinatory behaviors, these initial behavioral effects may be important first signs of the development of the later, more obviously "psychotic" (hallucinatory) behaviors. The exact nature of how stereotyped behavior patterns may progress into the more psychotic state is at present unknown, but may be of importance for understanding both amphetamine psychosis and schizophrenia (see also Lyon, 1979). It is of interest to note that in retrospective studies of the pathogenesis of schizophrenia, the gradual development of recognizable stages of behavioral changes was initially characterized by several amphetamine-like behavioral symptoms such as lack of sleep, focusing of attention on idiosyncratic aspects, and intensification of thought processes and attention (Bowers, 1968; Docherty et al., 1978). Similarly, in the experimental studies of amphetamine psychosis in humans, the initial acute drug effects (such as euphoria) were gradually replaced by dysphoric reactions before psychosis developed. It is thus possible that the initial acute effects of amphetamine in animals, i.e., stereotyped behaviors, may correspond to the initial phase of amphetamine's psychotomimetic effects. However, relatively few attempts have been made to incorporate the concept of stereotypy into a framework for understanding the organization and development of psychotic behavior, whether amphetamine psychosis or schizophrenia (see, however, Lyon, 1979; Lyon and Nielsen, 1979).

Although it will be important to explore pharmacological processes with respect to the development of psychotic behavior during continuous amphetamine treatment (see for example, Nielsen et al., 1980b), it will also be important to characterize the behavioral mechanisms which may underlie such processes. Thus, one may speculate that the continuous performance of stereotyped behavior, under the influence of amphetamine, would result in behavioral changes by means of learning. In this respect, it is perhaps important to keep in mind that the stereotypy-inducing properties of central stimulants may apply not only to the motor aspects of behavior, but equally well to perceptual-attentional aspects of behavior; these may play a major role in primates (and humans) in amphetamine effects—the induction of staring behavior by amphetamine in primates is a possible example hereof (see also Mathysse, 1977). Therefore, if indeed "hallucinatory" behavior as described in the present experiments reflects a genuine perceptual phenomenon, it could originate from the prolonged "locking in" of the animals' perception and direction of attention to certain restricted aspects of the visual field. A counterpart of such processes may be found in perceptual disturbances during extensive concentration on restricted visual fields (for example, radar screens), as has been reported in human experiments (Welford, 1976).

In summary, the present experiments identify hallucinatory behaviors in primates as a close analogue of amphetamine psychosis in humans. Furthermore, the results from the social family-group experiments indicate that the prolonged continuous presence of amphetamine can produce accumulating behavioral effects which may model similar gradual development of schizophrenic symptoms in humans. It is, however, important to realize that the present amphetamine regimens undoubtedly have several biochemical and behavioral effects that may be unrelated to psychosis in humans. Thus, while in drug models DA receptors have been implicated in schizophrenia, it should be kept in mind that only a localized subpopulation of dopaminergic receptors may be involved in the disease (Meltzer et al., 1981). However, with drugs such as amphetamine, many dopaminergic and nondopaminergic systems in the brain are activated. Therefore, the identification of specific pathways and associated behavioral effects involved in the psychotomimetic effects of amphetamine is an important task for future work in this area.

ACKNOWLEDGMENTS

The skillful technical assistance of Birgit Bager, Birthe Lehmann, and Robert Hughes is highly appreciated. Mogens Engelstoft, A/S Ferrosan, Denmark, kindly extracted the amphetamine base. This research was supported by grants from the Danish Medical Research Council No. 512-8908, the Danish Hospital Research Foundation for Greater Copenhagen, Faroe Islands, and Greenland No. 77/78, 17, NSF NATO No. MAR 1979, and the Wellcome Trust.

We wish to acknowledge the initial inspiration and collaboration on the present experiments with Dr. G. Ellison, UCLA, who assisted us in implementing the continuous drug-infusion technique via silicone capsules.

REFERENCES

Angrist BM, Gershon S (1970) The phenomenology of experimentally induced amphetamine psychosis—preliminary observations. Biol Psychiatr 2: 95–107

Angrist B, Sathananthan G, Wilk S, Gershon S (1974) Amphetamine psychosis: Behavioral and biochemical aspects. J Psychiatr Res 11: 13–23

Änggard E, Jönsson LE, Hogmark AL, Gunne LM (1973) Amphetamine metabolism in amphetamine psychosis. Clin Pharmacol Ther 14: 870–880

Bell DS (1973) The experimental reproduction of amphetamine psychosis. Arch of Gen Psychiatr 29: 35–40

Bowers MB (1968) Pathogenesis of acute schizophrenic psychosis. Arch of Gen Psychiatr 19: 348–355

Docherty JP, van Kammen DP, Siris SG, Marder SR (1978) Stages of onset of schizophrenic psychosis. Am J Psychiatr 135: 420–426

Ellinwood EH (1971) Effects of chronic methamphetamine intoxication in rhesus monkeys. Biol Psychiatr 3: 25–32

Ellison G, Nielsen EB, Lyon M (1981) Animal model of psychosis: Hallucinatory behaviors in monkeys during the late stage of continuous amphetamine intoxication. J Psychiatr Res 16: 13–22

Griffith JD, Cavanaugh JH, Held J, Oates JA (1970) Experimental psychosis induced by the administration of d-amphetamine. In: Costa E, Garatini S (eds) Amphetamines and related compounds. Raven Press New York pp 897–904

Huberman HS, Eison MS, Bryan KS, Ellison G (1977) A slow-release silicone pellet for chronic amphetamine administration. Eur J Pharmacol 45: 237–242

Janssen PAJ, Niemegeers CJE, Schellekens KHL, Lenaerts FM (1967) Is it possible to predict the clinical effects of neuroleptic drugs (major tranquilizers) from animal data? Arzneimittel Forschung 17: 841–854

Kramer JC, Fischman VS, Littlefield DC (1967) Amphetamine abuse. J Am Med Assoc 201: 305–309

Kupfer DJ, Wyatt RJ, Scott J, Snyder F (1970) Sleep disturbance in acute schizophrenic patients. Am J Psychiatr 126: 1213–1223

Lee T, Seeman P (1980) Elevation of neuroleptic/dopamine receptors in schizophrenia. Am J Psychiatr 137: 191–197

Lyon M (1979) Central stimulant drugs and the nature of reinforcement. In: Sjöden PO, Bates S, Dockens WS (Eds) Trends in behavior therapy. Academic Press New York pp 153–178

Lyon M, Nielsen EB (1979) Psychosis and drug-induced stereotypies. In: Keehn JD (Ed) Psychopathology in animals. Academic Press New York pp 103–143

Lyon M, Robbins T (1975) The actions of central nervous system stimulant drugs: A general theory concerning amphetamine effects. In: Essman W, Valzelli L (Eds) Current developments in psychopharmacology. Spectrum Publ New York pp 80–163

Mathysse S (1977) Animal models of human cognitive processes. In Hanin I, Usdin E (Eds) Animal models in psychiatry and neurology. Pergamon Press New York pp 75–82

Meltzer HY, Busch D, Fang VS (1981) Hormones, dopamine receptors and schizophrenia. Psychoneuroendocrinology 6: 17–36

Nausieda PA (1979) Central stimulant toxicity. In: Winken PJ, Bruyn GW, Cohen MM, Klawans HL (Eds) Intoxication of the nervous system. North-Holland Publ Comp Amsterdam pp 223–297

Nielsen EB (1981) Rapid decline of stereotyped behavior in rats during constant one week administration of amphetamine via implanted ALZET osmotic minipumps. Pharmacol Biochem Behav 15: 161–165

Nielsen EB, Lee TH, Ellison GD (1980a) After several days of continuous administration, d-amphetamine acquires hallucinogen-like properties. Psychopharmacology 68: 197–201

Nielsen EB, Lyon M (1982) Behavioral alterations during prolonged low level continuous amphetamine administration in a monkey family group *(Cercopithecus aethiops)*. Biol Psychiatr 17: 423–434

Nielsen EB, Nielsen M, Ellison G, Braestrup C (1980b) Decreased spiroperidol and LSD binding in rat brain after continuous amphetamine. Eur J Pharm 66: 149–154

Post RM, Lockfeld A, Squillace KM, Contel NR (1981) Drug-environment interaction: Context dependency of cocaine-induced behavioral sensitization. Life Sci 28: 755–760

Reisine TD, Rossor M, Spokes E, Iversen LL, Yamamura HI (1980) Opiate and neuroleptic alterations in human schizophrenic brain tissue. In: Pepeu G, Kuhar MJ, Enna SJ (Eds) Receptors for neurotransmitters and peptide hormones. Raven Press New York pp 443–450

Rosenberg DE, Wolbach HB, Miner EJ, Isbell H (1962) Observations on direct and cross tolerance with LSD and d-amphetamine in man. Psychopharmacologia 5: 1–15

Schechter MD, Cook PG (1975) Dopaminergic mediation of the interoceptive cue produced by d-amphetamine in rats. Psychopharmacologia 42: 185–193

Scheel-Krüger J (1971) Comparative studies of various amphetamine analogues demonstrating different interactions with the metabolism of the catecholamines in the brain. Eur J Pharm 14: 47–59

Schiorring E (1977) Changes in individual and social behavior induced by amphetamine and related compounds in monkeys and man. In: Ellinwood EH, Kilbey M (Eds) Cocaine and other stimulants. Plenum Press New York pp 481–522

Schiorring E, Hecht A (1979) Behavioral effects of low, acute doses of d-amphetamine on the dyadic interaction between mother and infant vervet monkey *(Cercopithecus aethiops)* during the first six postnatal months. Psychopharmacology 64: 219–224

Schlemmer RF, Tyler CB, Narasimhachari N (1979) The comparative effect of LSD, mescaline and DMT on primate social and solitary behavior. Federation Proc 37: 659

Seeman P (1981) Brain dopamine receptors. Pharmacol Reviews 32: 229–313

Segal DS, Janowsky DS (1978) Psychostimulant-induced behavioral effects: Possible models of schizophrenia. In: Lipton MA, DiMascio A, Killam KF (Eds) Psychopharmacology: A generation of progress. Raven Press New York pp 1113–1123

Segal DS, Weinberger SB, Cahill J, McCunney SJ (1980) Multiple daily amphetamine administration: Behavioral and neurochemical alterations. Science 207: 904–907

Siegel RK, Jarvik ME (1975) Drug-induced hallucinations in animals and man. In: Siegel RK, West LJ (Eds) Hallucinations: Behavior, experience and theory. John Wiley and Sons New York pp 71–161

Snyder SH (1973) Amphetamine psychosis: A "model" schizophrenia mediated by catecholamines. Am J Psychiatr 130: 61–67

Snyder SH, Banerjee SP, Yamamura HI, Greenberg D (1974) Drugs, neurotransmitters and schizophrenia. Science 184: 1243–1253

Trulson ME, Jacobs BL (1979) Long-term amphetamine treatment decreases brain serotonin metabolism: Implications for theories of schizophrenia. Science 205: 1295–1297

Welford AT (1976) Skilled performance: Perceptual and motor skills. Scott, Forestman and Co Glenview Illinois

West LJ, Janszen HH, Lester BK, Cornelisoon Jr FS (1962) The psychosis of sleep deprivation. Annals NY Acad Sci 96: 66–70

Wyatt RJ (1978) Is there an endogenous amphetamine? In: Wynne L, Cromwell R, Mathysse S (Eds) The nature of schizophrenia. John Wiley and Sons New York pp 125–166

Yokel RA, Wise RA (1975) Increased lever pressing for amphetamine after pimozide in rats: Implications for a dopamine theory of reward. Science 187: 547–549

Zarcone V, Azmui K, Dement W, Gulevich G, Kraemer H, Pivik T (1975) REM phase deprivation and schizophrenia. Arch of Gen Psychiatr 32: 1431–1436

Ethopharmacology: Primate Models of Neuropsychiatric Disorders, pages 101–135

Is There a Relationship Between Social Isolation, Cognitive Inflexibility, and Behavioral Stereotypy? An Analysis of the Effects of Amphetamine in the Marmoset

R.M. Ridley and H.F. Baker

Division of Psychiatry, Clinical Research Center, Harrow, Middlesex, United Kingdom

INTRODUCTION

We have been studying the behavioral effects of amphetamine treatment in a small New World primate, the marmoset (*Callithrix jacchus*), for the past 5 years. The effects of acute amphetamine administration have been assessed together with those of various centrally acting drugs in an effort to modify the amphetamine effects. We have also attempted to understand the nature of the major behavioral effect of amphetamine and have examined the progressive changes in behavior brought about by chronic administration of this drug.

Both acute and chronic treatments with amphetamine cause certain items of behavior to be repeated in a stereotyped form.

A series of experiments was carried out in which marmosets were trained on visual discrimination tasks, using either a rodent operant apparatus or a Wisconsin General Test apparatus, and the effect of amphetamine treatment on the learning and performance of these tasks was assessed. From these experiments, it became clear that marmosets demonstrated an inflexibility in their approach to solving problems under doses of amphetamine which were too low to elicit overt behavioral stereotypy.

We have also observed that marmosets treated with amphetamine show a reduction in social behavior, and further tests of this phenomenon are currently being developed.

At this stage, it is not clear just how these three facets of amphetamine-induced change are related although experiments using intracerebral cannulae are providing evidence that all three effects can result from the injection of amphetamine into one brain area, the ventral striatum (Annett and Ridley, 1982; Annett, personal communication), implying that they may be more than coincidentally related.

We are struck by the occurrence of stereotypy, cognitive inflexibility, and social isolation in infantile autism (Kanner, 1943) and in certain other conditions of profound behavioral disturbance (Ridley and Baker, 1982). The relationship of our findings to human mental disorders will be discussed at the end of this paper.

THE BEHAVIORAL EFFECTS OF ACUTE ADMINISTRATION OF AMPHETAMINE

The behavioral effects of acute amphetamine treatment have been studied in many primate species. Randrup and Munkvad (1967) have reported stereotyped behavior, which included rapid sideways movements, head bobbing, and visual "searching" in squirrel monkeys (*Saimiri sciureus*). These stereotypies were idiosyncratic, each animal reverting to its own particular form of stereotypy when injected again some months later. Idiosyncratic stereotypies such as staring at the hands, grasping movements, and rapid head movements have also been observed in vervet monkeys (*Cercopithecus aethiops*; Randrup and Munkvad, 1972). Amphetamine increases locomotion in owl monkeys (*Aotes trivirgatus*; Isaac and Troelstrup, 1969) but has been found to decrease locomotion in the rhesus (*Macaca mulatta*; Alexander and Isaac, 1965) and the squirrel monkey (Isaac and Troelstrup, 1969).

DIRECT OBSERVATION OF THE BEHAVIORAL EFFECTS OF AMPHETAMINE IN THE MARMOSET (*CALLITHRIX JACCHUS*)

Eight young marmosets (four male, four female), weighing 250–400 g each, were housed in individual cages (50 × 50 × 30 cm) containing food, water, and wooden perches in a room containing other caged marmosets. They were observed through a small aperture 3 m from the cages. With the aid of a metronome, behavior occurring every second over a period of 50 seconds was classified into the mutually exclusive categories: (1) inactivity: no discernible movement; (2) checking: rapid movement of the head only; (3) activities: movement of only part of the body, excluding the head only (this category included eating, drinking, manipulating parts of the cage, self-grooming, and scent-marking); (4) locomotion: displacement of the whole body.

Vocalization was not scored since this could occur concurrently with other categories, and social interaction could not be examined since the animals were individually housed. Four animals were tested concurrently. Amphetamine was given in increasing doses such that each animal received one dose of amphetamine per week (and one dose of apomorphine on a nonconsecutive day—see Ridley et al., 1980d).

The effect of 0–8 mg/kg d-amphetamine sulphate injected intramuscularly (im) can be summarized as follows (see Fig. 1): (1) a dose-dependent increase in checking with duration inversely related to dose; (2) a dose-dependent suppression of activities; (3) no change in locomotion; (4) a dose-dependent decrease in inactivity with duration inversely related to dose.

The inverse relation of the duration of increased checking and decreased inactivity to dose may be ascribed to the onset of severe stereotypy. At 4 and 8 mg/kg, this stereotypy was observed as very small movements of the whole body (postural adjustments), padding movements of the hands and feet, creeping movements with piloerection, and rigid immobility. Thus, severe stereotypy contributed to all four behavioral categories.

A comparison of the effects of the d- and l-isomers of amphetamine was made using another group of six adolescent marmosets housed together in a cage measuring 70 × 70 × 80 cm (Scraggs and Ridley, 1978). An additional category of contact consisting of any contact between two or more animals including touching, grooming, fighting, and playing was added to the behavioral categories already described. As before, behavior occurring every second in periods of 50 seconds was classified for each animal just prior to injection and at 12-minute intervals thereafter for 1 hour, followed by further readings at 2, 3, and 5 hours postinjection. The mean behavioral effects during the first hour are shown in Fig. 2, where it can be seen that the d-isomer is about twice as potent as the l-isomer in stimulating checking and decreasing inactivity. Additionally, a total suppression of activities and contact was produced by all doses of either isomer.

MODIFICATION OF THE BEHAVIORAL EFFECTS OF ACUTE AMPHETAMINE ADMINISTRATION BY OTHER DRUGS

Amphetamine administration has been shown to influence both dopaminergic and noradrenergic systems in the rat (Carlsson et al., 1966; Scheel-Kruger, 1971). In the first experiment in this series (Scraggs and Ridley, 1979) we chose to examine the way in which the dopamine antagonist, haloperidol, and the noradrenaline β-antagonist, propranolol, and the α-antagonist aceperone (Rolinski and Scheel-Kruger, 1973) might modify or influence the behavioral effects of acute amphetamine administration. We used the same animals and experimental design that were used to compare the isomers of amphetamine. Saline or the drug under test was administered 18 minutes after injection of amphetamine, the following doses being used:

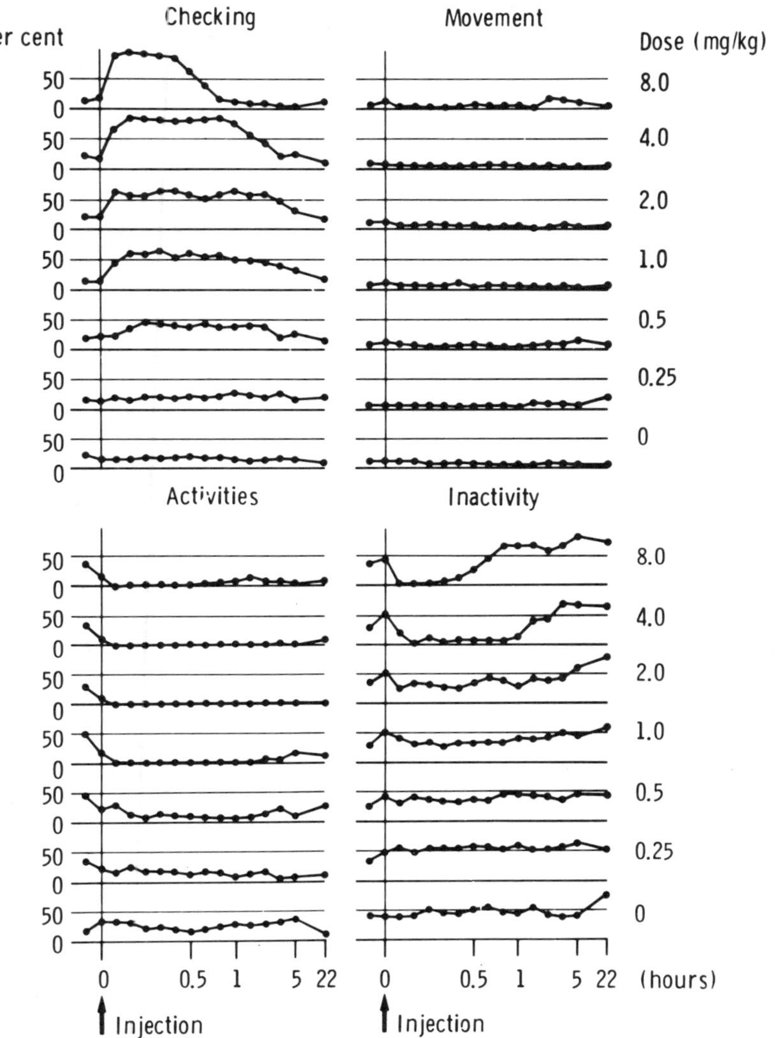

Fig. 1. The effect of 0 to 8.0 mg/kg d-amphetamine on checking, movement, activities, and inactivity. Graphs show mean proportion of each 50 sec reading spent in each behavioral category by eight marmosets. ● Indicates time when reading was taken. Note irregular time scale.

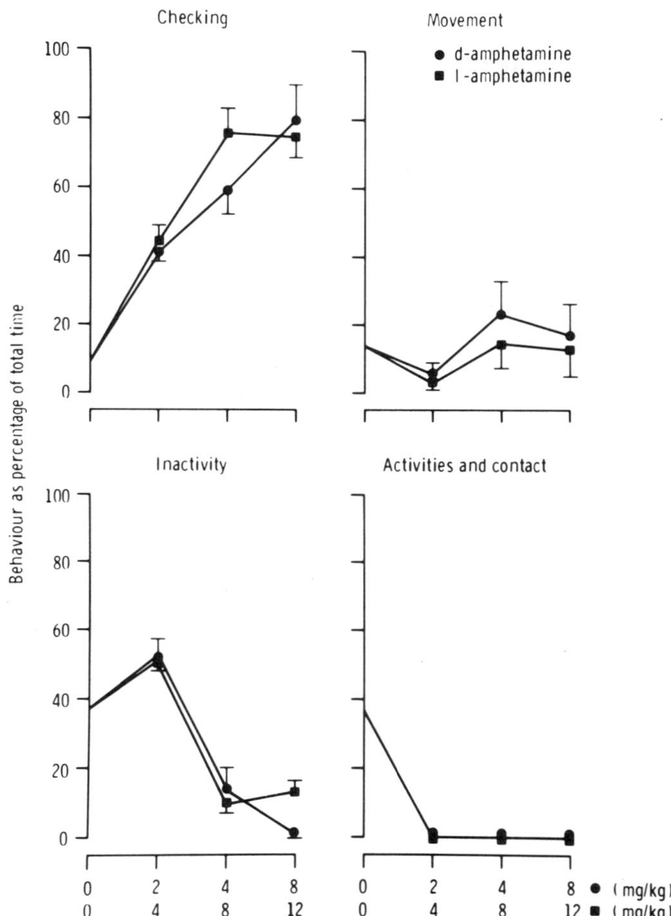

Fig. 2. Dose-dependent effects of d- and l-amphetamine averaged over five readings from 12 to 60 min post-injection in six marmosets. Note superimposition of abscissae for each isomer.

haloperidol 0.03–0.18 mg/kg, aceperone 10 mg/kg, propranolol 10 and 20 mg/kg. Haloperidol caused a dose-dependent suppression of amphetamine-induced checking and a dose-dependent increase in inactivity (Fig. 3). It should be noted that haloperidol has a suppressant effect in marmosets not treated with amphetamine, and that it does not reinstate the loss of activities and contact observed after amphetamine treatment. At the doses used propranolol was mildly sedative, whereas aceperone had no effect in ampheta-

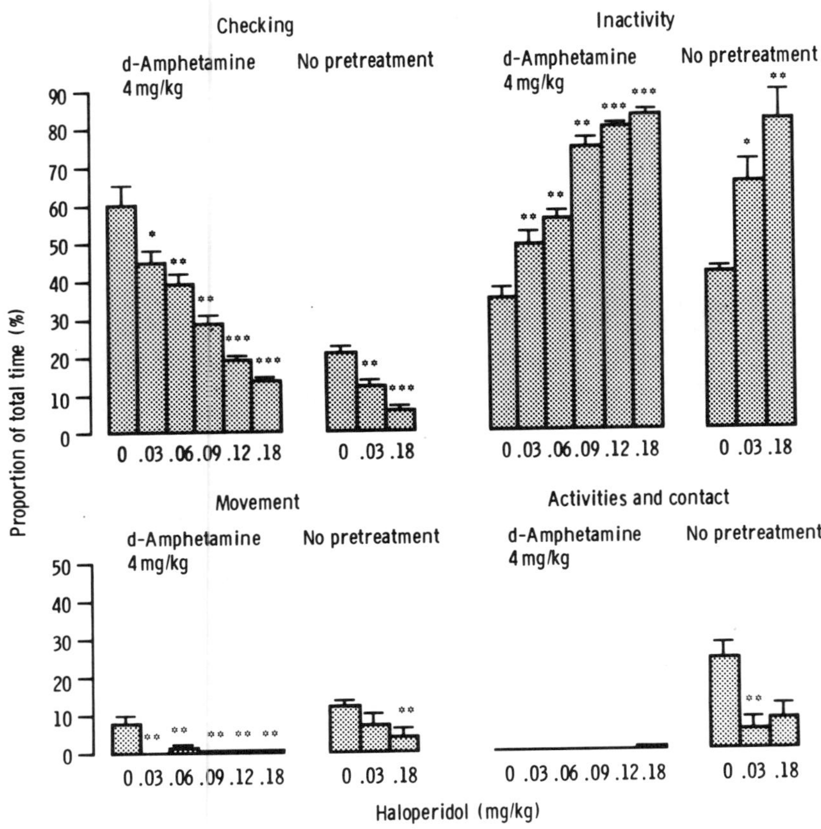

Fig. 3. Dose-dependent effects of haloperidol in marmosets pretreated with 4 mg/kg d-amphetamine or with no pretreatment over the period 18–66 min post injection (n=6). Ordinate shows behavior as mean % of time in six 50-sec observations. *p < 0.05, **p < 0.01, ***p < 0.001; two-tailed matched-pair t-test.

mine-treated animals. From these experiments we concluded that the behavioral effects of amphetamine are probably mediated by dopaminergic rather than noradrenergic systems.

In clinical practice, patients receiving dopamine-blocking neuroleptic therapy may show Parkinsonian side effects. In the treatment of the major psychoses it is a matter of some debate as to whether the efficacy of neuroleptics is necessarily correlated with extrapyramidal effects or whether the two actions of these drugs involve wholly separate neuronal systems (Chien and Dimascio, 1967). Sulpiride is reported to produce relatively few extrapyramidal side effects whereas metoclopramide and haloperidol may produce a high incidence of such symptoms (Meikle et al., 1977; Robinson, 1973; but see Ayd, 1978). We found that metoclopramide, in the dose range 0.75–3.0 mg/kg, antagonised amphetamine-induced behavior but was sedative in normal animals only at the highest dose (Ridley et al., 1980b), suggesting that its clinical assessment may be warranted where specifically mild and selective effects are desired. Sulpiride was very mildly sedative in both saline- and amphetamine-pretreated monkeys; it did not appear to antagonise specific amphetamine effects.

The existence in the rat of systems involving the neurotransmitter aminobutyric acid (GABA) which either augment or inhibit dopaminergic activity has been suggested by reports of a GABAergic striatonigral efferent pathway driven by dopaminergic striatal mechanisms (Garcia-Munoz et al., 1977) and of a GABAergic feedback loop, which inhibits nigrostriatal dopaminergic systems (Carpenter, 1976). A GABAergic accumbaltegmental pathway has also been reported by Waddington and Cross (1978).

We found that muscimol, a GABA agonist, when administered to amphetamine-pretreated marmosets, suppressed checking but induced a persistent, stereotyped gnawing, hitherto unseen (Ridley et al., 1979b). By comparison with experiments in rodents, we suggested that this stereotyped gnawing results from the synergistic effects of amphetamine in the nigrostriatal pathway and muscimol in the striatonigral pathway, and that muscimol suppresses amphetamine-induced checking by inhibiting extrastriatal dopaminergic mechanisms. Studies currently being pursued in this laboratory are providing evidence that checking is mediated by a site confined to the accumbal area (Annett and Ridley, 1982). The GABA analogue, baclofen, was found to be without specific effect on amphetamine-induced behavior (Ridley et al., 1980b). The l-isomer of baclofen was somewhat more sedative than the d-isomer, although this may have been due to the stereospecific inhibitory effect of the l-isomer on amino acid transmitter release (Olpe et al., 1978).

THE BEHAVIORAL EFFECTS OF CHRONIC ADMINISTRATION OF AMPHETAMINE

It is well known that chronic treatment with amphetamine leads to progressively more bizarre and restricted stereotypies in monkeys. For example, intense self-grooming and progressive fragmentation of behavior have been described in Old World monkeys (Utena et al., 1975; Ellinwood, 1971; Garver et al., 1975) while another prominent feature of chronic amphetamine treatment is social withdrawal (Machiyama et al., 1974; Garver et al., 1975; Schiorring, 1979; Schiorring and Hecht, 1979).

We administered amphetamine to a group of marmosets via their drinking water for a total of 16 weeks with additional haloperidol treatment during the middle 8-week period according to the regime in Fig. 4 (Ridley et al., 1979a).

In addition to the changes shown in Fig. 4, some changes in the quality of activities were observed. Initially, mixed activities which included normal grooming, scratching, manipulation of objects in the cage, and play gave way to bouts of intensive self-grooming of restricted parts of the body. Although this behavior did not bring out significant change in the activities score, phase 1 was terminated because some animals were developing sores and bald patches as a result of this excessive self-grooming.

Two effects of chronic treatment are of particular interest. When neuroleptic treatment was withdrawn checking rose abruptly, even though it had not been elevated when neuroleptic treatment began. This suggests that the decrease in checking during phase 1 was not due to neurotransmitter depletion (cf. Owen et al., 1981, for higher doses of amphetamine) but must have been due to a postsynaptic change. Secondly, contact between animals was decreased throughout the entire period of amphetamine treatment including a considerable proportion of time when no other active behavior was increased. This shows that the loss of social contact cannot be explained as consequence of increased behavior in other categories. Furthermore, this loss of social contact was not improved by haloperidol. Certain parallels might be drawn with the work of Angrist et al. (1980), who found an increase in emotional withdrawal in schizophrenic patients treated with amphetamine which was not alleviated by neuroleptic therapy, and Johnstone et al. (1978), who described the lack of effect of neuroleptics on the negative symptoms of schizophrenia.

IS CHECKING A FORM OF HYPERVIGILANCE?

Some workers have asserted that the rapid head movements (checking) observed in monkeys treated with amphetamine is attributable to hypervigilance (Garver et al., 1975; Randrup and Munkvad, 1972). We attempted to substantiate this assertion by investigating the behavior of individual marmosets placed in a diffusely lit plain drum containing four small windows which could be opened or closed. The drum was situated in the center of the monkey colony room so that an interesting environment was provided by looking through the windows. Marmosets injected with saline or amphetamine (0.25 mg/kg or 4.0 mg/kg) were placed in the drum. The proportion of

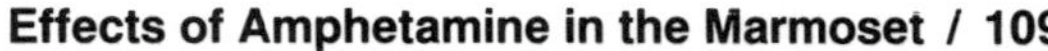

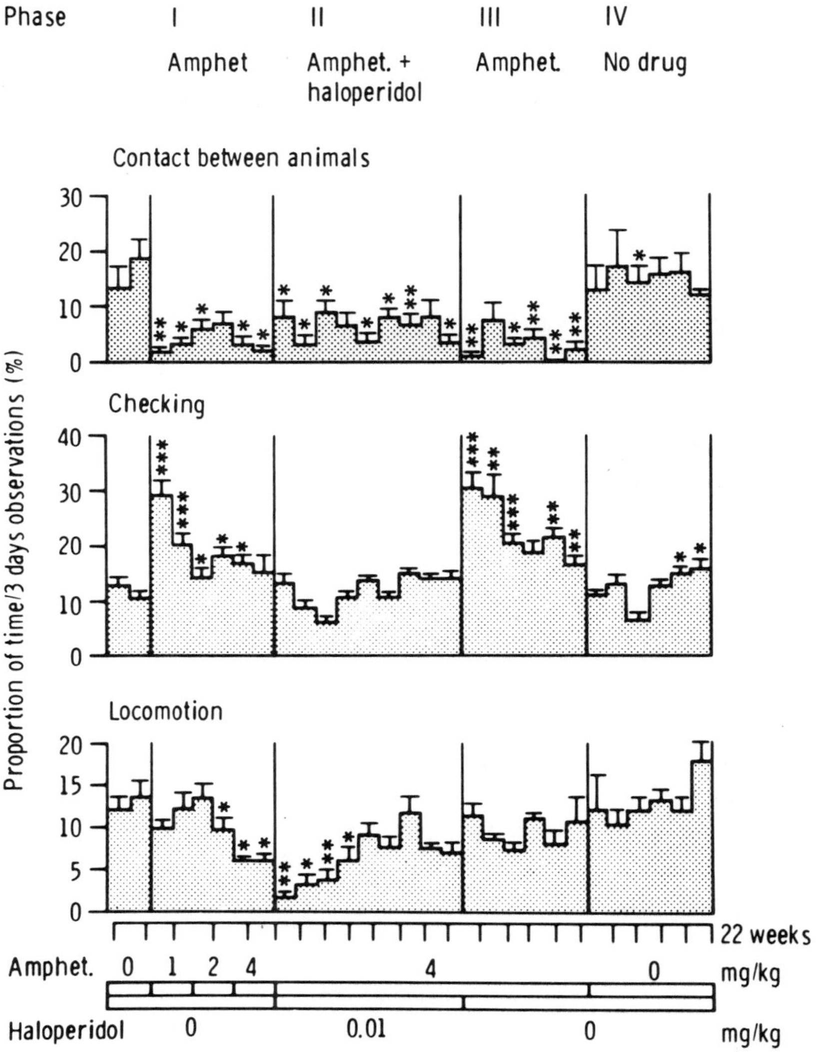

Phase I: Amphet | II: Amphet. + haloperidol | III: Amphet. | IV: No drug

Contact between animals

Checking

Locomotion

Proportion of time/3 days observations (%)

22 weeks

Amphet. 0 1 2 4 4 0 mg/kg

Haloperidol 0 0.01 0 mg/kg

Fig. 4. The effects of chronic amphetamine and haloperidol treatment on social contact, checking, and locomotion in a group of six marmosets. Ordinate shows the percentage of time averaged over 3 days observation spent in each behavioral category. Abscissa shows drug regime over time. Statistical comparison at each point of the histogram has been made against the point immediately preceding drug treatment using the matched pair t-test $^*p < 0.05$, $^{**}p < 0.01$, $^{***}p < 0.001$.

time spent at the windows, together with the duration of such visits, was measured over 1-minute periods at 5-minute intervals. The experiment was performed twice, once with the windows open and once with them closed. Fig. 5 shows that under saline control conditions, marmosets usually visit windows only when they are uncovered, indicating that this behavior is under visual stimulus control. At the lower dose of amphetamine (0.25 mg/kg), which does not stimulate checking, the behavior of the animals was the same as for the control conditions. At the higher dose, (4.0 mg/kg), which does stimulate checking, the time spent at open windows was suppressed. This suggests that checking movements are not directed toward visual stimuli and that checking is in fact largely incompatible with the performance of visually determined behavior.

Since we do not believe that checking is a form of hypervigilance, it may be asked why we still use this word to describe small head movements. First, the reference of this word to rapid head movements has not changed and is commonly understood, and second, this word could be understood to mean "stopping" or "arresting" a movement, which aptly describes the discontinuous head movements.

THE EFFECTS OF AMPHETAMINE ON PERFORMANCE OF VISUAL DISCRIMINATION TASKS

Having considered the effects of amphetamine on directly observable behavior, we turn now to a series of experiments designed to investigate the effects of very low doses of the drug (< 1 mg/kg) on psychological functions. At these low doses, overt behavior changes are not normally seen in marmosets. Our aim in these experiments is ultimately to relate the psychological effect of mild dopaminergic overactivity to the mental rather than to the subsidiary motor symptoms of psychosis. Our task is not yet completed although we believe that we are beginning to establish some links between psychotic symptoms and animal performance.

That amphetamine increases the probability of responding during nonreinforcement periods of a multiple operant schedule in rats has been known for some time (Clark and Steele, 1966). This tendency to overrespond after amphetamine is also found on DRL (differential reinforcement of low rate) schedules, where such behavior is disadvantageous to the animal (Kelleher and Coats, 1961), although correct performance on these schedules can be maintained under amphetamine if visual stimuli indicate when reinforcement is available (Heise and Lilie, 1970; Carey and Kritkausky, 1972). Thus,

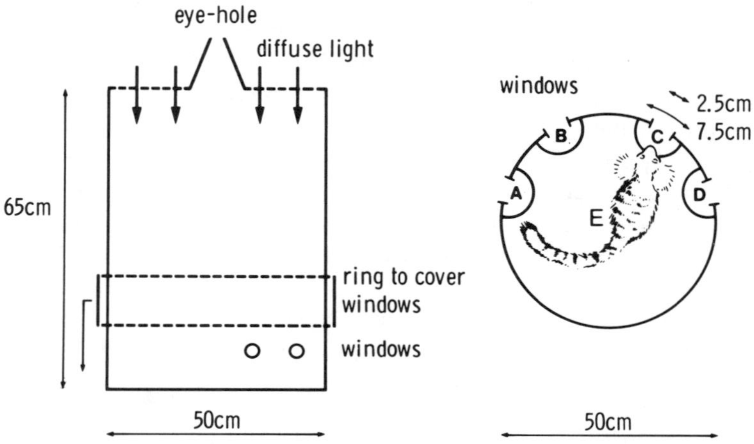

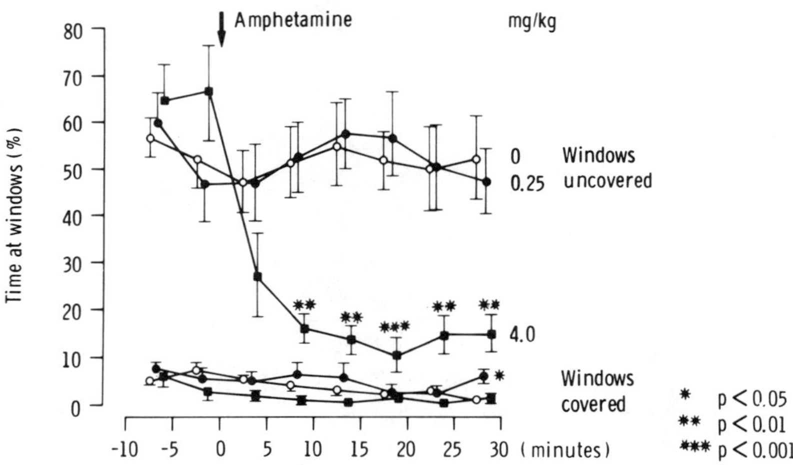

Fig. 5. The effect of amphetamine on the proportion of time spent at windows. Time spent at covered windows indicates amount of time at windows which is not under visual stimulus control, i.e., which occurs as a consequence of movement past each window (n=8).

stimulus control and response organization seem to be important factors in the modification of behavior under amphetamine.

In the first experiment of this series, we trained three marmosets to perform a red-white visual discrimination task in an operant test chamber originally designed for use with rats (Ridley et al., 1980a). In order to maintain motivational levels, the animals' normal daily diet was withheld until after their daily training sessions. They were not otherwise food-deprived. We used as reward freshly homogenized banana which was delivered using a dipper system in the center of the operant panel (see Fig. 6). A lever was positioned 9 cm to the left and another 9 cm to the right of this central food well. Two stimulus lights, one red and one white, were situated 5 cm above each lever.

We compared performance under amphetamine on two tasks: a simultaneous and a successive (or"go–no go") visual discrimination task. In the

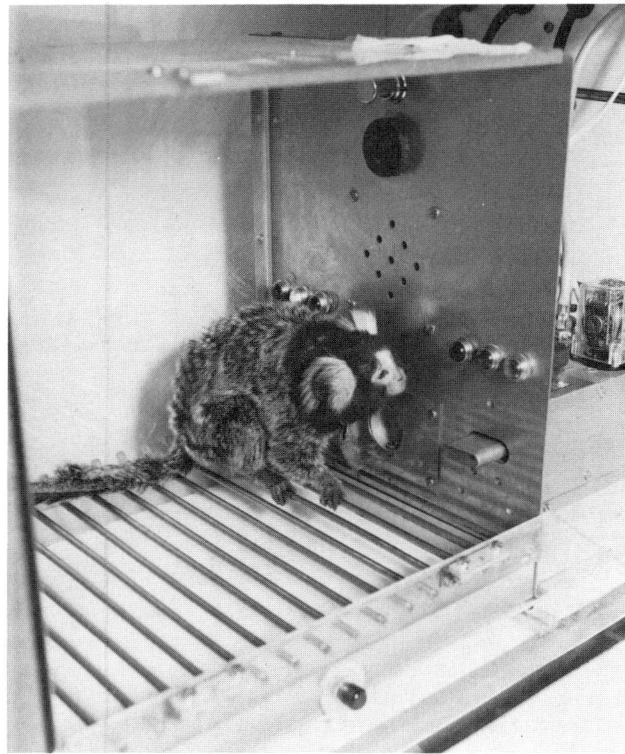

Fig. 6. Photograph of interior of operant chamber showing positions of stimuli, response levers, central banana reward dispenser, and marmoset.

simultaneous task, a red light appeared over one stimulus and a white light appeared over the other. If the lever below the red light was pressed the banana reward was immediately dispensed, but if the lever below the white light was pressed, no reward was given. After either lever was pressed, both lights were extinguished and both levers were inactivated for an intertrial interval of 8 sec. The left/right positions of the stimuli were determined by a pseudorandom schedule.

For the successive discrimination, one lever was removed. On each trial either a red or white light appeared over the remaining lever. After a red stimulus was presented, a lever press resulted in immediate reward and termination of the stimulus followed by an 8-sec intertrial interval. Such responses were scored correct. The white stimulus was presented for a maximum of 8 seconds during which a lever press would extinguish the light and deactivate the lever. Such a response was scored incorrect, and the unexpired portion of the trial was added to the intertrial interval.

Increasing doses of amphetamine progressively disrupted the performance of the successive version of the task but had no effect on performance of the simultaneous version (Fig. 7). All the errors under amphetamine were due to responding to the white stimulus.

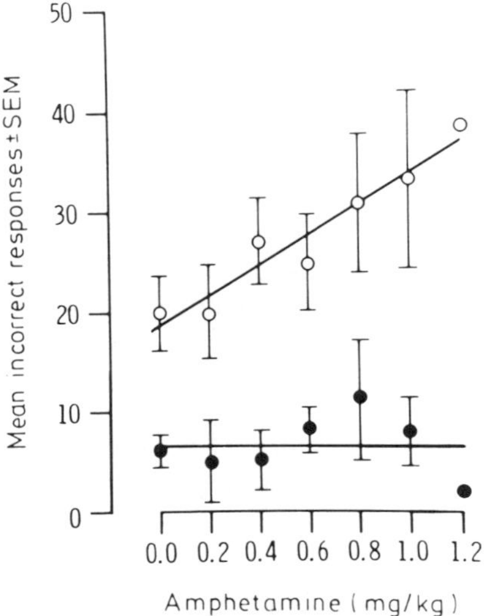

Fig. 7. Effects of 0–1.2 mg/kg d-amphetamine on successive (○) and and simultaneous (●) visual discrimination. n=3 except 1.2 mg/kg where n=2. Ordinate shows incorrect responses to white stimuli in 100 trials for each task at each dose. Maximum possible incorrect responses on successive task = 50. Chance performance on simultaneous task = 50 incorrect responses.

Although correct performance of the simultaneous task implies that the animals must have been able to perceive and discriminate between the stimuli and to perform the motor response, failure on the successive task could have been due either to difficulty in discriminating between stimuli when only one was presented (i.e., in the absence of a simultaneous comparison), or to difficulty in withholding a response when only the white stimulus was presented. We attempted to resolve this question by training the marmosets on a modified successive ("go here–go there") task (Ridley et al., 1980c). In this task, red or white stimuli are presented successively as in the previously described "go–no go" task, but in this task both levers are available. A response on the lever under a red stimulus was required in the usual way. When a white stimulus was presented, however, a response was required on the other lever. Correct performance of this task under amphetamine shows that animals are still able to discriminate between stimuli presented successively, suggesting that failure on the original "go–no go" task is due to an inability to refrain from responding. On the "go here–go there" task, responding under the white stimulus is inhibited at the behavioral level by responding on the other lever.

If marmosets treated with amphetamine do have difficulty in inhibiting certain responses, they may also be particularly susceptible to interference from extraneous events or from preceding trials. Where stimuli indicate that a response is required immediately as in simultaneous discrimination, direct stimulus control may prevent intrusion errors. Where the response is separated in time from stimulus presentation (as in the delayed-response task), scope for interference in the response may arise. We have been able to show that amphetamine does cause a mild impairment in the performance of a simultaneous, delayed-response task in which stimuli were presented for 4 seconds, while the levers became available for responding 0, 1, 2, or 3 seconds after the stimuli were switched off (Weight et al., 1980).

In summary, amphetamine seems to disrupt performance of tasks on which a degree of internal inhibition of responding is required and in which responding is not under direct and immediate stimulus control. These effects could be due either to a lowered threshold for the initiation of neural programs required to perform the response or to an alteration in the high-level programs controlling the choice of behavioral responses. In the next series of experiments, we directed our attention to the effects of amphetamine on choice behavior in the marmoset.

EFFECT OF AMPHETAMINE ON CHOICE BEHAVIOR IN DISCRIMINATION TASKS

We feel that an important distinction can be made between those processes which initiate and organize a motor response and those processes which are involved in the choice between possible behaviors. A simple suggestion from the observation of stereotyped behavior after large doses of amphetamine might be that motor programs are running on, uncontrolled by higher level behavior-organizing and -inhibiting systems. Similarly, the marmoset's impaired performance after amphetamine on previously learned discrimination tasks in an operant apparatus could be described as a failure of inhibitory mechanisms to keep inappropriate responding in check. Where direct and immediate stimulus control is available from the environment, these high-order systems may not be required and performance may be relatively unaffected by amphetamine. Although the experiments of the previous section show effects of amphetamine which are probably not the consequence of changes in the rate of responding, as may be the case in conventional operant schedules, the propensity to respond was clearly an important factor. We were therefore interested in tasks in which the choice of behavior could be separated from its performance, and to this end we turned to the Wisconsin General Test Apparatus (WGTA).

In the experiments to be described below we have shown that amphetamine can act on the nervous system in such a way as to maintain a neural program which represents stimulus-reward associations even when neural activity that determines stimulus choice and motor activity is changing. Since these neural programs are maintained in the face of contrary evidence from the environment, it is our belief that they may be equivalent to those which contribute to the maintenance of delusional beliefs in psychosis. Since we have also been able to show that these effects of amphetamine can be reversed by the dopamine-blocking neuroleptic, haloperidol, it would seem that these effects are mediated by dopamine. Thus, we have some evidence that neuroleptics may actually reverse the psychological processes maintaining delusions rather than acting at the level of motor output or arousal.

In the first experiment (Ridley et al., 1981c), animals were presented in the WGTA with a series of trials on which a screen was raised to reveal two small stimuli (plastic figures or junk objects approximately 5 cm high, mounted on white plastic disks) covering two small food wells (see Fig. 8). One food well contained a 3-mm cube of banana which the monkey could obtain by displacing the appropriate stimulus. Touching the other stimulus was not rewarded and was scored incorrect, and animals were allowed only one attempt at the correct response on each trial. The reward was always associated with the same stimulus, and the left-right position of this positive stimulus was determined by a pseudorandom schedule. Each trial lasted until the animal made a response.

Four experimentally sophisticated marmosets were first trained to discriminate between two stimuli, a toy ballerina (rewarded) and a toy Indian

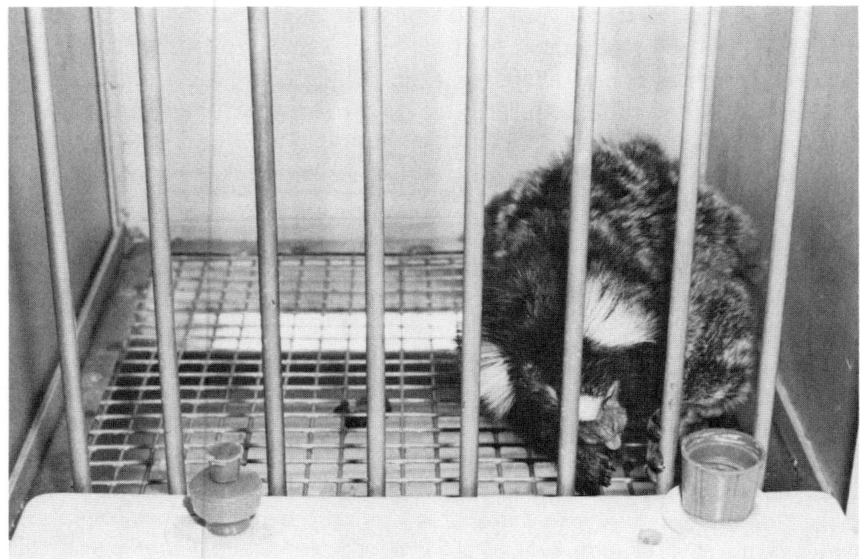

Fig. 8. Interior of Wisconsin General Test Apparatus showing marmoset performing junk object discrimination task.

(unrewarded), until they would reliably learn to choose the rewarded stimulus to a criterion of five consecutive correct responses within one training session whereupon the reward contingency was reversed (i.e., the Indian became rewarded and the ballerina unrewarded) and trial presentation continued until the animal learned to respond to the new rewarded stimulus to a criterion of five consecutive correct responses. Before drug testing began, training on the first task (learning) followed by the second (reversal) was continued for 12–15 days until the animals could perform both tasks to a criterion of five consecutive correct within one test session.

By the end of pretraining, learning scores (i.e., the number of trials up to, but not including, criterion trials) of about 20 were found for both learning and reversal tasks. The number of trials to criterion which would be expected on average if the choice of stimulus was random was found, by computer simulation, to be in excess of 60, suggesting that although the criterion used in these tasks was low, the animals were indeed learning. During drug testing each animal was presented with one task followed by its reversal on one day. The next day's training began with the task which each animal had performed last on the previous day. Amphetamine (0, 0.3, or 0.6 mg/kg) was given to the marmosets 20–30 min before training each day in ascending dose followed by descending dose order. Scores on the 2 days at each dose were summed for the learning task and the reversal task in an attempt to overcome any effects of drug order or daily variation. In a complementary experiment, 0.01 or 0.02 mg/kg haloperidol was given 10 minutes before amphetamine treatment, in a balanced design.

Under amphetamine the learning scores for task 2 (reversal) were increased though not for task 1 (see Fig. 9). It can also be seen that the number of trials up to but excluding two consecutive correct responses was also increased after amphetamine for task 2 but not for task 1. Pretreatment with haloperidol blocked the effect of amphetamine on reversal and this was particularly true of the perseverative responses made before two consecutive correct responses were made (Fig. 10). Thus, though amphetamine does not significantly affect the relearning of a task performed last on the previous day, it seriously disturbs the learning of a reversal task. Much of the effect of amphetamine can be described as the tendency for treated animals to make perseverative errors at the beginning of reversal—i.e., before two consecutive correct responses are made.

Since amphetamine-treated monkeys are not significantly impaired at learning the first task of each day, their difficulty on reversal cannot be ascribed to simple perceptual loss. Similarly, this difficulty cannot be due to the repetition or perseveration of a motor response since, in order to continue

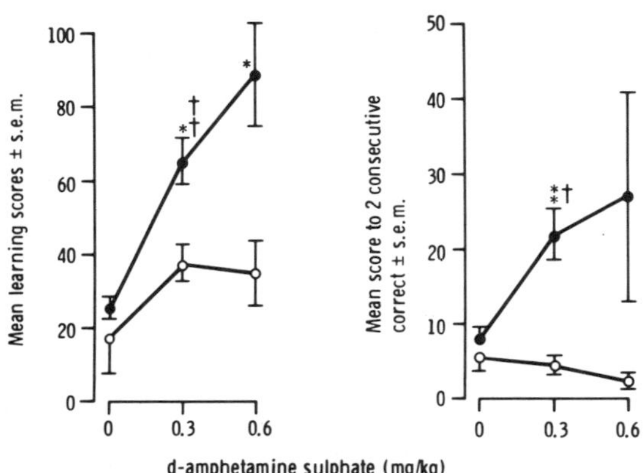

Fig. 9. Effect of amphetamine on learning scores (mean trials up to, but excluding, five consecutive correct responses) and mean trials up to but excluding two consecutive correct responses on ○ relearning (task 1) and ● reversal learning (task 2). *$p < 0.05$, **$p < 0.01$ comparing scores under amphetamine with relevant saline control. †$p < 0.05$, ‡$p < 0.01$ comparing scores on task 1 with task 2; two-tailed matched-pair t-test.

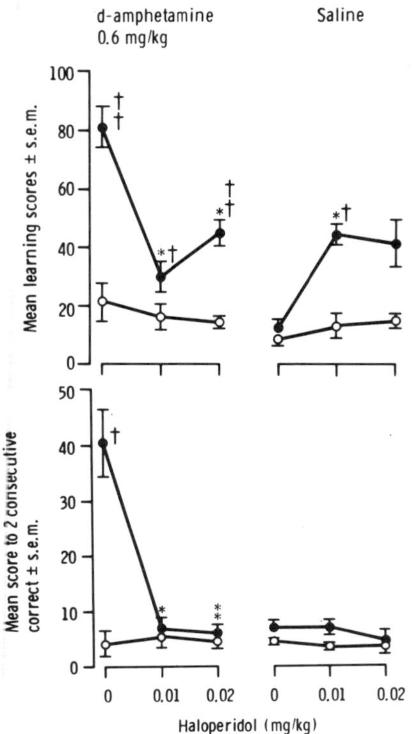

Fig. 10. Effect of haloperidol pretreatment on mean learning scores and mean scores to two consecutive correct (see Fig. 9) on ○ task 1 (relearning) and ● task 2 (reversal). Haloperidol given 30–40 min before testing, amphetamine 20–30 min before testing. *$p < 0.05$, **$p < 0.01$ comparing scores after pretreatment with haloperidol with the relevant amphetamine or saline condition. †$p < 0.05$, ‡$p < 0.01$ comparing scores on task 2 with task 1. Two-tailed matched-pair t-test.

to choose the previously rewarded object, the animal must make different left-right responses according to the pseudorandom schedule by which the stimuli change position. The impairment could, however, be due either to an inability to change a stimulus-choice habit (a higher-order response-organizing impairment) or to a failure to notice that the reward association of the stimuli had been reversed. Our analysis of the early trials of reversal suggests that, without amphetamine, well-trained marmosets are able to abandon a reward association after only one or two nonrewarded responses, although they may then need several more trials before reaching criterion. It is possible that two mechanisms are involved in reversal learning, one actively inhibiting an inappropriate reward association and the other acquiring the new association, and that after amphetamine, it is the inhibitory system which is impaired or overridden.

In a further experiment (Ridley et al., 1981b), we attempted to show that after amphetamine treatment marmosets would continue to choose an object which they preferred, presumably on the basis of its intrinsic qualities, despite contrary reward contingencies. Throughout this experiment novel objects—i.e., objects which the animals had never before encountered—were used as stimuli on each task. On each test day, animals were presented with two tasks. At the beginning and the end of each test session, animals were presented with ten practice trials of a well-learned task. On the first trial of each task, two novel objects were presented with either both or neither being rewarded. If the objects were rewarded on the first trial (task 1), the object which the monkey chose became the rewarded object in the following ten trials and the other object became unrewarded. If the objects were unrewarded on the first trial (task 2), the objects which the animal chose remained unrewarded and the other objects became rewarded (see Fig. 11). Thus in task 1, continued choice of the animal's preferred object was rewarded and

Task One

Trial 1	e.g.	Knob (rewarded)	vs	Button (rewarded)
		Animal chooses e.g. Knob		
Trial 2-11		Knob (rewarded)	vs	Button (unrewarded)

i.e. choice of animal's preferred object is rewarded

Task Two

Trial 1	e.g.	Pentop (unrewarded)	vs	Thimble (unrewarded)
		Animal chooses e.g. Pentop		
Trial 2-11		Thimble (rewarded)	vs	Pentop (unrewarded)

i.e. choice of animal's preferred object is unrewarded

Score on Task One - Task Two = tendency to continue choosing preferred object i.e. choice perseveration

Fig. 11. Design for novel object preference testing. See text for further explanation.

was scored correct, whereas in task 2 continued choice of the animal's preferred object was unrewarded and scored incorrect. In other words, if an amphetamine-treated animal's object preference on the first trial continued to affect performance on the subsequent ten trials (where only one object was rewarded) then a discrepancy between correct responses on task 1 and task 2 would be observed. That this is the case can be seen from Fig. 12. After amphetamine treatment, a significant difference between performance of tasks 1 and 2 emerges, a difference prevented by pretreatment with haloperidol.

This experiment shows that the perseverative tendency of amphetamine-treated marmosets to continue choosing a stimulus despite a changed reward contingency, which was found in the reversal experiment, also applies to idiosyncratic object preferences. In this case, however, the preference is not a simple reward association since the stimulus objects had never been encountered before the first trial, but may be related to the animal's previous experience of many objects, in and out of the test situation. This suggests that a reward association does not have to be made under the influence of amphetamine for it to be maintained in reversal under the drug.

It is possible, however, that a marmoset's initial choice of object is not based on object preference, but is essentially random, and that under amphetamine this choice is maintained. It was also not clear from the reversal

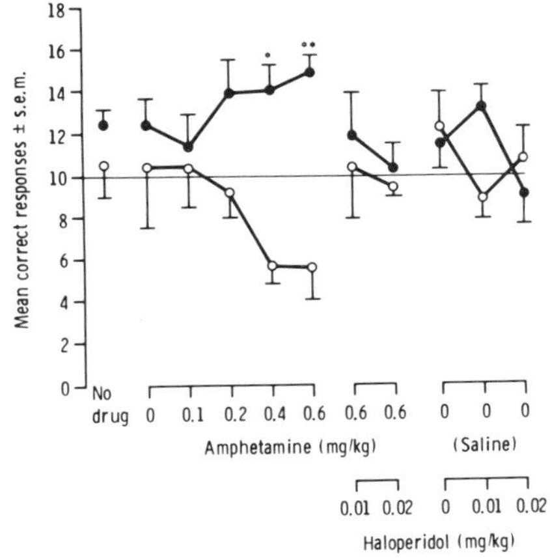

Fig. 12. Effect of increasing doses of amphetamine and haloperidol on choice behavior. Ordinate shows mean correct responses + s.e.m. on task 1 (●), where continued choice of the first object was scored correct, and task 2 (○), where continued choice of the first object was scored incorrect. n=5, *p < 0.02, **p < 0.005; two-tailed matched-pair t-test comparing performance on task 1 with task 2 at each dose.

experiment whether perseverative responding is due to continued reward association or to continued stimulus choice by force of habit. In the last and most difficult experiment of this series (Ridley et al., 1981a), we attempted to resolve these questions by dissociating the acquired stimulus-reward association from the motor responses which had been made to these stimuli. This was achieved by presenting animals on each task with five pretrials on which only one stimulus was presented over a central food well. Each animal was required to respond by displacing the object on all five trials before the test trials of each task began.

In conditions A and B, displacing the stimulus was rewarded; in conditions C and D, displacing the stimulus was not rewarded. On the subsequent ten trials of each task this initially encountered stimulus was paired with a novel object and only one was rewarded as in the conventional manner. In conditions A and C, the initially presented stimulus maintained its reward association (either positive or negative) in these discrimination trials, whereas in conditions B and D, the reward association of the initial stimulus was reversed on subsequent trials (see Fig. 13).

Trials 1-5	e.g.	Toy car (rewarded)			**A**
Trials 6-16		Toy car (rewarded)	vs	Cotton reel (unrewarded)	
Trials 1-5	e.g.	Doll (rewarded)			**B**
Trials 6-16		Clip (rewarded)	vs	Doll (unrewarded)	
Trials 1-5	e.g.	Hook (unrewarded)			**C**
Trials 6-16		Bottletop (rewarded)	vs	Hook (unrewarded)	
Trials 1-5	e.g.	Tube (unrewarded)			**D**
Trials 6-16		Tube (rewarded)	vs	Box (unrewarded)	

Task (A + C) - (B + D) = tendency for animal to preserve acquired reward association

Fig. 13. Design for acquired object-preference testing. See text for further explanation.

Thus in each condition, five responses were made to one of the two stimuli used in the discrimination trials, but in only two conditions, A and C, was the acquired reward association (either positive or negative) of use in the performance of these discriminations whereas in conditions B and D, the acquired reward association was contrary to the reward contingency of the subsequent ten trials. Thus if amphetamine-treated animals tend to carry over a previously acquired reward association, a discrepancy in the number of correct responses between the discrimination trials of A and C and those of B and D might become apparent. On the other hand, if animals treated with amphetamine tend to continue choosing the stimuli which they chose on the pretrials, irrespective of reward association, the performance on discrimination trials of A and D, where the previously encountered stimuli are both now rewarded, might be expected to be better than performance on the trials of B and C, where the previously encountered stimuli became unrewarded. It can be seen in Fig. 14 that there is a significant difference between correct performance of A and C and of B and D, a difference which becomes enhanced under amphetamine. From this experiment, we conclude that under amphetamine it is the reward association rather than the response tendency which perseverates.

RELATION OF AMPHETAMINE-INDUCED BEHAVIOR TO NEUROPSYCHOLOGY, MENTAL ILLNESS, AND BEHAVIORAL DISTURBANCE

Psychosis

Amphetamine has been of interest for many years, not only because it is a drug of abuse, but also because certain features of amphetamine-induced psychosis bear a marked resemblance to those associated with schizophrenia (Connell, 1958). Although amphetamine psychosis is usually found in chronic abusers, Kalant (1966) has described several cases of acute psychotic reactions and paranoid ideation after a single dose of the drug. Furthermore, Angrist et al. (1980) have demonstrated that amphetamine exacerbates psychotic symptoms in schizophrenics. Stereotypy or "punding" is often associated with amphetamine abuse although it can occur in the absence of other psychotic symptoms.

Segal et al. (1980) have suggested that the acute effects of amphetamine may be a better model of schizophrenia than the chronic syndrome, although this view is not shared by all (Ellison et al., 1981). We believe that the acute effects of low doses of amphetamine described in this chapter may be of relevance to the mental as opposed to the motor symptoms of schizophrenic

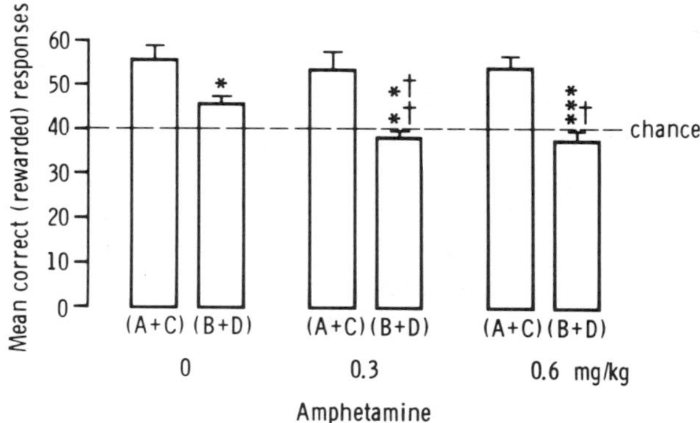

Fig. 14. Effect of amphetamine on combined scores on tasks (A and C) (meaning retained) and (B and D) (meaning changed) †$p < 0.05$, ‡$p < 0.01$ comparing amphetamine with saline on each task combination. *$p < 0.05$, **$p < 0.01$, ***$p < 0.001$ comparing scores on (A and C) with scores on (B and D) at each dose.

psychosis. In particular, we have demonstrated that choice behavior under amphetamine as measured in a WGTA is determined by previously acquired reward association or meaning rather than by an enhancement of motor habit. This distinction is important since the tendency to perform an action despite an appreciation of its inappropriateness could be construed as compulsive, while the inability to accept that behavior is inappropriate might be thought of as delusional. That neuroleptics can block the psychological effects of low doses of amphetamine is important since it suggests that, in clinical practice, neuroleptics may act directly on the psychological processes which underlie psychotic symptoms rather than acting nonspecifically by, for example, suppressing motor output. Despite the longevity of the dopamine hypothesis of schizophrenia (Randrup and Munkvad, 1967; Meltzer and Stahl, 1976) and the efficacy of dopamine-blocking neuroleptics in the treatment of this condition (Davis, 1975), there is, as yet, no clear psychological theory of the role of dopamine in brain function that is able to predict the occurrence of the symptoms of schizophrenia in states of dopaminergic overactivity.

Stereotyped behavior has always been recognized in schizophrenia (Kraepelin, 1971; Bleuler, 1950) although its importance is not emphasized in modern psychiatry. Neuroleptic treatment may prevent the development of such behavior, masking it with a general motor retardation or induce tardive dyskinesias, and, as a result, the diagnosis of movement disorders as primary symptoms of the disease may be obscured. Kraepelin (1971) described a wide variety of stereotypies in schizophrenia ranging from brief mannerisms and tics to complex patterns of behavior and movement resembling the stereotypies of mental defectives. Bleuler (1950), however, maintained that psychotic stereotypies could be understood in terms of the patients' preoccupations and attitudes. Such stereotypies appear to evolve in a manner comparable to the shortening and restriction of amphetamine-induced stereotypies in the course of chronic treatment in monkeys (Ellinwood et al., 1973).

We recently observed the evolution of stereotypy in a schizophrenic patient as we walked through the day hospital each morning. On admission, this distressed and tearful lady repeatedly asked those about her to take her home, holding up an envelope on which was written her address. She often sat by the door or window watching for the arrival of cars. Over the course of several weeks, this patient progressively restricted herself to one place in the room (by a window). She had by now lost her envelope but held up other pieces of paper or litter and she sat with the remnants of her wet handkerchief in the corner of her mouth. She was by this time largely mute and immobile and had stopped crying.

While the persistence of a delusional belief, and possibly the intrusions of overinclusive thinking, may be understood as a form of perseveration, schizophrenics do not necessarily show perseveration on cognitive tasks, although they often do. Thus Shakow (1962) has suggested that schizophrenics show a persistence in using a particular cognitive set when conditions demand a change, and Kay and Singh (1979) found some evidence of perseveration on a card-sorting test.

Self-mutilation is not uncommon in schizophrenics (Sweeney and Zamecnik, 1981) as well as in a variety of conditions of profound behavioral disturbance. Chamove and Anderson (1981) argue that a distinction can be drawn between self-aggression and self-injurious behavior, the latter being associated with stereotypy in monkeys. Self-aggression consists of threats and physical attacks directed toward the self, though not usually resulting in self-wounding (Anderson and Chamove, 1980, 1981). Such self-aggressive behavior may occur in instances of acute frustration of sexual or aggressive impulses toward other animals and may thus be regarded as inappropriately directed behavior rather than as inappropriate behavior per se. Self-injury, on the other hand, may result from the performance of stereotyped actions ranging, for example, from the minor damage caused by compulsive nail biting to the more serious effects of rocking and head banging seen in some mentally subnormal people. We have already referred to the development of bald patches and sores following prolonged bouts of stereotyped grooming in marmosets chronically treated with amphetamine (see above; Ridley et al., 1979a). The occurrence of both self-aggressive behavior and self-injurious stereotyped behavior is increased by rearing in isolation.

A distinction between aggression and self-injury can be seen in the effects of amygdalectomy. In monkeys, amygdalectomy caused a decrease in social aggression and produced "paradoxical tameness," but the appearance of self-injury in these animals was also reported (Kluver and Bucy, 1939). In humans, amygdaloid lesions have been found to decrease social aggression but to have little effect on self-inflicted injury (Kiloh et al., 1974). Amygdalectomized monkeys also show a tendency to put inedible objects into their mouths (Kluver and Bucy, 1939). While this may be a consequence of the visual agnosia or "psychic blindness" associated with this lesion, it may also be related to the pica and coprophagy sometimes observed in profound behavioral disturbances.

Perseveration and Frontal Lobe Function

It has been our observation that the effects of low doses of amphetamine on task performance in the marmoset bear a considerable resemblance to the effects of prefrontal cortical lesions in monkeys. For example, the impairment on performance of a successive but not simultaneous version of a visual discrimination task has been observed in monkeys with orbitofrontal lesions (Brutkowski et al., 1963) or lateral frontal lesions (Battig et al., 1962). Our experiment on higher-order choice mechanisms (Ridley et al., 1981b) resembles an experiment described by Mishkin (1964), who found that like marmosets treated with amphetamine, monkeys with lateral frontal ablations made many more errors on ten trial discrimination tasks where the rewarded object was their nonpreferred choice (based on first trial performance) than on ten trial tasks where the rewarded object was their preferred choice. This effect of preference was not seen in unoperated controls or animals with temporal lobe lesions. Similarly, Brush et al. (1961) found that if monkeys were presented with five trials of a single object (rewarded on some tasks and unrewarded on others) followed by ten trials of discrimination training using that object together with a novel object, monkeys with frontal lesions had particular difficulty on those tasks where the reward contingency of the first encountered object changed after five trials. This effect is essentially the same as we observed after amphetamine (Ridley et al., 1981a). The reversal impairment seen after amphetamine may also be induced after frontal lobe lesions (Gross, 1963; Mishkin, 1964) but can occur after lesions within the temporal lobe (Manning, 1972; Pribram et al., 1969). In the latter case, however, it was clear that most of the impairment was due to a prolonged period of responding at chance, whereas the frontal-lesioned animals made most errors at the beginning of each reversal such that performance was worse than chance (Gross, 1963). In this respect, the reversal performance of amphetamine-treated marmosets more closely resembles that of monkeys with frontal lesions than that of animals with lesions confined to the temporal lobe.

The most well-known effect of frontal lesions in monkeys is an impairment of performance on a delayed-response task (Jacobsen et al., 1935) although it was subsequently shown to be mainly the dorsolateral frontal rather than the orbitofrontal lesions which gave rise to this impairment (Brutkowski et al., 1960; described in Rosvold and Szwarcbart, 1964). Mishkin (1964) has argued that the principle effect of orbitofrontal lesions is perseveration of either object-reward associations or "central sets" of responding while the impairments following dorsolateral frontal lesions are due primarily to spatial difficulties which become apparent during the delay period. We believe that our results with low doses of amphetamine bear more resemblance to the effects of orbitofrontal than dorsolateral lesions, and this may explain the relatively mild impairment which we observed on delayed response performance (Weight et al., 1980).

Rosvold and Szwarcbart (1964) have proposed the existence of a neural "delayed-response system" which includes dorsolateral frontal cortex, caudate and subthalamic nuclei, and the substantia nigra, disruption of any of which may produce a delayed-response impairment. Similarly, the orbitofrontal cortex receives afferents from dorsomedial thalamus (Akert, 1964) and polysensory association cortex (Chavis and Pandya, 1976), while projecting to limbic cortex, striatum, and amygdala (Leichnetz and Astruc, 1975). Projections from the orbitofrontal areas seem to be particularly concentrated in the ventromedial portion of the striatum (Yeterian and van Hoesen, 1978), the area which, in the marmoset, is the most densely populated with dopaminergic nerve terminals (Schofield and Dixson, 1982). We have some preliminary evidence that the ventromedial striatum may be the most sensitive, behaviorally, to intracerebral injections of amphetamine (Annett and Ridley, 1982). Thus it seems likely that the rising dopaminergic pathway may exert an influence on behavior which is antagonistic to the tempering effects of descending influences from the orbitofrontal cortex, such that overactivity stimulated by amphetamine resembles the effects of lesions of this cortical region.

Social and Developmental Factors

Children who are born blind or severely mentally retarded may develop stereotyped rocking and twirling, unusual hand movements, and arm flapping (Keeler, 1958; Corbett et al., 1975; Berkson and Davenport, 1962). However, adults who become blind or who sustain incapacitating brain damage do not develop equivalent behaviors, suggesting that stereotyped behavior results from an abnormal maturational process in the brain. The exceptionally long period of development in humans may occur because the human nervous system is particularly dependent on sensory input to reach its full potential. Thelen (1979) has shown that, in the normal infant, repetitive behavior is exceedingly common but that this behavior is superseded, during early development, by a flexible responsiveness to the environment. Thus not only may the contents of stereotypies represent remnants of behavior appropriate to an earlier stage of development as suggested by Foley (1934) and Berkson (1967); the existence of stereotypy may also be indicative of a retardation in development.

Stereotypies are sometimes seen in children deprived of normal parental care at an early age (Spitz, 1945), although it would appear to be the environment into which a child is put, rather than the separation from the parents per se, which affects the development of these behaviors (Yarrow, 1964; Casler, 1968).

Stereotypy is an important and characteristic feature of early infantile autism (Kanner, 1943), and it is in this syndrome that the coexistence of social isolation, cognitive inflexibility, and behavioral stereotypy can be most clearly seen. These children are unable to make normal social relationships and may be distressed by provocative attempts to elicit social responses. They are frequently unable to master language even though they may show instances of very intelligent behavior and good memory. They often exhibit an "insistence on sameness" or acute distress if minor changes are made to their immediate surroundings (Kanner, 1943).

Hermelin and Frith (1971) have suggested that autistic children suffer from a higher-order perceptual deficit such that they are unable to construct meaningful events from sensory inflow. In particular, the interpretation and use of subtle social cues may be specifically affected (Eisenberg, 1956). Frith (1970a,b, 1972) has shown that autistic children may have difficulty in extracting features from sensory input in experiments on the production and recall of patterned sequences, while showing an abnormal tendency to impose pattern and structure on unstructured test material.

SYNTHESIS

We have attempted to show that under certain conditions stereotypy in both animals and man tends to occur in conjunction with social isolation and cognitive inflexibility, suggesting that these features of disturbed behavior are related, albeit in a complex way. We have argued that this triple syndrome occurs in monkeys treated with amphetamine and have emphasized its occurrence in the human amphetamine psychosis, in childhood autism, and in severely deteriorated schizophrenics. We would further suggest that such a constellation of symptoms will be found among the behavioral features of monkeys reared in social and sensory isolation, children reared in grossly inadequate circumstances, and in those children who, from birth, have been isolated from normal sensory input by virtue of sensory incapacity (e.g., blindness).

While we do not believe that there exists a biochemical equivalence between amphetamine treatment and the other conditions described (Owen et al., 1981), we do suggest that an understanding of amphetamine effects at the psychological level may illuminate the psychological processes underlying certain clinical conditions.

In our view, behavioral sterotypy is the end product of a variety of different pathways, and while the final neural mechanism underlying stereotypy may be common to all those conditions referred to above, we believe that the original clinical or social conditions which lead to this end state may be wholly separate. In particular, we regard infantile autism as a clinically distinct syndrome, unrelated either to schizophrenia or to conditions of upbringing.

We believe that the common thread which links these separate clinical syndromes and the effects of amphetamine treatment is the balance within the nervous system of internally and externally generated information which guides the choice of behavioral output.

There is a form of stereotypy, cage stereotypy (Hediger, 1955) and its human equivalent (which could be called constraint stereotypy), which we do not consider to be pathological. Cage stereotypies can develop in many animal species, including monkeys, as a result of continuous confinement in cages (Berkson et al., 1966; Meyer-Holzapfel, 1968). However, since these cage stereotypies can usually be broken by removing the animal from the cage (Berkson, 1967) and since they can develop at any age and not only during the period of the maturational processes of infancy, we believe that these behaviors represent the response of a normal nervous system to an abnormal environment. Similarly, the stereotyped pacing of humans under certain conditions of physical or social constraint (e.g., prisoners pacing their cells or expectant fathers pacing hospital waiting rooms) is not necessarily pathological and is abandoned as soon as the constraint is removed. It might be argued, however, that the internal drive to act exceeds the environmental opportunity for action, resulting in the repetition of a limited repertoire.

The normal nervous system is designed to be responsive to the external environment. Neurophysiological studies of the visual system have shown that the capacity for responsiveness of visual neurons is determined largely by previous sensory input (Held and Hein, 1963). A critical or sensitive period is said to exist in very early infancy during which sensory input permanently affects subsequent activity of neurons (Bateson, 1964).

Early sensory input may markedly affect the functioning of the central nervous system as a whole such that a very wide range of behavior may be permanently influenced by the conditions of rearing. We believe that behavioral stereotypy can be regarded as evidence that the nervous system is not responding to external events. Where clinical conditions are present from birth, the normal maturational processes, which are themselves responses to sensory input, may be distorted. In schizophrenia, the nervous system may have become damaged, possibly as a consequence of a viral infection (Crow et al., 1979; Tyrrell et al., 1979) so that it is no longer able to respond to the environment but generates fragmentary and largely meaningless or inappropriate behavior.

In primates, including man, responses are not linked to sensory stimuli by simple stimulus-response bonds, but are normally related in a flexible manner via complex, cognitive, mediating processes. Cognitive flexibility may itself be determined by a rich and variable sensory input during the critical period of early infancy, and it may degenerate if the meaning-content of sensory input is lost in schizophrenic psychosis.

During high-dose amphetamine treatment in monkeys, one simple behavioral pattern occurs to the exclusion of other behaviors. This could be due to a motor program being stimulated to the detriment of other motor programs or because the behavior has been initiated before other neural programs have been able to exert an influence. The latter suggestion is strengthened by the resemblance of the effects of amphetamine treatment to those of frontal lobe lesions. The frontal lobes could be regarded as making a contribution to the decision to act based on factors outside the immediate situation—for example, by inhibiting a response tendency during reversal learning. Low doses of amphetamine, which do not induce stereotypy behavior, do induce a state of cognitive inflexibility. In this state, responses are based on previously acquired reward association (i.e., information already existing within the nervous system) rather than being adapted to new sensory input from a changed environment.

The therapeutic implications of the suggestion that stereotypy exists in conditions of nonresponsiveness to the environment are clear. Conditions of profound behavioral disturbance, associated with stereotypy, are likely to be exacerbated in situations of enforced idleness, poor institutional care, confinement, and, particularly, solitary confinement. In view of the relationship between stereotypy and self-injurious behavior, a similar exacerbation might be expected in those individuals suffering from behavioral disturbances including self-mutilation, self-abuse, and parasuicide. For example, Wilmanns (1940) has argued that the high incidence of schizophrenia among prisoners serving long sentences occurs because the criminal act is related to their schizophrenic constitution but that their psychosis becomes manifest only after a period of confinement. It is our view that while confinement of behaviorally disturbed individuals may be necessary it will in fact contribute to their deterioration unless accompanied by opportunities for responsive behavior—e.g., retraining of life skills and social performance.

Social performance cannot be regarded as separate from the interaction of an individual with the environment since so much of this environment consists of other individuals. This social environment changes constantly in a way in which the inanimate environment does not, so that social relationships may be seen as the most complex interaction between an individual and his surroundings. It is thus to be expected that when an individual's ability to respond appropriately to circumstances is gravely impaired, social skills will be the most severe casualty. Since social interaction in humans is greatly dependent on the use of language, it is not surprising that the development of language skills has a beneficial effect on a wide variety of behavioral problems (Brown, 1960).

It is our hope that an appreciation of the underlying maturational and biological factors which result ultimately in the development of behavioral stereotypy will contribute to the ability of those concerned to devise a more suitable therapeutic approach to this unfortunate form of behavior.

ACKNOWLEDGMENTS

We would like to thank R. Scraggs, M. Weight, T. Haystead, P. Bowes, and L. Annett for undertaking much of the care, observation, and training of the animals.

The following figures were reprinted with permission: Figs. 1, 5 from "Amphetamine and related stimulants: chemical, biological, clinical and sociological aspects" Ed. J. Caldwell; copyright The Chemical Rubber Co., CRC Press, Inc. Fig. 2 from Psychopharmacology 59, 242–245 (1978). Fig. 3 from Psychopharmacology 62, 41–45 (1979). Fig. 7 from Psychopharmacology 67, 241–244 (1980). Fig. 12 from Psychopharmacology 72, 173–177 (1981). Fig. 14 from Psychopharmacology 75, 283–286 (1981). Psychopharmacology is published by Springer-Verlag, Heidelberg. Fig. 4 from Biological Psychiatry 14, 753–765 (1979) published by Plenum Publishing Corp.,

New York. Figs. 9, 10 from Pharmacology, Biochemistry and Behavior 14, 345–351 (1981) published by ANKHO International Inc.

REFERENCES

Akert K (1964) Comparative anatomy of frontal cortex and thalamofrontal connections. In: Warren JM, Akert K (eds) The Frontal Granular Cortex and Behavior. McGraw-Hill, New York, pp 372–396

Alexander M, Isaac W (1965) Effect of illumination on the activity of the rhesus macaque. Psychol Rep 16: 311–313

Anderson JR, Chamove AS (1980) Self-aggression and social aggression in laboratory-reared macaques. J Ab Psychol 89: 539–550

Anderson JR, Chamove AS (1981) Self-aggression behavior in monkeys. Current Psycho Rev 1: 139–158

Angrist B, Rotrosen J, Gershon S (1980) Differential effects of amphetamine and neuroleptics on negative versus positive symptoms in schizophrenia. Psychopharmacol 72: 17–19

Annett LE, Ridley RM (1982) Behavior after intra-accumbens and caudate amphetamine in a primate species. Brit J Pharmacol 75: 106P

Ayd FJ Jr (1978) Haloperidol: Twenty years' clinical experience. J Clin Psychiatr 39: 807–814

Bateson PPG (1964) An effect of imprinting on the perceptual development of domestic chicks. Nature (London) 202: 421–422

Battig K, Rosvold HE, Mishkin M (1962) Comparison of the effects of frontal and caudate lesions on discrimination learning in monkeys. J Comp Physiol Psychol 55: 458–463

Berkson G (1967) Abnormal stereotyped motor acts. In: Zubin J, Hunt HF (eds) Comparative Psychopathology. Grune and Stratton, New York, pp 76–94

Berkson G, Davenport RK (1962) Stereotyped movements of mental defectives. I. Initial survey. Am J Ment Deficiency 66:849–852

Berkson G, Goodrich J, Kraft I (1966) Abnormal stereotyped movements of marmosets. Perceptual Motor Skills 23: 491–498

Bleuler E (1950) Dementia Praecox or the Group of Schizophrenias (Transl. Zinkin J) International Universities Press, New York

Brown JL (1960) Prognosis from presenting symptoms of pre-school children with atypical development. Am J Orthopsychiatr 30: 382–390

Brush ES, Mishkin M, Rosvold HE (1961) Effects of object preferences and aversions on discrimination learning in monkeys with frontal lesions. J Comp Physiol Psychol 54: 319–325

Brutkowski S, Mishkin M, Rosvold HE (1960) The effect of orbital and dorsolateral frontal lesions on conditioned inhibitory reflexes in monkeys. Acta Physiol Polon 11: 664–666 (In Polish)

Brutkowski S, Mishkin M, Rosvold HE (1963) Positive and inhibitory motor CR's in monkeys after ablation of orbital or dorsolateral suraces of the frontal cortex. In: Gutman E (ed) Central and Peripheral Mechanisms of Motor Functions. Academy of Sciences Czechoslovakia

Carey RJ, Kritkausky RP (1972) Absence of a response rate-dependent effect of d-amphetamine on a DRL schedule when reinforcement is signalled. Psychonom Sci 26: 285–286

Carlsson A, Fuxe K, Hamberger B, Lindquist M (1966) Biochemical and histochemical studies on the effects of imipramine-like drugs and (+)-amphetamine on central and peripheral catecholamine neurons. Acta Physiol Scand 67: 481–497

Carpenter MB (1976) Anatomy of the basal ganglia and related nuclei: A review. In: Eldridge R, Fahn S (eds) Advances in Neurology. Raven Press, New York, 14: 7–48

Casler L (1968) Perceptual deprivation in an institutional setting. In: Newton S, Levine S, Thomas CC (eds) Early Experience and Behavior: Psychological and Physiological Effects of Early Environmental Variation. Charles C Thomas, Springfield Illinois pp 573–626

Chamove AS, Anderson JR (1981) Self-aggression, stereotypy and self-injurious behavior in man and monkeys. Current Psychol Rev 1: 245–256

Chavis DA, Pandya DN (1976) Further observations on corticofrontal connections in the rhesus monkey. Brain Res 117: 369–386

Chien CP, DiMascio A (1967) Drug-induced extrapyramidal symptoms and their relations to clinical efficacy. Am J Psychiatr 123: 1490–1498

Clark FC, Steele BJ (1966) Effects of d-amphetamine on performance under a multiple schedule in the rat. Psychopharmacol 9: 157–169

Connell PH (1958) Amphetamine Psychosis. Maudsley Monograph No 5 Chapman and Hall, London

Corbett JA, Harris E, Robinson R (1975) Epilepsy. In: Wortis J (ed) Mental Retardation and Developmental Disabilities Vol 7. An annual review. Brunner/Mazel, New York, pp 79–111

Crow TJ, Ferrier IN, Johnstone EC, MacMillan JF, Owens DG, Parry RP, Tyrrell DAJ (1979) Characteristics of patients with schizophrenia or neurological disorder and virus-like agent in cerebrospinal fluid. Lancet i: 842–844

Davis JM (1975) Overview: maintenance therapy in psychiatry: I. Schizophrenia. Am J Psychiatr 132: 1237–1245

Eisenberg L (1956) The autistic child in adolescence. Am J Psychiatr 112:607–612

Ellinwood EH Jr (1971) Effect of chronic methamphetamine intoxication in rhesus monkeys. Biol Psychiatr 3: 25–32

Ellinwood EH Jr, Sudilovsky A, Nelson LM (1973) Evolving behavior in the clinical and experimental amphetamine (model) psychosis. Am J Psychiatr 130: 1088–1093

Ellison G, Nielsen FB, Lyon M (1981) Animal model of psychosis: hallucinatory behaviors in monkeys during the late stage of continuous amphetamine intoxication. J Psychiatr Res 16: 13–22

Foley JP (1934) First year development of a rhesus monkey (*M. mulatta*) reared in isolation. J Genet Psychol 45: 39–105

Frith U (1970a) Studies in pattern detection in normal and autistic children. I. Immediate recall of auditory sequences. J Abnormal Psychol 76: 413–420

Frith U (1970b) Studies in pattern detection in normal and autistic children. II. Reproduction and production of color sequences. J Exper Child Psychol 10: 120–135

Frith U (1972) Cognitive mechanisms in autism: experiments with color and tone sequence production. J Autism Childhood Schizophren 2: 160–173

Garcia-Munoz M, Nicolaou NM, Tulloch IF, Wright AK, Arbuthnott GW (1977) Feedback loop or output pathway in striato-nigral fibers? Nature 265: 363–365

Garver D, Schlemmer F, Maas J, Davis J (1975) A schizophreniform behavioral psychosis mediated by dopamine. Am J Psychiatr 132: 33–38

Gross CG (1963) Discrimination reversal after frontal lesions in monkeys. J Comp Physiol Psychol 56: 52–59

Hediger H (1955) Studies of the Psychology and Behavior of Captive Animals in Zoos and Circuses. Criterion Press, New York

Heise GA, Lilie NL (1970) Effects of scopolamine, atropine and d-amphetamine on internal and external control of responding on non-reinforced trials. Psychopharmacol 18: 38–49

Held R, Hein A (1963) Movement produced stimulation in the development of visually guided behavior. J Comp Physiol Psychol 56: 872–876

Hermelin B, Frith U (1971) Psychological studies of childhood autism. Can autistic children make sense of what they hear? J of Special Ed 5: 1107–1117

Isaac W, Troelstrup R (1969) Opposite effect of illumination and d-amphetamine upon activity in the squirrel monkey (*Saimiri*) and the owl monkey (*Aotes*). Psychopharmacol 15: 260–264

Jacobsen CF, Wolfe JB, Jackson TA (1935) An experimental analysis of the functions of the frontal association area in primates. J Nerv Ment Dis 83: 1–4

Johnstone EC, Crow TJ, Frith CD, Carney MWP, Price JS (1978) Mechanism of the antipsychotic effect in the treatment of acute schizophrenia. Lancet i: 848–851

Kalant OJ (1966) The Amphetamines: toxicity and addiction. Brookside Monograph No 5, University of Toronto Press

Kanner L (1943) Autistic disturbance of affective contact. Nerv Child 2: 217–250

Kay SR, Singh MM (1979) Cognitive abnormality in schizophrenia: a dual process model. Biol Psychiatr 14: 155–176

Keeler WR (1958) Autistic patterns and defective communication in blind children with retrolental fibroplasia. In: Hoch PH, Zubin J (eds) Psychopathology of Communication. Grune and Stratton, New York, pp 64–83

Kelleher RJ, Coats L (1961) Effects of d-amphetamine, meprobamate, phenobarbital, mephenasin or chlorpromazine on DRL and FR schedules of reinforcement with rats. J Exper Anal Behav 4: 327–330

Kiloh LG, Gyre RS, Rushworth RG, Bell DS, White RT (1974) Stereotactic amygdaloidotomy for aggressive behavior. J Neurol Neurosurg Psychiatr 37: 437–444

Kluver H, Bucy PC (1939) Preliminary analysis of functions of the temporal lobes in monkeys. Arch Neurol Psychiatr 42: 979–1000

Kraepelin E (1971) Dementia Praecox and Paraphrenia. Barclay RM (transl) Livingstone, Edinburgh

Leichnetz GR, Astruc J (1975) Efferent connections of the orbitofrontal cortex in the marmoset (*Saguinus oedipus*) Brain Res 86: 169–180

Machiyama Y, Hsu SC, Utena H, Katagiri M, Hirata A (1974) Aberrant social behavior induced in monkeys by the chronic methamphetamine administration as a model of schizophrenia. In: Mitsuda H, Fukuda T (eds) Biological Mechanisms of Schizophrenia and Schizophrenia-Like Pyschosis. Igaku Shoin, Tokyo, pp 97–105

Manning FJ (1972) Serial reversal learning by monkeys with inferotemporal or foveal prestriate lesions. Physiol Behav 8: 177–181

Meikle DH, Gallant DM, Kessler C (1977) An evaluation of a unique new antipsychotic agent sulpiride: effects on serum prolactin and growth hormone levels. Am J Psychiatr 134: 1371–1375

Meltzer HY, Stahl SM (1976) The dopamine hypothesis of schizophrenia: a review. Schizophren Bull 2: 19–76

Meyer-Holzapfel M (1968) Abnormal behavior in zoo animals. In: Fox MW (ed) Abnormal Behavior in Animals. W.B. Saunders, Philadelphia, pp 476–503

Mishkin M (1964) Perseveration of central sets after frontal lesions in monkeys. In: Warren JM, Akert K (eds) The Frontal Granular Cortex and Behavior. McGraw-Hill, New York, pp 219–241

Olpe HR, Demieville H, Baltzer V, Bencze WL, Koella WP, Wolf P, Haas HL (1978) The biological activity of d- and l-baclofen (Lioresal). Eur J Pharmacol 52: 113–136

Owen F, Baker HF, Ridley RM, Cross AJ, Crow TJ (1981) Effect of chronic amphetamine administration on central dopaminergic mechanisms in the vervet. Psychopharmacol 74: 213–216

Pribram KH, Douglas RJ, Pribram BJ (1969) The nature of non-limbic learning. J Comp Physiol Psychol 69: 765–772

Randrup A, Munkvad I (1967) Stereotyped activities produced by amphetamine in several animal species and man. Psychopharmacol 11: 300–310

Randrup A, Munkvad I (1972) Influence of amphetamines on animal behavior: stereotypy, functional impairment and possible animal-human correlations. Psychiatr Neurol Neurochir 75: 193–202

Ridley RM, Baker HF (1982) Stereotypy in monkeys and humans. Psychol Med 12: 61–72

Ridley RM, Baker HF, Crow TJ (1980d) Behavioral effects of amphetamines and related stimulants; the importance of species differences as demonstrated by a study in the marmoset. In: Caldwell J (ed) Amphetamines and Related Stimulants: Chemical, Biological, Clinical, and Sociological Aspects. CRC Press, Florida, pp 97–116

Ridley RM, Baker HF, Haystead TAJ (1981a) Perseverative behavior after amphetamine: dissociation of response tendency from reward association. Psychopharmacol 75: 283–286

Ridley RM, Baker HF, Scraggs PR (1979a) The time course of the behavioral effects of amphetamine and their reversal by haloperidol in a primate species. Biol Psychiatr 14: 753–765

Ridley RM, Baker HF, Weight ML (1980a) Amphetamine disrupts successive but not simultaneous visual discrimination in the monkey. Psychopharmacol 67: 241–244

Ridley RM, Haystead TAJ, Baker HF (1981b) An involvement of dopamine in higher order choice mechanisms in the monkey. Psychopharmacol 72: 173–177

Ridley RM, Haystead TAJ, Baker HF (1981c) An analysis of visual object reversal learning in the marmoset after amphetamine and haloperidol. Pharmacol Biochem Behav 14: 345–351

Ridley RM, Scraggs PR, Baker HF (1979b) Modification of the behavioral effects of amphetamine by a GABA agonist in a primate species. Psychopharmacol 64: 197–200

Ridley RM, Scraggs PR, Baker HF (1980b) The effects of metoclopramide, sulpiride and the stereoisomers of baclofen on amphetamine-induced behavior in the marmoset. Biol Psychiatr 15: 265–274

Ridley RM, Weight ML, Haystead TAJ, Baker HF (1980c) "Go here–go there" performance after amphetamine: the importance of the response requirement in successive discrimination. Psychopharmacol 69: 271–273

Robinson OPW (1973) Metoclopramide—side effects and safety. Postgraduate Med J 49: Suppl 4: 77–80

Rolinski Z, Scheel-Kruger J (1973) The effect of dopamine and noradrenaline antagonists on amphetamine-induced locomotor activity in mice and rats. Acta Pharmacol Toxicol 33: 385–399

Rosvold HE, Szwarcbart MK (1964) Neural structures involved in delayed-response performance. In: Warren JM, Akert K (eds) The Frontal Granular Cortex and Behavior. McGraw-Hill, New York, pp 1–15

Scheel-Kruger J (1971) Comparative studies of various amphetamine analogues demonstrating different interactions with the metabolism of the catecholamines in the brain. Eur J Pharmacol 14: 47–59

Schiorring E (1979) Social isolation and other behavioral changes in groups of adult vervet monkeys (*Ceropithecus aethiops*) produced by low, non-chronic doses of d-amphetamine. Psychopharmacol 64: 297–302

Schiorring E, Hecht A (1979) Behavioral effects of low, acute doses of d-amphetamine on the dyadic interaction between mother and infant vervet monkeys (*Cercopithecus aethiops*) during the first six post-natal months. Psychopharmacol 64: 219–224

Schofield SP, Dixson AF (1982) Distribution of catecholamine and indoleamine neurons in the brain of the common marmoset (*Callithrix jacchus*). J Anatomy 134: 315–338

Scraggs PR, Ridley RM (1978) Behavioral effects of amphetamine in a small primate: relative potencies of the d- and l-isomers. Psychopharmacol 59: 243–245

Scraggs PR, Ridley RM (1979) The effect of dopamine and noradrenaline blockade on amphetamine-induced behavior in the marmoset. Psychopharmacol 62: 41–45

Segal DS, Weinberger SB, Cahill J, McCunney SJ (1980) Multiple daily amphetamine administration: behavioral and neurochemical alterations. Sci 207: 904–907

Shakow D (1962) Segmental set. A theory of the formal psychological deficit in schizophrenia. Arch Gen Psychiatr 6: 17–33

Spitz RA (1945) Hospitalism. An enquiry into the genesis of psychiatric conditions in early childhood. Psychoanalytic Stud Child 1: 53–74

Sweeney S, Zamecnik K (1981) Predictors of self-mutilation in patients with schizophrenia. Am J Psychiatr 138: 1086–1089

Thelen E (1979) Rhythmical stereotypies in normal human infants. Animal Behav 27: 699–715

Tyrrell DAJ, Parry RP, Crow TJ, Johnstone EC, Ferrier IN (1979) Possible virus in schizophrenia and some neurological disorders. Lancet i: 839–841

Utena H, Machiyama Y, Hsu SC, Katagiri M, Hirata A(1975) A monkey model for schizophrenia produced by methamphetamine. Contemp Primatol (5th In Congr Primatol), pp 502–507

Waddington JL, Cross AJ (1978) Neurochemical changes following kainic acid lesions of the nucleus accumbens: implications for a GABAergic accumbal-ventral tegmental pathway. Life Sci 22: 1011–1014

Weight ML, Ridley RM, Baker HF (1980) The effects of amphetamine on delayed response performance in the monkeys. Pharmacol Biochem Behav 12: 861–864

Wilmanns K (1940) On murder in the prodromal stage of schizophrenia. Z Ges Neurol Psychiatr 170: 583–662 (In German)

Yarrow JL (1964) Separation from parents during early childhood. In: Hoffman ML, Hoffman LNW (eds) Review of Child Develolpment Research. Russell Sage Foundation, New York, pp 89–136

Yeterian EH, Van Hoesen GW (1978) Cortico-striate projections in the rhesus monkey: the organization of certain cortico-caudate connections. Brain Res 139: 43–63

Ethopharmacology: Primate Models of Neuropsychiatric Disorders, pages 137–155

Ethological Analysis of Amphetamine Action on Social Behavior in Squirrel Monkeys (*Saimiri sciureus*)

Klaus A. Miczek and Lisa H. Gold

Department of Psychology, Tufts University, Medford, Massachusetts 02155

THE RATIONALE FOR THE STUDY OF DRUG EFFECTS IN GROUPS OF MONKEYS

Most primate species, including humans, are social in nature; yet behavioral, neurophysiological, and neurochemical effects of drugs are routinely studied in single animals. Primates that are removed from their social context may in fact represent unusual biological entities.

Among the many valid reasons for studying drug effects in socially intact primates, two appear particularly important. First, the effects of drugs on behavioral, neurochemical, and other physiological processes appear to be determined by the role, status, or rank an animal occupies in a social group. Second, many types and facets of social behavior are the primary targets of drug action. This rationale needs comment and illustration.

Social interactions in primate groups follow predictable patterns which in many species result in a clearly identifiable hierarchical organization. Success in competitive agonistic behavior leads to a stratification of group members which in the most simple cases can be portrayed as a linear hierarchy. However, in many primate species triangular and probabilistic relationships may lead to a more complex organization. In addition to obvious species differences, there are important genealogical, ecological, and situational variables which may determine a particular social organization.

For example, in groups of squirrel monkeys (*Saimiri sciureus*) of Peruvian and Colombian origin, living in captivity, a clear and stable social stratification is apparent (Miczek and Gold, in press). Figure 1 illustrates the sociograms for three groups of monkeys, excluding the interactions with infants and juveniles. The frequency of grasping, displacing, and displaying the genitals was tallied according to who initiated the behavior and who received it in dyadic interactions. At the top of the sociogram are monkeys that initiated a high number of agonistic behaviors and which received few; these monkeys are referred to as dominant. Monkeys of an intermediate status

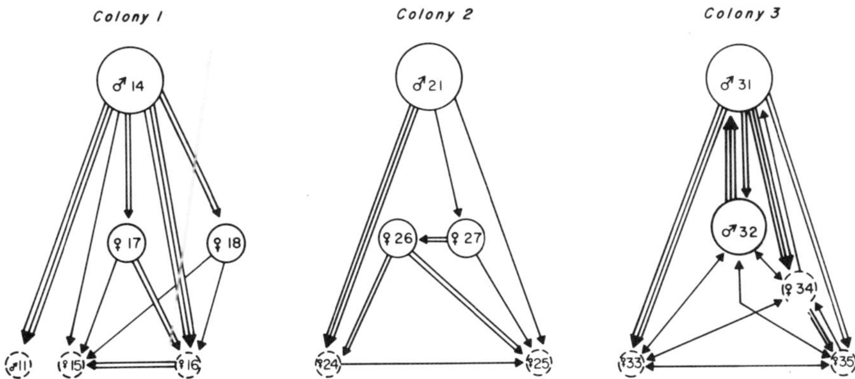

Fig. 1. Sociograms of three colonies of squirrel monkeys in March and April 1981. The size of the circle represents the number of agonistic behaviors which an animal initiated as compared to those which it received; the larger the circle, the greater the difference between the number of behaviors sent and received—i.e. the difference score, D. The dashed circles refer to animals with a negative difference score—i.e. animals that are primarily recipients of agonistic behaviors. The arrows indicate the direction of agonistic interactions; the number of lines in the arrows portrays the frequency of these interactions. One line symbolizes 1-5 interactions; 2 lines, 6–10 interactions; 3 lines, more than 10 interactions (from Miczek and Gold, 1983).

include those that initiated only slightly more agonistic behavior than they received; these monkeys are considered subdominant. Monkeys on the bottom tier were primarily recipients of agonistic interactions, and they are called submissive.

Status in the social hierarchy may determine several effects of psychoactive drugs. It appears that there are status-linked behavioral, physiological, and possibly neurochemical characteristics which are substrates of drug action. Support for this conclusion is already accruing. Significant differential changes in catecholamine synthesis have been noted in dominant and subordinate tree shrews (Raab and Oswald, 1980); dominant macaque monkeys also differ from lower-ranking animals in gonadal and adrenal hormone secretion (Sassenrath, 1970; Rose et al., 1971; Sapolsky, 1982; Stecklis et al., 1982).

Haber and associates (1981) analyzed the effects of chronically administered amphetamine on the social rank of rhesus monkeys (*Macaca mulatta*) belonging to two colonies. Amphetamine caused no significant changes in submissive or threatening behavior when these two behavior categories were examined by themselves; however, when submissive reactions by amphetamine-treated subordinate monkeys were grouped together with threats by amphetamine-treated dominant animals, a significant amphetamine effect became apparent: The rank-characteristic agonistic behavior of dominant and subordinate monkeys was amplified by chronic low amphetamine doses.

In female stumptail macaques (*Macaca arctoides*) d-amphetamine effects on submissive behavior appeared to be influenced by hierarchical rank (Schlemmer and Davis, 1981, and this volume). d-Amphetamine, 1.6 mg/kg, b.i.d., increased submissive gestures such as lip smack and submissive present in high-ranking females; by contrast, females designated delta and epsilon failed to show an amphetamine effect (see Figure 4 in Schlemmer and Davis, this volume). It is tempting to relate the rank-related amphetamine effects on submissive responses that occur out of appropriate context in macaques to the sources of individual variation in drug response in humans (Schlemmer and Davis, 1981).

A recent example of amphetamine effects on elements of motor activity in squirrel monkeys (*Saimiri sciureus*) highlights social status as an important

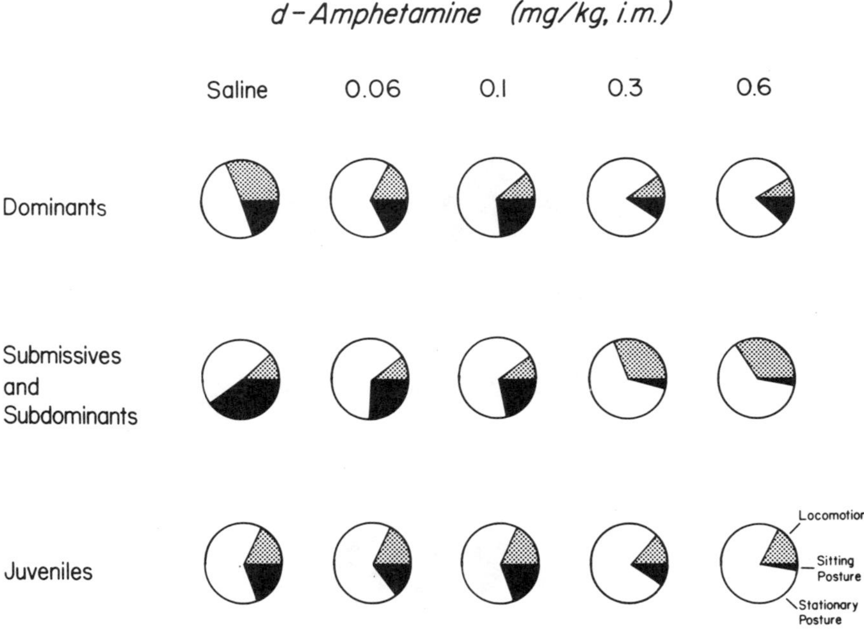

Fig. 2. Activity budget analysis of d-amphetamine (i.m.) on dominant (top row), subdominant and submissive (center row), and juvenile monkeys (bottom row). Columns refer to different doses of d-amphetamine. The proportions of time spent in locomotion, sitting posture, and stationary posture are portrayed as segments of a circle.

determinant of drug action (Miczek and Gold, in press). Figure 2 portrays the results of an activity budget analysis focusing on three types of motor behavior: locomotion, sitting posture, and stationary posture (Fig. 3).

Members of three independent colonies of monkeys were individually administered with d-amphetamine, and the frequency and duration of the

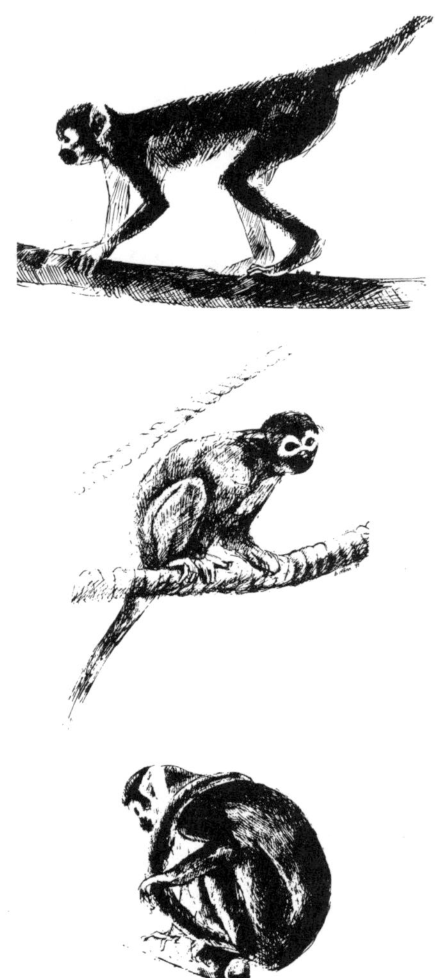

Fig. 3. Three elements of solitary or self-directed motor activity in squirrel monkeys: locomotion (top), stationary posture (center), sitting (bottom). The drawings are based on photographs, prepared by Bonnie Dann (from Miczek and Yoshimura, 1982).

treated monkey's behavior were recorded using the focal animal technique. As shown in Figure 1, the adult population of each colony was differentiated according to how much and how successfully each member engaged in agonistic interactions. In addition to obvious differences in social behavior, dominant monkeys also differed from subdominant and submissive monkeys in how much time they allocated to certain kinds of motor activity. As indicated in the "Saline" column, dominant and juvenile monkeys engaged in a high level of locomotor behavior as compared to subdominant and submissive monkeys. The time spent in the relaxed sitting posture was substantially longer for subdominant and submissive animals than for dominant and juvenile members of the colonies.

A range of amphetamine doses (0.06–0.6 mg/kg, i.m.) was selected which extended to those inducing motor sterotypies. Dominant monkeys differed from subdominants and submissives not only in the magnitude but also in the direction of amphetamine effects on locomotor responses. With increasing amphetamine doses locomotion was progressively decreased in dominant monkeys, whereas an increase was observed in subdominant and submissive monkeys. Locomotor behavior of juvenile monkeys was not significantly altered in this dose range. In all types of monkeys the time allocated to the sitting posture declined with increasing amphetamine doses; this effect was particularly striking in subdominant and submissive monkeys that assumed the sitting posture for long periods during control observations.

The initial attempt to analyze just three distinctly different types of motor activity revealed that the history of social behavior significantly predicts how amphetamine affects the way animals allocate time to nonsocial behavior. The three postures and movements were selected for the activity analysis, because they account for more than 90% of the total observation time. A more extensive and comprehensive analysis of the behavioral repertoire is expected to uncover shifts in additional classes of behavior due to amphetamine action.

The rationale for the study of drug effects on groups of primates gains further significance because various types of social behavior are selectively and specifically altered by several drugs. In contrast to the extensive pharmacological investigations into conditioned performance measures, motor sterotypies, and behavioral indices of memory and perception, little is known about drug effects on the rich repertoire of social interactions. It may be that investigators with expertise in the analysis of primate social behavior are prejudiced against experimental work involving drugs (i.e., drugs are "dirty"), and, conversely, many pharmacologists exhibit a cavalier attitude toward detailed quantitative measurements of complex patterns of social behavior in groups of primates. Many investigators also believe that drugs affect conditioned behavior more readily than unconditioned behavior patterns.

Experimental protocols have been developed in several primate species which permit the study of drug effects on maternal behavior, juvenile play, social interactions among adult group members, and competitive behavior, as well as attack and threat toward unfamiliar intruders. A few selected examples will illustrate these efforts.

Schiørring and Hecht (1979) studied the interactions between mother and infant vervet monkeys (*Cercopithecus aethiops*) and found severe social withdrawal after low, acute doses of d-amphetamine (0.1, 0.15, 0.2 mg/kg, s.c.) were administered to the mother. Amphetamine treatment of the mother led to a lack of the ventral-ventral posture and eye contact, normally shown toward the infant. The amphetamine-treated mother actively rejected the approaching infant and failed to groom him. When separated by a clear fiberglass screen, mother and infant normally spent more than 90% of the total observation time close to the screen in an attempt to establish the closest possible contact. After administration of 0.2 mg/kg d-amphetamine s.c., the mother was near the separating screen less than 9% of the time; instead she engaged in continuous motor stereotypies. Social withdrawal and failure to respond to socially relevant stimuli in the mother-infant pair of vervet monkeys parallel similar phenomena in humans following amphetamine administration.

In a group of juvenile stumptail macaques (*Macaca arctoides*) intragastric administration of amphetamine (0.5 mg/kg) greatly suppressed play behavior (Schlemmer et al., 1976). The most significant aspect of this behavioral effect of amphetamine was the nearly complete elimination of solitary play; less marked decreases were observed in social play such as rough-and-tumble play and invitation to play. Another form of social behavior, huddling, actually increased after the first dose of amphetamine, and this increase persisted for 4 weeks of daily drug administration. The authors noted that the "paradoxical" quieting effect of amphetamine on juveniles' motor activity contrasts sharply with opposite effects in adult macaques. Failure to respond to invitations to social activities and to initiate play behavior in juvenile macaques parallels similar amphetamine effects in adults.

Juvenile squirrel monkeys strongly affiliate with their mothers, particuarly when threatened. We studied the effects of amphetamine and other psychoactive drugs on affiliative behavior in these monkeys under varied social conditions (Miczek et al., 1981). Affiliative behavior was measured in a specially designed apparatus, which is illustrated schematically in Figure 4. In brief, a juvenile monkey and his mother were placed into opposite ends of

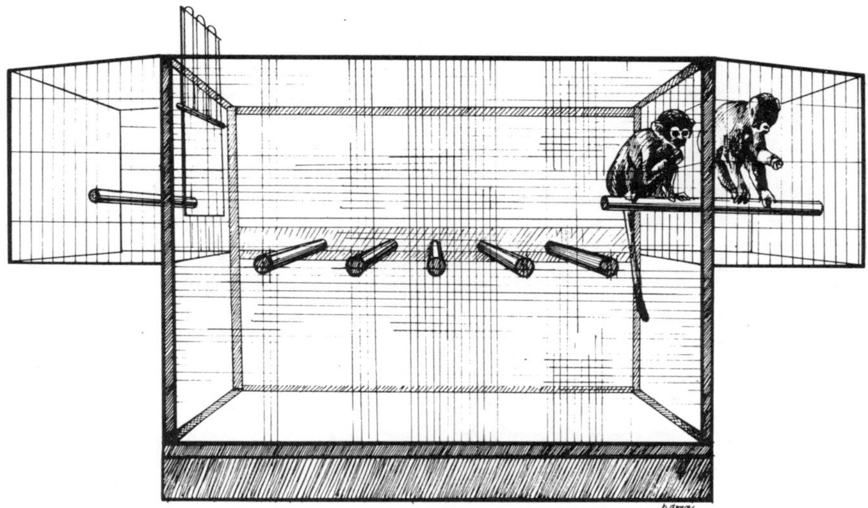

Fig. 4. Schematic of apparatus used for measuring affiliative behavior. The drug-treated monkey is placed into the starting cage on the left; the door to the center compartment is then opened allowing access to the center compartment for 5 min. The drawing portrays a saline-treated monkey, perching next to a nontreated group member confined in the small cage on the right. Drawing by Bonnie Dann (from Miczek and Yoshimura, 1982).

a three-compartment apparatus. A test began by providing the juvenile monkey access to the large center compartment which was equipped with six equally spaced perches. Under control conditions the juveniles spent about 37% of the total observation time on the perches closest to their mothers (Fig. 5A). d-Amphetamine (0.3, 1.0 mg/kg, i.m.) severely decreased the time spent close to the mother.

In a second phase of the experiment, a cage containing an unfamiliar adult male monkey was added to the apparatus. The physical proximity of the unfamiliar monkey greatly altered the affiliative behavior of the juveniles toward their mothers and the effects of amphetamine: The time spent near to the mother doubled, amounting to 73% of the total observation period; administration of d-amphetamine, even up to 1.0 mg/kg, remained ineffective in modifying the strong affiliative response toward the mother. The sharp contrast of amphetamine effects in the presence versus absence of an unfamiliar adult male highlights the importance of social context as a determinant of drug action.

Interactions among adult members of primate groups are readily altered by d-amphetamine. Recently, we studied the effects of acute administration of d-amphetamine on agonistic behavior in three groups of squirrel monkeys

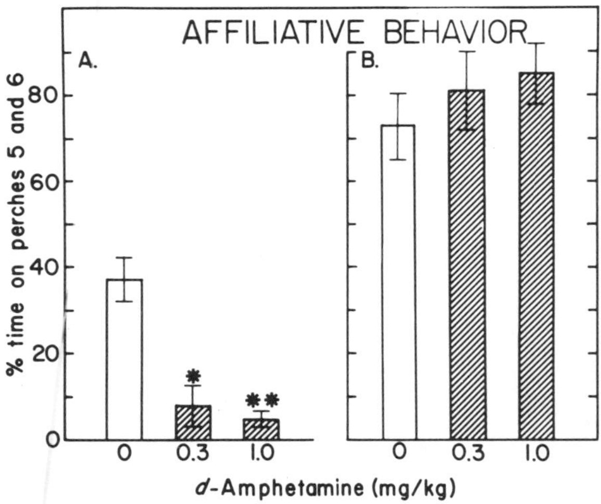

Fig. 5. The effects of saline vehicle (0) and d-amphetamine (0.3, 1.0 mg/kg) on the percent of time spent on perches 5 and 6 as an index of affiliation. (A) Assessment of affiliative responses by juvenile squirrel monkeys toward their mothers. (B) Assessment of affiliative responses by juvenile squirrel monkeys toward their mothers in the presence of an unfamiliar adult male monkey. Statistically significant differences between saline vehicle and amphetamine treatment are identified by asterisks: $*P < 0.05$, $**P < 0.01$. Vertical lines in each bar represent $\pm$ 1 SEM (from Miczek et al., 1981).

(Miczek and Gold, in press). After identifying the social status of each group member (see Fig. 1), d-amphetamine (0.1–1.0 mg/kg, p.o.; 0.06–0.6 mg/kg, i.m.) was administered to one animal in each group at a time, and the incidence of several salient agonistic behaviors was recorded. These behaviors included grasping (Fig. 6), displacing (Fig. 7), and displaying the genitals toward other monkeys (Fig. 8).

The effects of d-amphetamine on agonistic behavior depended on the social status of the individual monkeys within their group. Low doses of d-amphetamine (0.1, 0.3 mg/kg, p.o.) caused dominant monkeys to engage less frequently in agonistic behavior; higher doses (0.6, 1.0 mg/kg) completely reversed the typical pattern of agonistic behavior in dominant monkeys (Fig. 9, top row). Amphetamine-treated dominant monkeys failed to display toward other group members, or displace or grasp them. They became primarily recipients of agonistic behavior, paralleling the pattern characteristic of submissive animals.

When amphetamine was administered to subdominant monkeys, complete social isolation resulted; these monkeys did not initiate any agonistic behavior, nor were they the target of these actions (Fig. 9, center row). Submissive

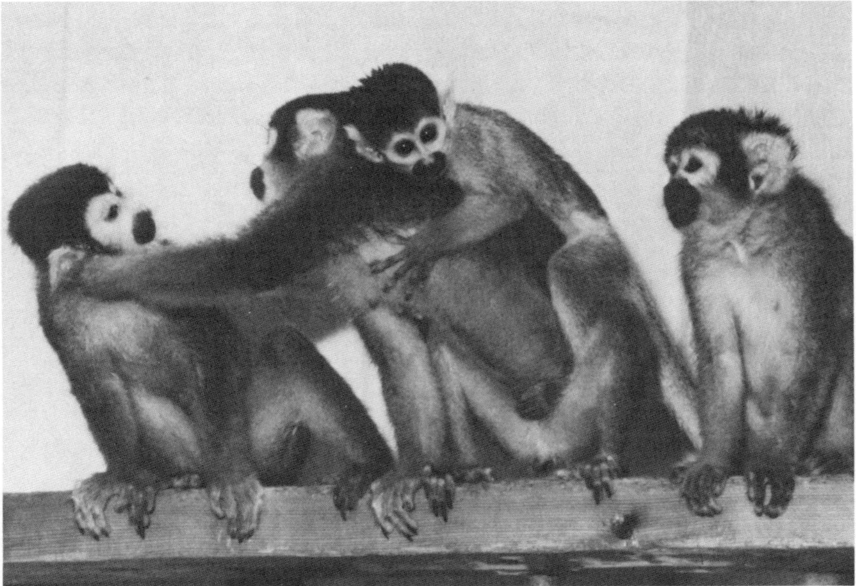

Fig. 6. One adult female squirrel monkey grasps another adult female. Photograph by C. Miczek.

monkeys rarely directed any agonistic behavior toward other group members; they were primarily the recipients of these behaviors. Amphetamine, even up to the 1.0 mg/kg dose, did not alter the characteristic pattern of agonistic behavior in submissive monkeys. Poignant and Avril (1978) also observed a complete suppression of social initiatives after amphetamine treatment (0.6 mg/kg, p.o.) of a dominant female in an all-female group of squirrel monkeys.

The suppression of agonistic behavior in dominant squirrel monkeys lasted for more than 1½ hours after an acute amphetamine administration (0.3 mg/kg, i.m.; Fig. 10, bottom). Curiously, the incidence of olfactory marking was not affected by this dose of d-amphetamine (Fig. 10, top). Regardless of the treatment condition, the return to the colony after the injection procedure always resulted in a large bout of olfactory marking. This large injection artifact obscured any potential effect of low, acute amphetamine doses on olfactory behavior.

The remarkable sensitivity of dominant monkeys to the actions of d-amphetamine may reflect a characteristic functional activity in the mediating neurochemical systems. We have postulated that the behavioral changes after challenge with amphetamine may indicate status-linked differences in the dynamics of catecholamine systems (Miczek and Gold, in press).

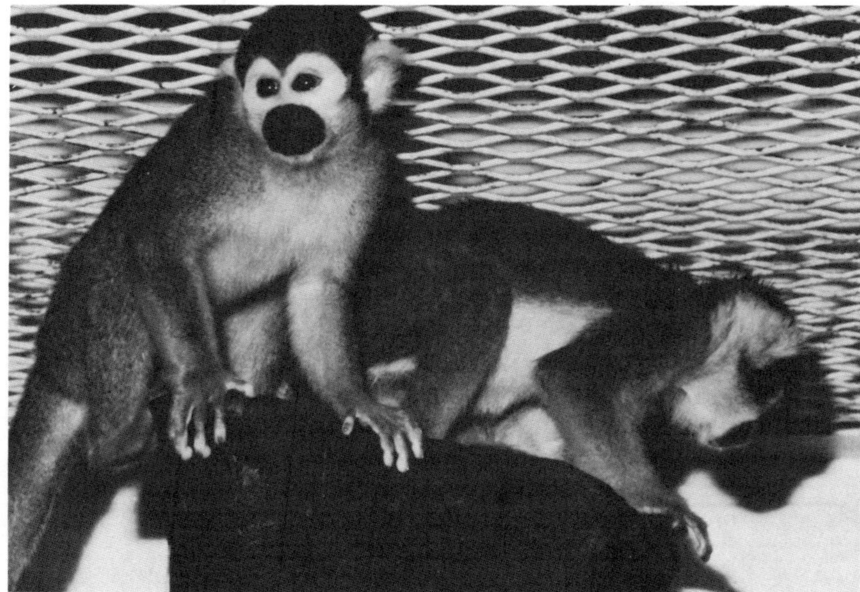

Fig. 7. The alpha male squirrel monkey in colony 1 displaces a submissive male from a preferred resting site. Photograph by C. Miczek.

SQUIRREL MONKEYS AS SUBJECTS OF ETHOPHARMACOLOGICAL STUDIES

Squirrel monkeys have become a frequently used primate species in laboratory research on the behavioral analysis of drug action (e.g., Hanson, 1968; Barrett, in press). Several considerations may be significant in the choice of an appropriate primate species for ethopharmacological studies, ranging from the purely pragmatic to historical and theoretical issues.

Comments on the squirrel monkey have to begin with the perceptive observations of the French naturalist Comte de Buffon who wrote in his "Histoire naturelle" some 200 years ago: "From the gracefulness of its movement, the smallness of its size, the brilliant colour of its hair, the largeness and vivacity of its eyes, and its round visage, the Saimiri has uniformly been preferred to all other sapajous [Editor's note: capuchins]: it is indeed the most beautiful of this tribe." This description was complemented by an exquisite illustration which is reproduced in Figure 11. A comprehensive account of the biology of the squirrel monkey has been edited by Rosenblum and Cooper (1968), and an update is currently being prepared.

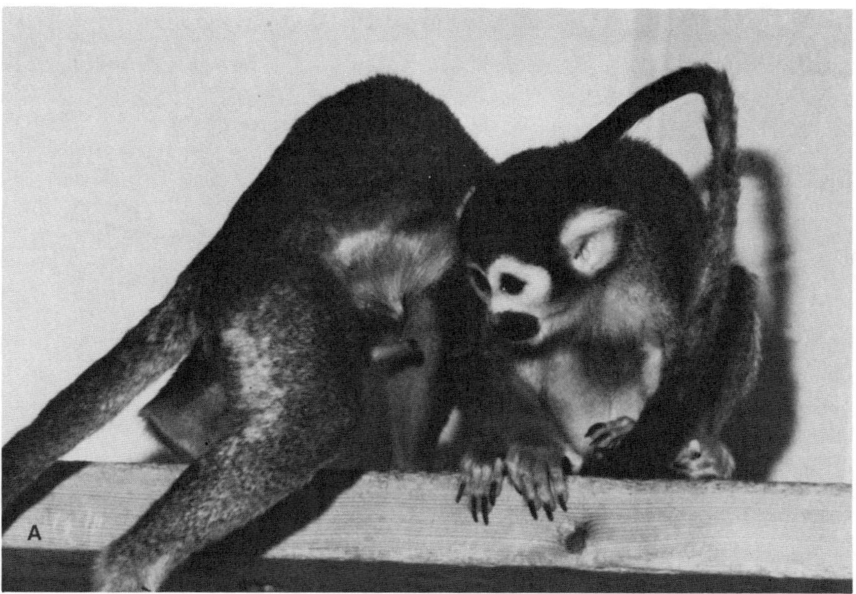

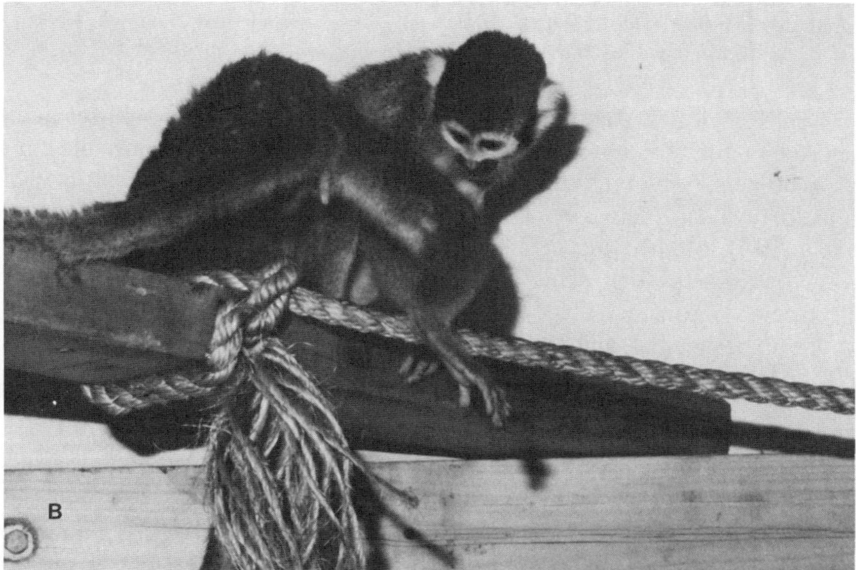

Fig. 8. A) An adult male squirrel monkey exhibiting a close penile display toward a young adult male. B) An adult female squirrel monkey shows a close clitoral display toward another adult female. Photographs by C. Miczek.

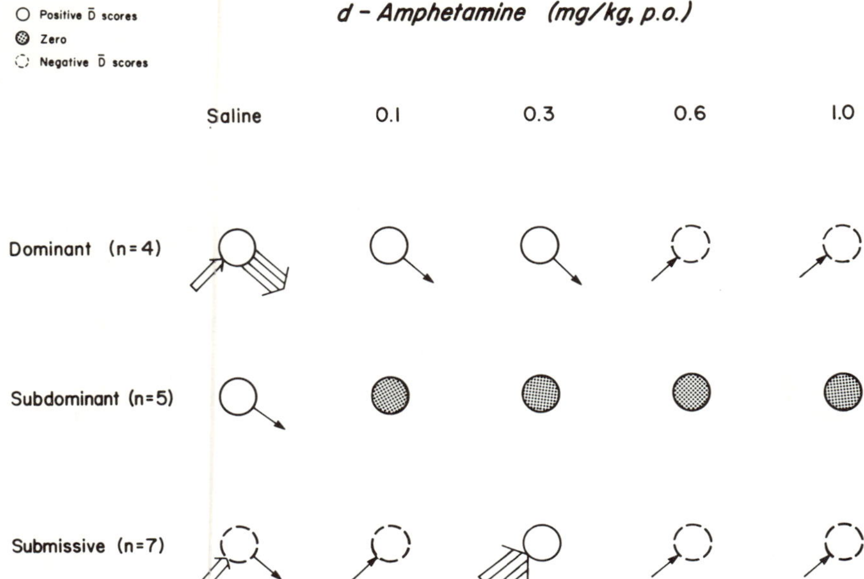

Fig. 9. Effects of d-amphetamine on agonistic behavior in dominant, subdominant, and submissive monkeys. The format of circles and arrows parallels that of Fig. 1. Negative difference scores are portrayed as dashed circles (from Miczek and Gold, in press).

A most significant issue for pharmacological studies is the squirrel monkey's elaborate repertoire of social behavior. More than 100 identifiable units of social behavior have been defined in the context of mother-infant interactions, play and affiliative behavior, sexual and agonistic behavior (e.g., Hopf et al., 1974). Methods for quantitative measurement of behavioral units have been developed which achieve a high degree of reliability and accuracy. Electronic data collection devices afford complete and uninterrupted focus on the experimental animals and enable virtually error-free data analysis (e.g., Miczek and Gold, in press; Dubach and Bowden, this volume; Smith and Byrd, this volume; Reite and Short, this volume).

When social relationships in groups of squirrel monkeys have stabilized, agonistic interactions are confined to a few episodes during the course of the day, and individual members typically retain their social status over consecutive years. Since squirrel monkeys breed on a seasonal basis, there are annual peaks in hormone-dependent social behavior such as agonistic, copulatory, and maternal behavior, even in captive conditions in the northern hemisphere (Rosenblum, 1968; Kaplan, 1977).

The implications for pharmacological studies are significant. The elaborate repertoire of social behavior in squirrel monkeys demands thoroughly

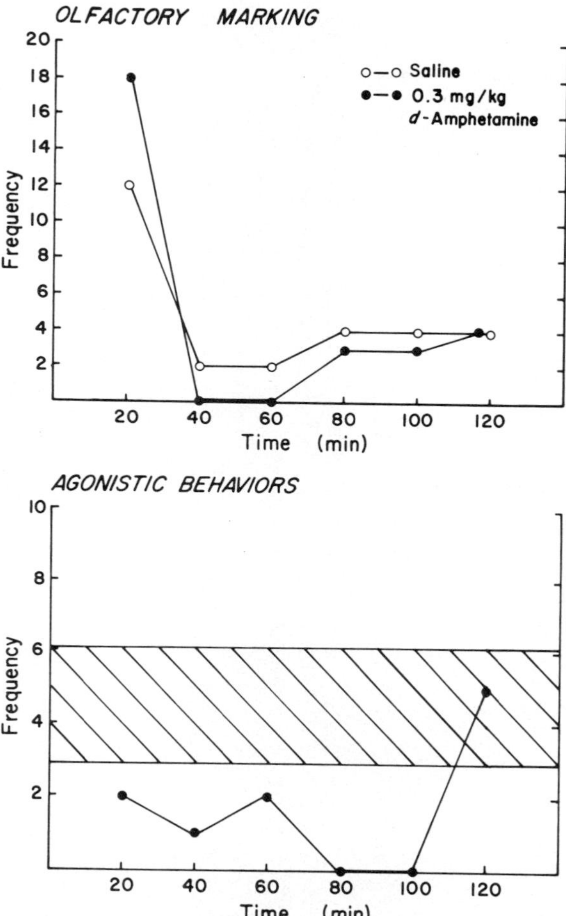

Fig. 10. Effects of 0.3 mg/kg d-amphetamine on olfactory marking (top) and agonistic behaviors (bottom) in a representative dominant male (31) over 2 hours. Twenty-minute totals of olfactory marking from amphetamine and saline control experiments are illustrated (top). The range of control values for agonistic behavior during the saline session is indicated by the shaded area (bottom). (From Miczek and Gold, in press.)

familiar observers equipped with satisfactory recording devices. Pharmacological manipulations are bound to interact with seasonal and circadian hormonal fluctuations and consequent changes in the levels of social behavior. The episodic nature of social behavior within groups of squirrel monkeys requires special research protocols which permit the transient actions of drugs to coincide with the occurrence of the behavior of interest. We have attempted to arrange the environmental and social conditions so that compet-

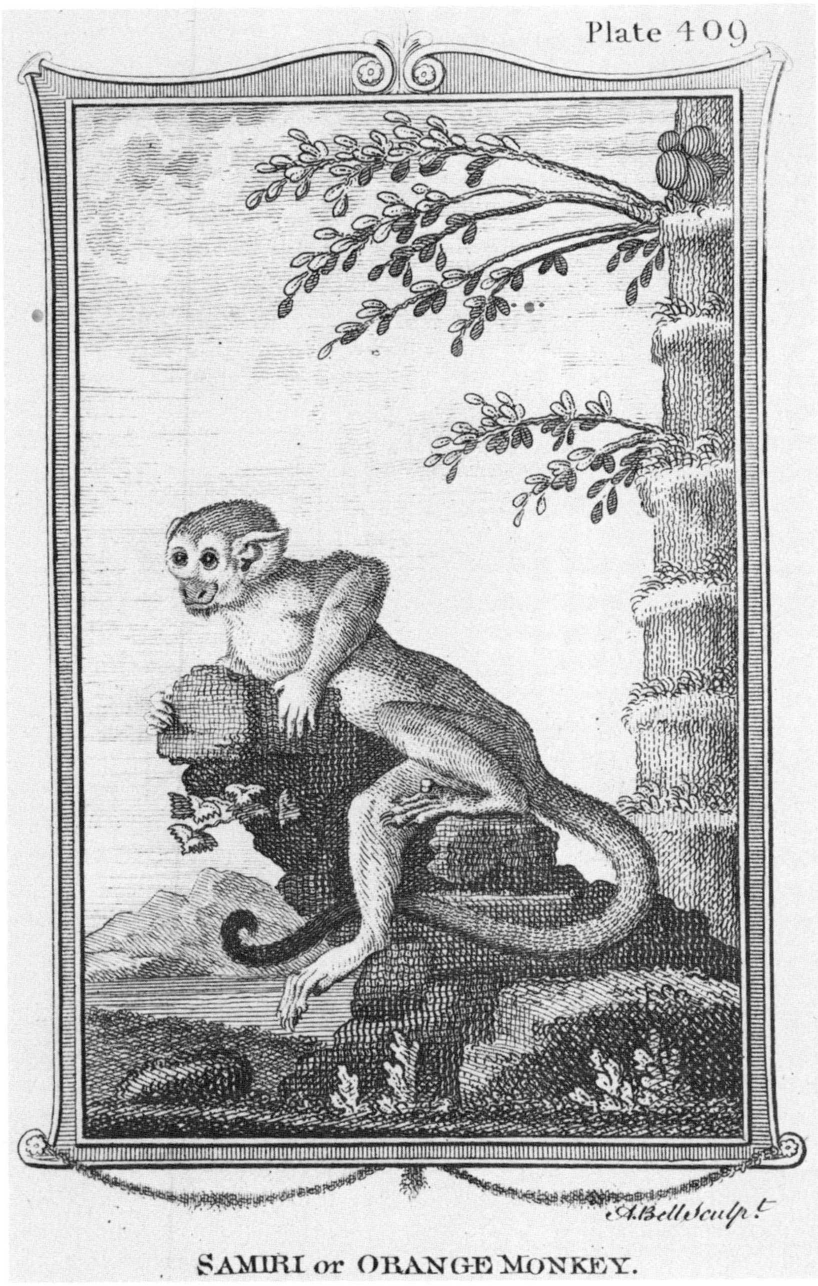

Fig. 11. Reproduction of plate 409, entitled "Samiri or Orange Monkey," showing a squirrel monkey, from "Histoire naturelle, générale et particulière, avec la description du cabinet de Roi" by Comte de Buffon, 1749–1803.

itive as well as affiliative activities within the group, and also attack and threat toward intruders occur in a reliable and predictable manner (Miczek, 1978; Miczek et al., 1981).

Pragmatic considerations often influence the choice of species. The squirrel monkey's small size, ease of handling, and relative availability contributed to its widespread and long-standing use in behavioral pharmacology and endocrinology (Hanson, 1968; Barrett, in press; Dews, 1972; Rosenblum and Coe, in press). Many essential details for satisfactory care and clinical management of squirrel monkeys are known, most significantly a diet high in protein and vitamins, especially C and D3 (Kelleher et al., 1963; Lang, 1968).

Starting in the 1950s squirrel monkeys were selected by researchers in academic and industrial laboratories as subjects for the experimental analysis of drug action on operant behavior (e.g., Kelleher et al., 1963; Dews, 1972). All major classes of psychoactive drugs have been and continue to be investigated in squirrel monkeys whose behavior is under the control of schedules of reinforcement and punishment (Barrett, in press). By contrast, very little is known about the effects of drugs on facets of social behavior in squirrel monkeys, and systematic studies have only recently begun (e.g., Jones et al., 1974; Poignant and Avril, 1978; Plotnik et al., 1975; Miczek, 1978; Miczek et al., 1981; Miczek and Yoshimura, 1982; Miczek and Gold, in press).

LIMITATIONS OF STUDYING DRUG EFFECTS ON SOCIAL BEHAVIOR IN PRIMATES

One of the most significant issues in ethopharmacological studies is that of experimental control. In contrast to the well-defined and tightly controlled variables of the experimental situations which have been most often used in behavioral pharmacology (e.g., Kelleher and Morse, 1968), research protocols for the study of drug action on primate social behavior resemble those for field research and typically do not stipulate experimental control over the behavioral measures. The frequency, intensity, and temporal distribution of various types of social behavior in a group of monkeys depend on a host of variables such as the evolutionary stage of the selected species, and its adaptation to captive conditions; the nature, variety and quantity of food, particularly if provisioned; the season and climate; the group composition; the history of each individual group member and its genealogical relationship to other members; the opportunity for group members to spatially separate. These and other variables, although very influential, usually remain nonmanipulated in ethopharmacological studies. This approach differs from the research strategy that follows the principles and practices of pharmacological studies of experimentally conditioned behavior. For example, it is possible to cause squirrel monkeys to bite inanimate objects by using various protocols of food and electric shock presentation in a tightly controlled test environment (e.g., Azrin et al., 1964; DeWeese, 1977), a behavioral measure of high internal validity, but without proven external validity.

The subtle nature of many types of social behavior often precludes experimental interventions. An appropriate research method must not destroy the social process it purports to study (Altmann, 1974). Captivity in itself may lead to a loss of significant portions of the behavioral repertoire; bizarre behavioral routines may emerge, and substantial changes in aggressive and reproductive behavior may occur. The proximate causes of social interactions remain to be elucidated; for example, the sudden threat, pursuit, and attack by one group member toward another often occurs without readily identifiable cause, and the episodic nature of such behavioral sequences is labeled as "spontaneous." The question persists as to what accounts for the moment-to-moment changes in social interactions in terms of situational events and biological processes.

Altmann (1974) suggests employing nonmanipulative controls which will not infringe upon the social behavior that is under study. Comparing data that are collected from different but related groups of subjects, or from the same groups at different times and locales, may allow quasi-experimental designs.

Another possible research strategy for ethopharmacological studies relies on the use of stimulus situations which ethologists have identified as "releasers." Presentation or removal of biologically relevant events have already been investigated as reliable methods of engendering intense and frequent social behaviors suitable for the study of drug action—for example, the separation from the mother which leads to profound changes in the physiology and behavior of infants (e.g., Reite and Short, this volume; Kraemer et al., this volume); the appearance of an intruder which produces threat displays, culminating in attack bites (e.g., Miczek, 1978).

A further strategy for enhanced experimental control focuses on social behavior evoked by electrical brain stimulation. This was one of the earlier research strategies, stemming mainly from work with cats and rodents, and leading to a few spectacular observations in primates (e.g., Delgado, 1966; Ploog and MacLean, 1962; Perachio and Alexander, 1975). Only a few pharmacological studies have been performed with primate social behavior that is evoked by brain stimulation (e.g., Apfelbach and Delgado, 1974). The exact nature of the behavior that is actually elicited by localized delivery of electrical impulses to brain structures depends on the social and environmental conditions that prevail at the time of the stimulation. It has been argued that aggressive, defensive, and flight behavior evoked by electrical brain stimulation may be due to the aversive properties of the electrical impulses (Plotnick, 1974).

Data acquisition based on direct observation is an essential and also critical issue for ethopharmacological studies. Accurate, objective, and reliable records of behavioral events have become the hallmark of behavioral pharmacology, and most researchers rely on automatic measuring devices (e.g., Dews, 1972). Direct observation is prone to observer bias, interpretative, inaccurate, selective, and subjective records, possibly to a larger degree than other methods. Observation is also time-consuming; it requires dedicated, keen, and well-trained researchers, and rarely lends itself to automation, although it may be supplemented with automatically recorded events such as telemetered movement indices and vocalizations.

In spite of the potential pitfalls, the observational method is also the strength of ethopharmacological studies. Instead of relegating the observational method to a preliminary step in dealing with a research question, the most profitable strategy is to employ techniques that eliminate observer bias, ensure accurate, objective, and reliable records, and enhance sensitivity so that it is comparable to more experimental and manipulative research. Such techniques are already available and are continuously improving (e.g., Altmann, 1974; Sackett, 1978). The increasing use of portable microprocessors that are dedicated to data acquisition eliminates many problems in the process of recording, transferring, and analyzing observational data (e.g., Miczek and Yoshimura, 1982; Miczek, 1982; Miczek and Gold, in press; Dubach and Bowden, this volume; Smith and Byrd, this volume).

Focusing on the specific patterns of social interactions in a given species of primates prompts the question to what extent the behavioral effects of amphetamine or other agents in groups of primates are relevant to the human situation. As illustrated by the contributions to the present volume, a variety of Old World and New World primates are studied, and the relative advantages of each species become apparent. At the present stage of investigation it seems most profitable to advocate investigations in a large variety of species and situations since no species is a clearly superior model case of human behavior. The study of primate social behavior offers unique opportunities for pharmacological and biochemical questions. Nearly all information on biochemical mechanisms is based on experiments in rodents; yet the range, subtlety, and complexity of primate behavior promises to be the most appropriate source for behavioral data.

ACKNOWLEDGMENTS

Preparation of this chapter and the research were supported by U.S.P.H.S. grants DA-02632 and AA-05122.

REFERENCES

Altmann J (1974) Observational study of behavior: Sampling methods. Behaviour 49: 227–267

Apfelbach R, Delgado JMR (1974) Social hierarchy in monkeys (*Macaca mulatta*) modified by chlordiazepoxide hydrochloride. Neuropharmacology 13: 11–20

Azrin NH, Hutchinson RR, Sallery RD (1964) Pain-aggression toward inanimate objects. J Exper Anal Behav 7: 223–228

Barrett JE (in press) The behavioral pharmacology of the squirrel monkey. In Rosenblum LA, Coe C (Eds.) The Handbook of Squirrel Monkey Research. New York: Plenum

Buffon GLL Comte de (1812) Histoire naturelle, générale et particulière, avec la description du cabinet de roi. Paris: De l'Imprimerie royale. Translated with notes and observations by William Smellie. London: T. Cadell and W. Davies

Delgado JMR (1966) Aggressive behavior evoked by radio stimulation in monkey colonies. Amer Zoologist 6: 669–681

DeWeese J (1977) Schedule-induced biting under fixed-interval schedules of food or electric-shock presentation. J Exper Anal Behav 27: 419–431

Dews PB (1972) Assessing the effect of drugs. In Myers RD (Ed) Methods in psychobiology. Vol. 2. London: Academic Press, pp 83–124

Haber S, Barchas PR, Barchas JD (1981) A primate analogue of amphetamine-induced behaviors in humans. Biol Psychiat 16: 181–196

Hanson HM (1968) Use of the squirrel monkey in pharmacology. In Rosenblum LA, Cooper RW (Eds.) The Squirrel Monkey. New York: Academic Press, pp 365–392

Hopf S, Hartmann-Wiesner E, Kühlmorgen B, Mayer S (1974) The behavioral repertoire of the squirrel monkey (*Saimiri*). Folia Primatologica 21: 225–249

Jones BC, Clark DL, Consroe PF, Smith HJ (1974) Effects of (−) delta-9 trans tetrahydrocannabinol on social behavior of squirrel monkey dyads in a water competition situation. Psychopharmacologia 37: 37–43

Kaplan J (1977) Breeding and rearing squirrel monkeys in captivity. Lab Animal Sci 27: 557–567

Kelleher RT, Gill CA, Riddle WC, Cook L (1963) On the use of the squirrel monkey in behavioral and pharmacological experiments. J Exper Anal Behav 6: 249–262

Kelleher RT, Morse WH (1968) Determinants of the specificity of behavioral effects of drugs. Ergeb Physiol Biol Chem Exp Pharmakol. 60: 1–56

Lang CM (1968) The laboratory care and clinical management of *Saimiri* (squirrel monkeys). In Rosenblum LA, Cooper RW (Eds.) The Squirrel Monkey. New York: Academic Press, pp 393–416

Miczek KA (1978) Δ^9−Tetrahydrocannabinol: Antiaggressive effects in mice, rats, and squirrel monkeys. Science 199: 1459–1461

Miczek KA (1982) Ethological analysis of drug action on aggression, defense, and defeat. In Spiegelstein MY and Levy A (Eds.) Behavioral Models and the Analysis of Drug Action. Amsterdam: Elsevier Scientific, pp 225–239

Miczek KA, Gold LH (1983) d-Amphetamine in squirrel monkeys of different social status: Effects on social and agonistic behavior, locomotion, and stereotypies. Psychopharmacology (in press)

Miczek KA, Woolley J, Schlisserman S, Yoshimura H (1981) Analysis of amphetamine effects on agonistic and affiliative behavior in squirrel monkeys (*Saimiri sciureus*). Pharmacol Biochem Behav 14 (Suppl 1): 103–107

Miczek KA, Yoshimura H (1982) Disruption of primate social behavior by d-amphetamine and cocaine: Differential antagonism by antipsychotics. Psychopharmacology 76: 163–171

Perachio AA, Alexander M (1975) The neural bases of aggression and sexual behavior in the rhesus monkey. In: Bourne GH (ed) The Rhesus Monkey, Vol 1. New York: Academic Press, pp 381–409

Ploog DW, MacLean PD (1962) Display of penile erection in squirrel monkey (*Saimiri sciureus*). Animal behavior 11: 32–39

Plotnik R (1974) Brain stimulation and aggression: Monkeys, apes, and humans. In Holloway RL (Ed.) Primate Aggression, Territoriality, and Xenophobia. New York: Academic Press, pp 389–415

Plotnik R, Mollenauer S, Gore W, Popov A (1975) Comparing the effects of scopolamine on operant and aggressive responses in squirrel monkeys. Pharmacology Biochem Behav 3: 739–748

Poignant JC, Avril A (1978) Pharmacological studies on drugs acting on social behaviour of the squirrel monkey—Effects of amineptine, piribedil, d-amphetamine and amitriptyline. Arzneimittel-Forschung 28: 267–271

Raab A, Oswald R (1980) Coping with social conflict: Impact on the activity of tyrosine hydroxlase in the limbic system and in the adrenals. Physiology and Behavior 24: 387–394

Rose RM, Holaday JW, Bernstein IS (1971) Plasma testosterone, dominance rank and aggressive behaviour in male rhesus monkeys. Nature 231: 366–368

Rosenblum LA (1968) Some aspects of female reproductive physiology in the squirrel monkey. In Rosenblum LA, Cooper RW (Eds.) The Squirrel Monkey. New York: Academic Press, pp 147–169

Rosenblum LA, Coe C (in press) The Handbook of Squirrel Monkey Research. New York: Plenum

Sackett GP (Ed) (1978) Observing Behavior. Vol. 1 and 2. Baltimore: University Park Press

Sapolsky RM (1982) The endocrine stress-response and social status in the wild baboon. Hormon Behav 16: 279–292

Sassenrath EN (1970) Increased adrenal responsiveness related to social stress in rhesus monkeys. Hormones and Behavior 1: 283–298

Schiørring E, Hecht A (1979) Behavioral effects of low, acute doses of d-amphetamine on the dyadic interaction between mother and infant vervet monkeys (*Cercopithecus aethiops*) during the first postnatal months. Psychopharmacology 64: 219–224

Schlemmer RF Jr, Casper RC, Siemens FK, Garver DL, Davis JM (1976) Behavioral changes in juvenile primate social colony with chronic administration of d-amphetamine. Psychopharmacol Comm 2: 49–59

Schlemmer RF Jr, Davis JM (1981) Evidence for dopamine mediation of submissive gestures in the stumptail macaque monkey. Pharmacol Biochem Behav (Suppl 1) 14: 95–102

Steklis HD, Brammer GL, Raleigh MJ, McGuire MT (1982) Serum testosterone, male dominance, and aggression in captive groups of vervet monkeys (*Cercopithecus aethiops sabaeus*). Int J Primatol 3: 337

Ethopharmacology: Primate Models of Neuropsychiatric Disorders, pages 157–184

Response to Intracerebral Dopamine Injection as a Model of Schizophrenic Symptomatology

Mark F. Dubach and Douglas M. Bowden

Regional Primate Research Center and Department of Anthropology (M.F.D.), and Department of Psychiatry and Behavioral Sciences (D.M.B.), University of Washington, Seattle, Washington 98195

INTRODUCTION

Clinical approaches to both schizophrenia and Parkinson's disease have for many years been closely interrelated with basic research on the basal ganglia, and particularly with research on the dopamine (DA) systems within the basal ganglia. While the involvement of DA neurons in Parkinsonism is substantiated by histological and histochemical observations (Hornykiewicz, 1966; Carlsson, 1974), the link between DA and schizophrenia is more tenuous.

The evidence for this link is pharmacological. Drugs used to treat schizophrenia in humans have been shown to block DA receptors in rodents, and in fact, their clinical potency is proportional to their affinity for DA receptors (Creese and Snyder, 1978; Seeman et al., 1978). This by no means demonstrates that shizophrenia is caused by a general increase in DA transmission (Iversen, 1978). It does draw attention to the basal ganglia, however, because most of the brain's DA receptors are located there. This attention is heightened by the observation that common symptoms of schizophrenia such as apathy, dementia, and attentional deficits frequently occur in other neurological syndromes that involve lesions of the basal ganglia (Bowman and Lewis, 1980).

Animal models have contributed substantially to the development of clinical approaches to schizophrenia (Randrup and Munkvad, 1967; Kokkinidis and Anisman, 1980). A prominent example is the rodent's stereotypic response to peripherally administered stimulants that release DA. This model has proven useful in the development of antipsychotic DA antagonists. The low cost and convenience of rodent models based on the systemic injection of a drug ensure their continued importance, both in pharmaceutical engineering and in basic biomedical research. Nevertheless, the behavioral analogy between the gnawing, licking rodent and the schizophrenic human is limited. An animal model that allows more detailed analysis of neural mechanisms and that involves more human-like behavioral patterns could lead to clinically important insights into the biological nature of schizophrenia.

One important element of such a model that has been explored in the rat is the injection of DA agonists into specific areas of the brain. This method has been applied most successfully to the nucleus accumbens (Jackson et al., 1975; Grabowska and Anden, 1976; Pijnenburg and van Rossum, 1973), but the common effect at this site in the rat is increased locomotor activity, which is not a familiar symptom of schizophrenia. Thus, the use of a behaviorally more appropriate species is a key element required for a detailed model of schizophrenia. In other areas of reasearch on the basal ganglia, such as anatomy and physiology, much of the most exciting recent work has been done in primates (e.g. Iansek and Porter, 1980; Goldman-Rakic, 1982; Van Hoesen et al., 1981). The closer phylogenetic, behavioral, and neuroanatomical relations between monkeys and humans are good reasons for this emphasis. The use of a primate for intracerebral injections represents an advance in the development of an important new animal model for schizophrenia (Dill et al., 1979; Dubach and Bowden, 1980).

In this chapter we describe for the first time reliable effects of discrete intracerebral dopamine (IC-DA) injections on the social behavior of an Old World monkey, the long-tailed macaque. The injections were made in a ventral striatal site including a large part of the nucleus accumbens and also the ventromedial edge of the caudate nucleus. The effects on behavior were reminiscent of the social withdrawal and affective neutrality that are common symptoms of schizophrenia. Furthermore, in this chapter we outline methods developed for the use of intracerebral injections to explore other discrete sites in the DA terminal areas of the monkey brain. The effects elicited at the site reported here are not regarded as a detailed or complete animal model of schizophrenia, but they do represent a promising step toward that goal.

BACKGROUND

Intracerebral Injections in Primates

In the last few years, great advances have been made toward an understanding of the neuroanatomy, histology, neurotransmitter physiology, and receptor pharmacology of neural systems involving DA (Lindvall and Björklund, 1978; Pasik et al., 1979; DeLong and Georgopoulos, 1979; Glowinski, 1981; Titeler and Seeman, 1980). But the role that DA systems play in ongoing patterns of behavior is not clear, and progress on this front has been slow. A review of attempts to understand the functions of the neostriatum, the largest DA terminal area, found current theories "remarkably diverse and often vaguely stated" (Divac and Öberg, 1979). The behavioral aspect of research on the functions of DA systems is critically important if the impressive advances in our understanding of DA anatomy and pharmacology are to be made clinically useful with regard to schizophrenia.

If neuroleptics reduce the diverse symptoms of schizophrenia by a blockade of DA receptors, then it is reasonable to suppose that specific symptoms of the syndrome might involve excessive DA function in particular DA terminal areas (Snyder, 1976; Carlsson, 1978). The possibility that some DA areas, especially the nucleus accumbens, are more affected in schizophrenia than other areas has often been suggested (Hökfelt et al., 1974; Stevens, 1979; Matthysse, 1981). Nevertheless, it is not currently possible to account for the diversity of schizophrenic symptoms by reference to the detailed behavioral anatomy of DA areas. One way to fill this gap in our understanding may be an extensive exploration of the behavioral effects of IC-DA in various discrete brain sites in a primate.

The advent of neurotransmitter receptor pharmacology in the last ten years has brought with it an increasing interest in the use of intracerebral injections of neurotransmitter agonists and antagonists to address this problem (Fog et al., 1971; Fuxe and Ungerstedt, 1976; Pijnenburg et al., 1976). Intracerebral injections offer a unique combination of benefits. Relatively specific agonists and antagonists of certain receptors can be used to activate restricted sets of neural elements, and because the effects are largely reversible, the same animals can be used for multiple experiments and as their own controls. Monkeys offer several advantages for this technique not available in rodents: (1) they are phylogenetically closer to humans, so that neuropharmacologic information gained is likely to be more relevant to the human; (2) the behavioral repertoire of the primate is larger, allowing for more detailed distinctions to be made between the effects of different intracerebral treatments; and (3) the volume of the neostriatum is much greater in the monkey, allowing for treatment restricted to more circumscribed anatomical locales.

Nevertheless, investigators in research involving IC-DA have generally used rodents as subjects. They have focused on locomotor hyperactivity and stereotypic motor behavior. Locomotion has been measured by activity meters, and sterotypies have usually been quantified by the use of rating scales that assign numerical values along a single intensity continuum to such behaviors as sniffing, head bobbing, repetitive limb movements, biting, licking, and gnawing (Pijnenburg et al., 1976; Costall et al., 1977). In rodents, IC-DA typically elicits hyperactivity from the nucleus accumbens and sterotypy from the caudate-putamen (Jackson et al., 1975; Grabowska and Anden, 1976; Pijnenburg and van Rossum 1973). But a wide variety of other DA agonists have also been tested, and some can produce opposite results, namely hyperactivity from the head of the caudate and stereotypy from the nucelus accumbens (Costall et al., 1974, 1975; Cannon et al., 1977). Our own experiments in rats (C. Liles, unpublished observations) have shown that even DA itself, when injected with tranylcypromine into the caudate, can elicit hyperactivity as well as stereotypy. In a few recent studies in the rat, distinctions have been made between dorsal and ventral or lateral and medial sections of the striatum. Such studies have produced somewhat different behavioral results depending on the locus of the injection (Costall et al., 1980; Joyce et al., 1981).

The intracerebral injection technique in rodents has been very promising. However, a single injection in the caudate-putamen of the rat ordinarily involves at least half the volume of the total nucleus, which is roughly 4 mm in diameter. The caudate-putamen in a macaque occupies approximately 15 times the volume of the analogous structure in the rat. Clearly, there is much more opportunity in the monkey to analyze which parts of the neostriatum contribute to various components of the multiple behavioral effects of DA stimulation. Because of the technical difficulties involved, the use of primates in such studies has not previously been pushed to its full advantage.

Behavioral effects of IC-DA in the striatum of a nonhuman primate were observed in a pilot study that preceded the work reported here (Dubach and Bowden, 1980), and in experiments conducted by Dill and associates (Dill et al., 1979; Jones et al., 1981). The results described in the present chapter confirm our pilot findings for IC-DA injections into the ventral striatum. Dill's group also made injections in and near the nucleus accumbens of a New World monkey, the squirrel monkey (*Saimiri sciureus*), and consistently observed an increase in activity after a delay of more than one hour. These results from two laboratories clearly showed that IC-DA was effective in eliciting behavioral changes in nonhuman primates.

Neuroanatomy

Interpretation of the results of IC-DA treatments reported here and of the work cited above requires an understanding of the structures involved. Recent reviews on this subject are available (Graybiel and Ragsdale, 1979; Dray, 1980; Féger, 1981; Kitai, 1981). The term "basal ganglia" is used here to represent the following subcortical areas: (1) the striatum, which includes the structures that we have injected; (2) substantia nigra and the ventral tegmental area; (3) globus pallidus and substantia innominata; and (4) subthalamus. Each set of structures has cytological, physiological, and pharma-

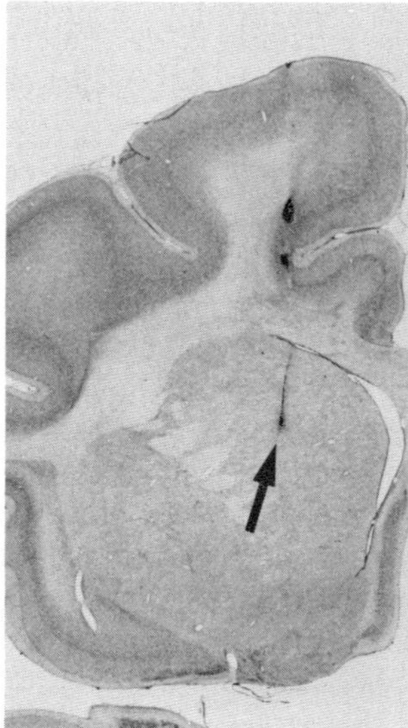
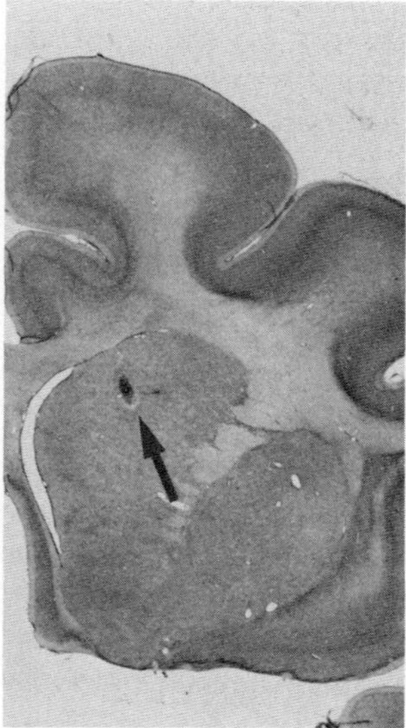

Fig. 2. Injection site in dorsal striatum (arrows) of monkey A2.

When this injection method was used, more than 85% of detectable injected DA remained within a 1.5 mm radius of the center of the injection site for at least an hour (Dubach and Bowden, in preparation). This was determined by making a series of injections of tritiated DA into different parts of the striatum of a test monkey, using a punch technique to remove small cylinders of tissue at variable distances from the injection site, and measuring the radiolabeled DA in a scintillation counter.

Some control trials involved the intracerebral injection of saline (1 μl), acidified with HCl to match the pH of the DA injections; other control trials involved only sham injections, in which no needles were actually put into the brain. No differences were observed between the two types of control.

The VS site (Fig. 1) was centered 1–1.3 mm rostral to the anterior edge of the anterior commissure, 2.5–3.0 mm from the midline, at a depth varying between those of the dorsal and ventral boundaries of the commissure. Based on the atlas of Shantha et al. (1968), injections of 1.5 mm radius centered at this location involved the posterior-dorsal portion of the nucleus accumbens, along with small portions of the ventral caudate nucleus and the bed nuclei of stria terminalis and anterior commissure.

The DS site (Fig. 2) was located in a rostrodorsal part of the caudate nucleus, centered 4.5–5.5 mm from the midline, at a depth of 0.5–3 mm below the ventral edge of the corpus callosum. This control site was about 7 mm distant from the VS injection site, thereby representing a nearby but nonoverlapping location in a DA terminal area.

Trial Schedule

Each trial began at 2 p.m. Before the trial, the two monkeys were given 2-minute injections simultaneously. The injection needles remained in place for an additional 2 minutes, and then were removed. The platform caps were replaced, and the monkeys were released into a small carrying cage and brought together to the door of the experimental cage. Five minutes after removal of the needles, the door was opened by remote control and the animals entered the experimental cage.

The cage, 113 cm wide, 125 cm deep, and 143 cm high, had a front of tempered glass. The video camera was located a few feet away, mounted above curtains that surrounded a one-way glass window concealing the human observer. A 52 × 52 cm shelf was located in the rear left corner of the cage, 68 cm above the floor. A white cardboard box under the shelf contained a rubber ball and ring. A toy rubber snake was fastened to one side of the cage.

From the moment the monkeys entered the cage, data were recorded continuously on video tape for 36 minutes. Only the first 18 minutes of each video recording were actually used for data analysis, because the marked changes in behavior were evident from the beginning of the trial.

Each pair of monkeys was tested for three weeks for each site. As shown in Fig. 3, the first week consisted of pretreatment control trials on Monday, Wednesday, and Friday. The next week included two IC-DA trials, on Tuesday and Friday, and two interim control trials on Wednesday and Thursday. The third IC-DA trial came on Monday of the third week, followed by three post-treatment control trials.

Data Acquisition and Analysis

For this project we developed a comprehensive data acquisition system for coding and analyzing monkey behavior from videotape recordings. Given

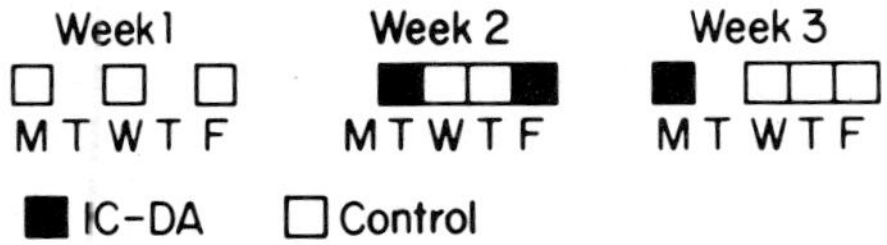

Fig. 3. Trial schedule. For each site in each pair of monkeys, the series of behavioral trials lasted three weeks. Within these three weeks, IC-DA and control trials were made on the indicated days; on remaining days, the monkeys were not treated or removed from their home cages.

the rich functional diversity likely to be found in DA terminal areas, there could be a variety of behavioral effects elicited by treatment of different sites in the striatum. In order to miss as little as possible, we needed a system that allowed simultaneous recording of several aspects of behavior and that was flexible enough to accommodate rare and novel behaviors as they occurred. To meet these needs, we developed software that adapted a digitizer and a microcomputer for use as an ethological recording device.

Behaviors were defined along three principal dimensions—activity, posture, and object (Table I). Within each dimension, definitions were exhaustive and mutually exclusive. The activity dimension included all distinguishable combinations of manual, oral, and visual behaviors. Eight stationary postures were defined. When the monkeys were at rest, the distinction between posture and activity was meaningful and useful; when they were in locomotion, the distinction was no longer relevant. The various forms of locomotion labeled by superscript "a"s under activities were therefore included both in the activity and posture dimensions. Objects associated with the activities included loose objects provided in the cage, parts of the cage itself, and various parts of the two monkeys. Handedness of manual activities was also recorded.

The digitizer (Talos model 622 Cybergraph) consisted of a reinforced glass tablet 22 inches square, and a small cursor held by hand flat against the table and moved around at will. The cursor emitted a signal that was picked up by thin wires embedded in the tablet and sent to an Imsai 8080 microcomputer, giving it the X and Y coordinates of the location of crosshairs fixed to the cursor. The computer was programmed to poll the digitizer every 0.1 second.

By the use of a plastic overlay and software to match, the tablet surface was divided into a large number of squares that were defined to code for as many aspects of behavior as necessary. Any new behavior could easily be assigned to a position on the tablet as it occurred. At the beginning of each successive 30-second segment of the 18-minute videotape, the observer placed the cursor in the box on the digitizer tablet representing the appropriate activity. The observer pressed a button on the cursor to start both the videorecorder (Sony Betamax) and the timer in the computer simultaneously, and held it down keeping the cursor in place, until the activity, the posture, the object, or the handedness changed. At this point a behavioral event was completed, and the observer released the button to stop the timer and recorder. Other sets of boxes on the tablet were used to inform the computer of the posture, object, and handedness of the completed event. Then the observer brought the cursor to the next appropriate activity box and pressed the button, starting the timer and the videotape again.

TABLE I. Principal Dimensions Used to Record Behavior of Experimental Monkeys

Activities		
Examine	Social groom	4—Walk[a]
Examine—touch	Self-groom	2—Walk[a]
Examine—hold	Self-scratch	4—Walk, crouched[a]
Sniff	Attempt to mount	2—Walk, crouched[a]
Sniff—touch	Mount	4—Walk, backwards[a]
Sniff—hold	Sit, present neck for grooming	Run[a]
Lick	Stand, present	Climb up[a]
Lick—touch	Crouch, present	Climb down, tail first[a]
Lick—hold	Mutual sniff and kiss	Climb down, head first[a]
Nibble	Mutual hug and lip	Jump up[a]
Nibble—touch	Beg	Jump down[a]
Nibble—hold	Evade (monkey)	Jump orient[a]
Gnaw	Bat away (monkey)	Stay in transfer cage
Gnaw—touch	Pull (monkey)	Rest
Gnaw—hold	Snap (at monkey)	Lookout
Touch, not looking	Head twist	Flinch
Hold, not looking	Lipsmack	Wet dog
Knock aside	Threat	Arm Wave
Drop	Grimace	
Break	Yawn	
Eat		

Postures	Objects
Sit	Body parts (self)
4—Stand	Body parts (other)
2—Stand	Cage parts
Lie	Package
Hang	Box
Cling	Paper
Crouch	Ball
2—Stand with support	Ring
Locomotion[a]	Rubber snake
	Small thing—can't be seen
	No object

[a]See text.

Analysis consisted of summarizing the duration and frequency of each event along the three dimensions described for the 18-minute trial.

For an independent measure of locomotor patterns, the digitizer was also used to trace the progress of each monkey as it moved around the cage. For this purpose a large television monitor was placed behind the transparent digitizer tablet and another program was used to translate the location of the crosshairs on the digitizer into the location of the monkey in the cage. In this way, the rate of locomotion in each episode, the distance covered, the path, and the timing relative to movements of the other animal could be monitored, as well as the location and distance between the monkeys at all times.

RESULTS

Differences between behavior in the pretreatment control trials and in the IC-DA trials for the VS series are shown in Fig. 4. The ordinate of each graph represents the number of seconds (out of 18 minutes) spent in a given activity. The four subjects, three experimental (A1, A2, and B1) and one unilateral control (B2), are represented on the abscissa. Data from each experimental monkey are presented together, with three open bars to the left representing the control trials and three shaded bars to the right representing the IC-DA trials. For the unilateral control animal, all six trials are represented by open bars. The probability under each animal's code represents the results of a one-tailed t-test comparing the mean from control trials with the mean from DA trials for that animal. (The one-tailed test was used because the direction of behavioral change was predicted on the basis of results of the pilot project (Dubach and Bowden, 1980)).

The significance level (P) shown above each graph was derived by applying the chi-square test for the joint probability of the results from the three experimental animals (Winer, 1971). Because the first two p-values were based on a pair of monkeys tested together and thus were not fully independent, they were averaged. The test then consisted of adding the negative logarithms of the independent p-values, one for pair A and one for monkey B1, then multiplying by 2. The result is distributed as a chi-square with 4 degrees of freedom.

The interobserver reliability estimate accompanying each figure is based on three 18-minute trials in which the behavior of one monkey was recorded both by the principal observer and by a student observer trained for two weeks on the system. For each trial, the absolute value of the difference between the two observers' totals for a given behavior was calculated. These differences were summed over the three trials and taken as a percentage of the principal observer's total over the three trials, then subtracted from 100%.

The most salient effect of DA injections into the VS site was the virtual elimination of social grooming, a very common behavior that occupied more than one-third of each monkey's time during control trials (Fig. 4a). Self-grooming, although less common than social grooming in the control trials, was also drastically reduced (Fig. 4b). The loss of grooming was balanced

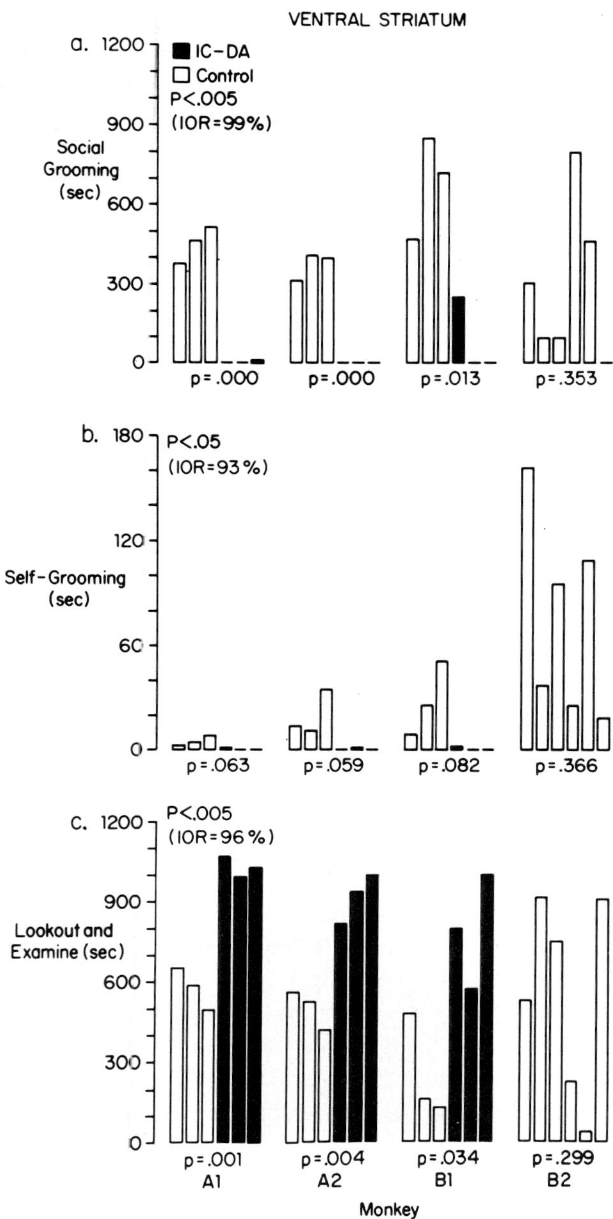

Fig. 4. Effects of bilateral IC-DA in ventral striatum on grooming and looking behaviors. a: Social grooming was virtually eliminated. In the frequent cases of no social grooming, the histogram is represented simply by a bar at the bottom. b: Self-grooming was greatly reduced; in some cases, it was eliminated completely. The total duration of self-grooming in control trials was much lower than that of social grooming (note the difference in scale on the ordinate). c: "Lookout" and "Examine" became the predominant activity of the monkeys in IC-DA trials. P, joint probability; IOR, interobserver reliability (see text).

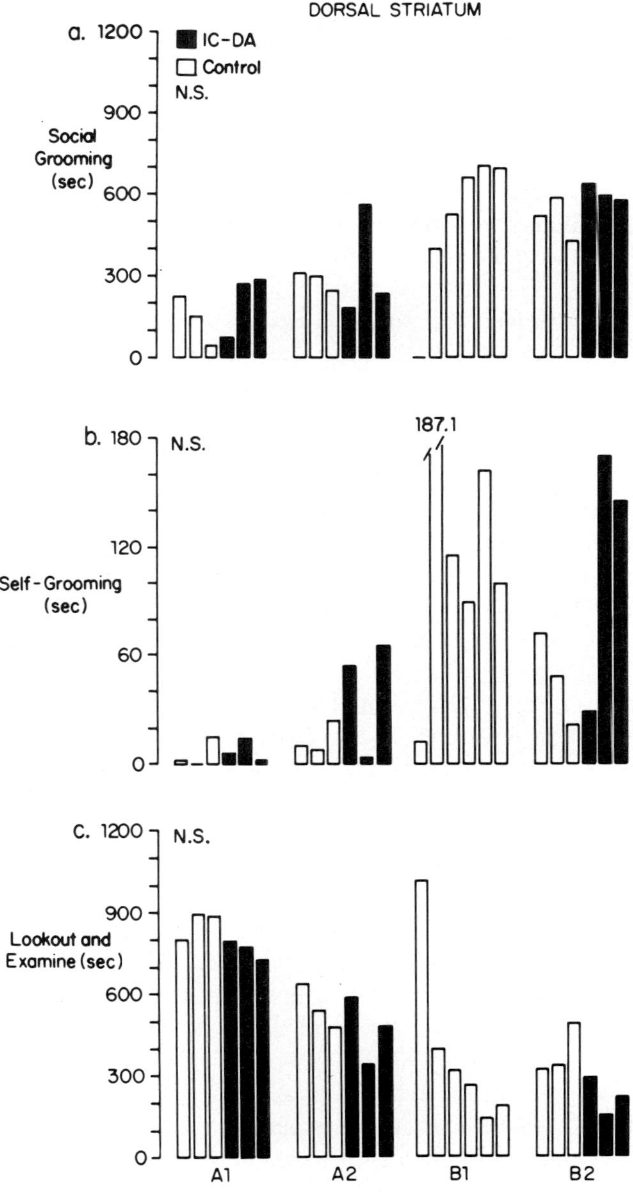

Fig. 5. IC-DA in the dorsal striatum had no effect on social grooming (a), self-grooming (b) or looking behaviors (c), behaviors that were altered by treatment of the ventral striatal site. The unilateral control animal for this site was monkey B1.

by an increase in the time spent at Lookout and Examine (Fig. 4c). "Lookout" was defined as looking in a series of directions with no nearby object as a focus of attention. "Examine" was defined as looking at an object within 18 inches. Taken together, these comprised a very common behavior, partly because when one monkey was engaged in social grooming, the monkey being groomed was engaged in Lookout behavior. Given the sizable contribution of being groomed to Lookout in the control trials, the increase in Lookout and Examine in the absence of grooming was all the more striking.

The neuroanatomical specificity of the effects was tested by comparing this behavioral picture with that seen following DA injections into the DS control site. Fig. 5 displays the total durations of the same three behavioral measures in three animals with bilateral injections at this site and one unilateral control, monkey B1. Clearly, the elimination of grooming and the increase of looking behavior seen after DA injection into the VS site did not occur after similar treatment in the DS site. These results were also consistent with those of the pilot study.

The pharmacological specificity of the effects was tested by a trial on one pair of monkeys in which 10 μg of haloperidol, a relatively specific DA receptor antagonist, were injected into the VS site 10 minutes before the DA injection. As shown in Fig. 6, the distinct behavioral effects of 45 μg of DA were reversed by haloperidol.

The behavioral effects of DA injections into the VS site persisted beyond the day of treatment, as illustrated by data from pair A (Fig. 7). The data for interim control trials (the days between the two DA trials of the second week) show that social grooming was diminished and looking was usually enhanced as compared with pretreatment controls. The three post-treatment control trials showed a gradual return toward pretreatment levels over a period of a few days after the last treatment.

It is unlikely that the decreased grooming seen after injection of DA into the VS site was due to general sedation. The postural data showed that time spent in restful positions (Sit and Lie) was no different during the treatment trials (Fig. 8a). Furthermore, the DA injections did not influence the amount of time spent in locomotion (Fig. 8b).

Another interpretation of the elimination of social grooming could be that injection of DA into the VS site exerted a general suppressive effect on all prehensile or manipulative behavior. The data, however, showed no significant effect on climbing or clinging on vertical supports or the ceiling. In fact, the trend was toward an increase in these behaviors during IC-DA trials (Fig. 9a). Object manipulation was also not significantly affected (Fig. 9b).

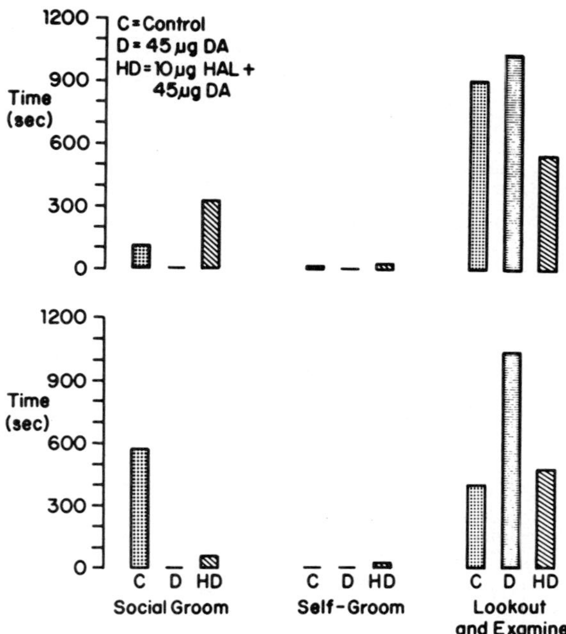

Fig. 6. Effects of haloperidol blockade in monkeys A1 (above) and A2 (below). Each set of three histograms in these figures represents the total duration of the indicated behavior in a control trial (C), and IC-DA trial 8 days later (D), and, after another 10 days, an IC-DA trial in which the DA injection was made 10 minutes after a 10-μg injection of haloperidol at the same site (HD). For all three behaviors, the effect of IC-DA was reversed by haloperidol.

The reluctance of the monkeys to groom one another suggests that they withdrew socially after IC-DA treatment. This avoidance of normal social interaction is reminiscent of autistic withdrawal or of the flattened affect often observed in schizophrenia. It must be recognized, however, that characterization of the VS-DA syndrome as social withdrawl may be too general, because grooming is only one aspect of social interaction. DA injections into the VS site did not significantly affect mounting behavior by the dominant animal or presenting to be groomed by either animal (Fig. 10). Mounting is generally an assertive behavior, and presenting for grooming is also more commonly a behavior displayed by the higher-ranking member of a male-male pair (Turillazzi et al., 1982). It may be that only friendly or giving interactions, but not assertive interactions, are eliminated by DA at the VS site.

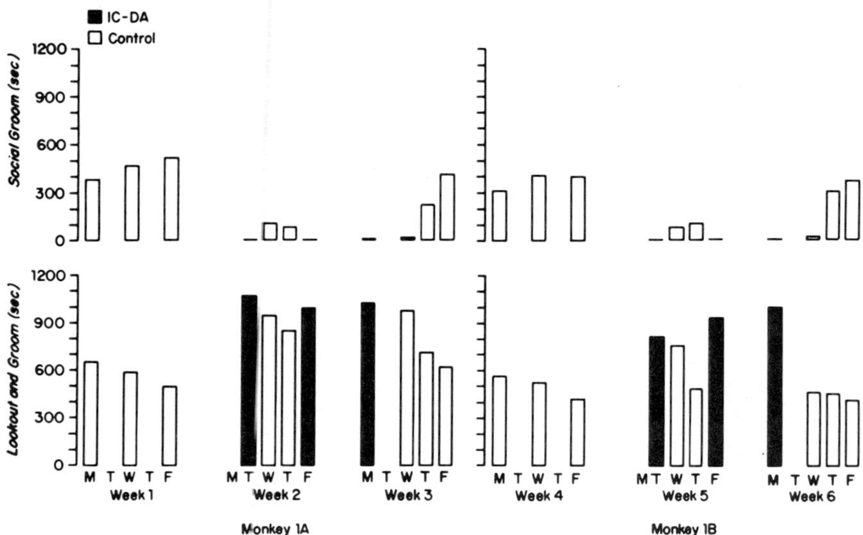

Fig. 7. Behavior during pretreatment, interim, and post-treatment control trials. Letters represent days of the week. Data shown in the three pretreatment control trials to the left (M, W, F) and in the three shaded IC-DA trials (T, F, M) are the same as in Fig. 4. Interim controls (W & T of Week 2) and post-treatment controls (W, T, & F of Week 3) show the effects of IC-DA that persisted for a day or two after the treatment.

DISCUSSION

The syndrome produced by local injection of DA into a ventrostriatal site consisted of the elimination of grooming and an increase in looking behavior. These results represent the first data on the effects of IC-DA on primate social behavior. They indicate that intracerebral injection provides a promising approach to fundamental issues of basal ganglia function and dysfunction. The striatum, in particular, has a complex and puzzling organizaiton that is beginning to be revealed by modern techinques. For example, a single injection of radiolabeled amino acid at a given site in the cortex labels an extensive, irregularly shaped band of striatial tissue extending rostrocaudally to cover most of the length of the caudate or the putamen (Goldman and Nauta, 1977; Yeterian and Van Hoesen, 1978). Such bands overlap extensively with the projection areas of other distant but interconnected cortical sites.

Structural evidence of intricate overlapping of such inputs and outputs is consistent with the complex integrative role that has often been suggested for the striatum (Divac and Öberg, 1979). The results reported here show that local DA injections in the monkey are a useful way of exploring the relevance of this integrative function to the behavior of the animal as a whole.

The integrative role of the nucleus accumbens in particular has received a great deal of attention in recent years because of its association with the limbic system via hippocampal and temporal lobe afferents (Heimer and Wilson, 1975; Swanson and Cowan, 1975, 1977; DeFrance et al., 1980; Newman and Winans, 1980; Chronister et al., 1981; Hemphill et al., 1981; Groenewegen et al., 1981; Krayniak et al., 1981). This nucleus has been

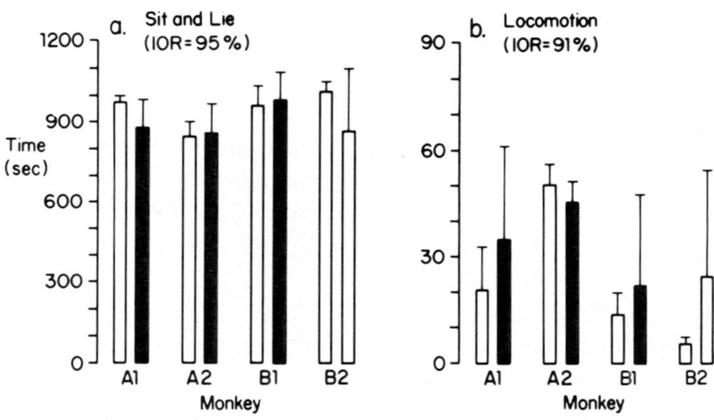

Fig. 8. Lack of significant sedative effect of IC-DA in ventral striatum on restful postures (a) or total locomotion (b). Each bar represents, for one animal, the mean and standard deviation of the values for the control trials (open bar) or the IC-DA trials (shaded bar).

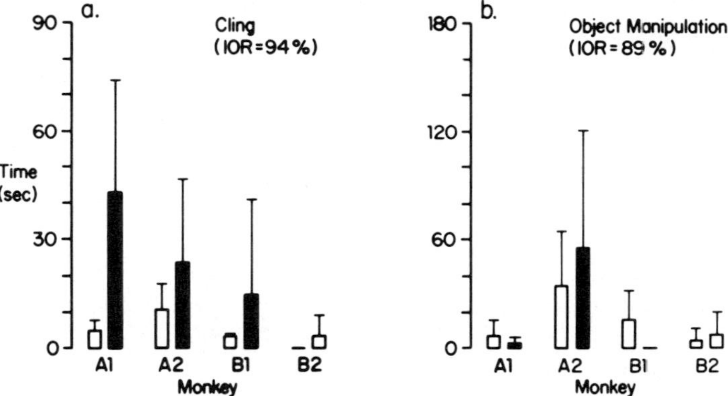

Fig. 9. Lack of significant effect of IC-DA in ventral striatum on manual behaviors including prehensile posture and locomotion (a) and manipulation of objects (b).

characterized as an interface between limbic and motor systems (Mogenson et al., 1980), and has been referred to as a possible source of schizophrenic disorders (Matthysse, 1981). It is particularly significant, therefore, that our injection in the VS, which involved a dorsal, caudal part of the nucleus accumbens most heavily, also resulted in a specific elimination of social grooming behavior. It is reasonable to interpret this effect as analogous to the affective neutrality or social withdrawal commonly observed in schizophrenia.

The persistence of decreased levels of grooming for as long as 48 hours after the injection may be due to relatively long-term changes in the neurophysiology of local dopaminergic mechanisms. The nature of such changes produced by IC-DA injections could be of considerable interest. Alternatively, however, the persisting behavioral changes may also be caused by state-dependent learning, encompassing different areas of the brain. It would be useful in this context to inject DA and return the animals immediately to their home cages the first day, then observe social interaction 24 and 48 hours later. If reduced grooming were observed under these circumstances, long-term local changes, such as the storage of large amounts of DA in nerve terminals, would be implicated.

Several laboratories have reported the effects of DA injected into the nucleus accumbens of the rat. The result most consistently observed is an increase in locomotor activity, although the use of other DA agonists at this site has also produced stereotypies (Costall et al., 1977). Neill (1981) reported that locomotor hyperactivity was also elicited from the rat by injections in the ventral caudate just above the nucleus accumbens. In contrast, our injections in a VS site in *M. fascicularis* produced no locomotor effect. There are a number of possible explanations for this difference.

The most important is the species difference. Several major differences between rodent and primate brains involve the basal ganglia. Some of these relate specifically to the VS, the focus of the present study. The structure directly underlying the nucleus accumbens, the olfactory tubercle, is entirely different in the two species (Heimer et al., 1977). In the rat, it is a prominent bulge at the base of the brain, a partially laminated structure that receives massive input from the olfactory bulb; its olfactory input may be important for the rat's locomotor exploration of its environment, a behavior that is usually accompanied by sniffing. The superficial laminated portion of the olfactory tubercle, which is not considered part of the striatum, intervenes between VS and the base of the brain. In the monkey, by contrast, the bulge is replaced by the anterior perforated substance. As clarified by Heimer et al. (1977), this area does not receive any significant olfactory bulb input, and

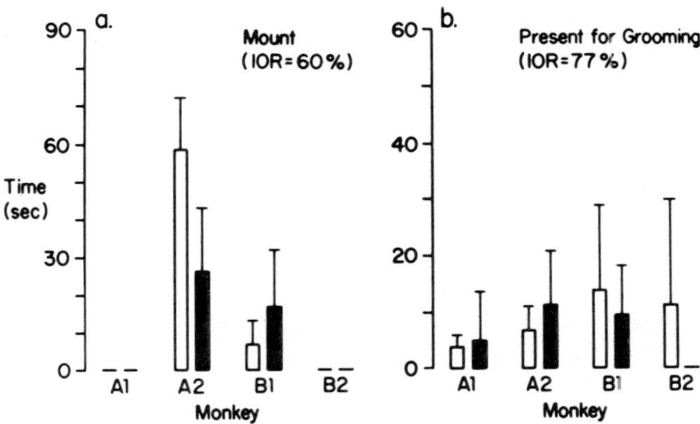

Fig. 10. Lack of effect of IC-DA in ventral striatum on mounting (a) and presenting (b) behaviors.

the olfactory tubercle homologue defined by such input is restricted to a small rostral area near the olfactory tract. Little if any lamination can be seen in the anterior perforated substance. The VS of the primate extends all the way to the base of the brain.

In both rats and monkeys, the most prominent descending afferents to the nucleus accumbens are from the temporal cortex, including the entorhinal area and the subiculum of the hippocampus. The exact source of these afferents is not well established in either species, although several studies have addressed this issue (Newman and Winans 1980; Hemphill et al., 1981; Krayniak et al., 1981). Thus, detailed interspecific comparisons cannot be made at this time. However, hippocampal and temporal lobe morphologies of the two species are quite dissimilar, given the tremendous expansion of the temporal neocortex and the rostroventral relocation of these structures in the primate. Differences in the internal organization of these areas have accompanied the morphological changes (Van Hoesen et al., 1979; Rosene and Van Hoesen, 1981), so that input to the nucleus accumbens can hardly be said to be the same in the two species.

More general species differences derive from the expansion of the cortex in primate evolution. Projections to the striatum from secondary sensory and association cortices, which hardly exist in the rat, are extensive in the monkey. Cortical connections to and from subcortical structures, which in the rat pass through the striatum in small scattered bundles, are collected into the internal capsule in primates, dividing the striatum into caudate and putamen. A cytoarchitectonic pattern of cell clusters surrounded by capsules containing axons and glial cells has been reported for the monkey; such structuring, which may be related to the distribution of internal capsule fibers in the striatum, has been observed in a very different form in the rodent (Goldman-Rakic, 1982).

The entopeduncular nucleus in the rat is almost entirely enclosed in the cerebral peduncle, but in the monkey it is aligned with the rest of the globus pallidus and known as the internal segment of that structure. The very large, acetylcholinesterase-positive cells of the basal nucleus of Meynert, which coexist with cells of the substantia innominata in both species, also invade most of the globus pallidus and some of the entopeduncular nucleus in the rat. In the monkey, on the other hand, they are arranged in orderly layers around the internal segment and in the lamina between the internal and external segments, but not in the globus pallidus itself (Divac, 1975; Parent et al., 1979). Layering of afferents to the globus pallidus from the subthalamus is also seen in monkeys but not in rats (Nauta and Cole, 1978).

The functional significance of most of these anatomical differences remains to be seen, but it would be unwise to assume that they have none. The manifold differences in spontaneous and learned behavior of rats and monkeys must have some neuroanatomical basis. The proposal that neuroanatomical differences may lead to different responses to IC-DA is a reasonable one.

The observation that squirrel monkeys differ from long-tailed macaques in their responses to IC-DA in the VS may also be explained in part by species differences. Injection of DS into the nucleus accumbens and olfactory tubercle also produced hyperactivity of various kinds in the squirrel monkey (Dill et al., 1979; Jones et al., 1981). Increased activity was observed in Dill's experiments after a latency of one to two hours. This effect was measured by a photocell activity meter and by direct observation, which revealed intense self-grooming, juvenile posturing, and occasionally exaggerated startle responses, as well as "intense searching activity" (Dill et al., 1979). In our project, in contrast to both rat and squirrel monkey studies, the only consistent effect in *M. fascicularis* was the elimination of grooming and the increase in looking behavior. Even two hours after the IC-DA injection, no sign of hyperactivity was noted.

The colloquial word "monkey" actually embraces two very different groups of species. *Saimiri sciureus* is a platyrrhine or New World monkey. Phylogenetically, the platyrrhine line of descent is thought to have separated roughly 50 million years ago from the catarrhine line of descent, which includes Old World monkeys, apes, and humans (Goodman, 1975; Pilbeam, 1972). Therefore, the ancestors of squirrel monkeys, on one hand, and long-tailed macaques, on the other, have been genetically separate for about 50 million years. Even though both are called monkeys, major differences in the behavioral organization of the brain should not be too surprising. The divergence of the two lines that led to *M. fascicularis* and to *Homo sapiens* took place, by comparable estimates, about 40 million years ago. Therefore, the genetic distance between New World and Old World monkeys is actually greater than the genetic distance between Old World monkeys and humans.

Species differences alone may account for the differences between our results and those observed in rats and squirrel monkeys. In addition, however, major technical differences, particularly the size and location of the injection site, may also have played a role. Injections of the same volume in rats (e.g., Jackson et al., 1975) presumably spread at least as far as our own, but in the much smaller rat brain this would involve a much larger functional area. Our site was restricted to an area within the dorsal and caudal part of the nucleus, also touching on the ventral caudate and perhaps the bed nuclei of the stria terminalis and the anterior commissure. In the rat, comparable injections probably reach the entire nucleus accumbens, also encroaching on these neighboring structures. It is well known that local treatments of closely apposed structures in the brain may have very different effects. A relevant example in the present context comes form a study by Kozlowski and Marshall (1980) showing that unilateral injection of gamma-aminobutyric acid antagonists in substantia nigra can produce turning in either direction, depending on whether pars compacta or pars reticulata receives the injection. The projections from various sources to the nucleus accumbens do not reach all parts of it in equal density, and some cytoarchitectural diversity can also be seen in the nucleus (Chronister et al., 1981). The effects we observed may be specific to the particular area injected rather than to the nucleus accumbens or the VS as a whole.

With respect to work in the squirrel monkey, the injection site described by Jones et al. (1981) was slightly more ventral than our own, and the site described by Dill et al. (1979) was considerably more so. Furthermore, their injection methods involved the permanent implantation at the site of 26-ga injection tubing, and the injection of 2 μl of DA solution followed by 2 μl of saline before each trial (Dill, 1977; Jones et al., 1981). Because the squirrel monkey is smaller then the long-tailed macaque, while the injection volumes were four times as large as ours, the total functional area treated was probably considerably larger.

Finally, differences in the animals' environments during the experiments may have contributed to differences in results. Rats are typically treated alone in small cages rather than in open fields. Similarly, squirrel monkeys were observed singly in small (30 $\times$ 28 $\times$ 60 cm) cages. Our experiment was conducted in a larger cage, with two animals present, so that social contact and considerably more room for locomotion were available.

Even the present experiment, however, was conducted in a rather limited enivronment and therefore leaves open some important behavioral questions. If the treated animal were observed in a larger setting with more places to go, would it withdraw physically from the other animals? In a larger social group with both sexes, several age groups, and normal dominance hierarchy, would the treated animal's relations with various companions be affected in different ways? If a greater variety of objects were available, would effects on object handling be observed? Would feeding and drinking be affected if food and water were available? Would a female be affected by the treatment in a different way? The nucleus accumbens receives input from cortical and subcortical limbic structures, and its output to motor and autonomic effectors is indirect. It is therefore unlikely to be simply a "grooming center" or a "locomotor center." It may be able to affect a number of different behaviors under different circumstances. To test this interpretation, it would be necessary to perform similar experiments in different social and physical environments.

The pharmacological analysis initiated in this study was very limited, but the blockade of IC-DA effects by a single dose of haloperidol was promising. Furthermore, in preliminary efforts we determined that grooming was eliminated by both 45 μg and 90 μg of DA. Haloperidol at a dose of 10 μg did not affect the response to 90 μg of DA, but completely reversed the response to 45 μg. Together, these results suggest that the effect is dose-related and mediated by DA receptors. Further pharmacological analysis of IC-DA effects in the monkey could yield important information on the physiology of the striatum as it relates to behavior.

CONCLUSIONS

The data presented here are consistent with the idea that the nucleus accumbens plays a role in schizophrenic behavior. The elimination of active social grooming from the monkeys' behavioral repertoire may be a change related to the affective neutrality often seen in schizophrenia. As such, it provides a closer parallel to this illness than the increased locomotion observed after similar treatment in the rat. The methods developed in this project represent a promising new approach to the detailed modeling of schizophrenia and to the study of the behavioral organization of the striatum.

ACKNOWLEDGMENTS

We thank Ms. Kim Grant, Ms. Linda Hayward, and Dr. Robert Dealy for their assistance during experimental sessions in the pilot project, and Mr.

John Cobb for his contribution in coding behaviors on the computer system for the purpose of making interobserver reliability estimates. We also thank Smith Kline & French Laboratories, Philadelphia, for providing Tranylcypromine for this project.

The research was supported by the Graduate School Research Fund at the University of Washington, and by USPHS grants RR00166 and MH14062 to the University of Washington.

REFERENCES

Bowman M, Lewis MS (1980) Sites of subcortical damage in diseases which resemble schizophrenia. Neuropsychol 18:597–601

Björklund A, Lindvall O (1975) Dopamine in dendrites of substantia nigra neurons: suggestions for a role in dendritic terminals. Brain Res 83:531–537

Cannon JG, Lee T, Goldman HD, Costall B, Naylor RJ (1977) Cerebral dopamine agonist properties of some 2-aminotetralin derivatives after peripheral and intracerebral administration. J Med Chem 20:1111–1116

Carlsson A (1974) Brain monoamines in basal ganglia disease. In: Current Concepts in the Treatment of Parkinson's Disease. Yahr MP (ed) Raven Press New York pp 133–140

Carlsson A (1978) Does dopamine have a role in schizophrenia? Bio Psychiatr 13:3–21

Carpenter MB, Nakano D, Kim R (1976) Nigrothalamic projections in the monkey demonstrated by autoradiographic technics. J Compar Neurol 165:401–416

Cheramy A, Leviel V, Glowinski J (1981) Dendritic release of dopamine in the substantia nigra. Nature 289:537–542

Chronister RB, Sikes RW, Trow TW, DeFrance JF (1981) The organization of nucleus accumbens. In: The Neurobiology of the Nucleus Accumbens. Chronister RB, DeFrance JF (eds) Haer Institute Brunswick Maine pp 97–146

Clavier RM, Atmadja S, Fibiger HC (1976) Nigrothalamic projections in the rat as demonstrated by orthograde and retrograde tracing techniques. Brain Res Bull 1:379–384

Costall B, DeSouza CX, Naylor RJ (1980) Topographical analysis of the actions of 2-(N,N-dipropyl)amino-5,6-dihydroxytetralin to cause biting behavior and locomotion hyperactivity from the striatum of the guinea pig. Neuropharmacol 19:623–631

Costall B, Naylor RJ, Cannon JG, Lee T (1977) Differentiation of the dopamine mechanisms mediating stereotyped behavior and hyperactivity in the nucleus accumbens and caudate-putamen. J Pharm Pharmacol 29:337–342

Costall B, Naylor RJ, Neumeyer JL (1975) Differences in the nature of the stereotyped behavior induced by aporphine derivatives in the rat and in their action in extrapyramidal and mesolimbic brain areas. Eur J Pharmacol 31:1–16

Costall B, Naylor RJ, Pinder RM (1974) Design of agents for stimulation of neostriatal dopaminergic mechanisms. J Pharm Pharmacol 26:753–762

Creese I, Snyder SH (1978) Behavioral and biochemical properties of the dopamine receptor. In: Psychopharmacology: A Generation of Progress. Lipton A, DiMascio A, Killiam KF (eds) Raven Press New York pp 377–388

DeFrance JF, Marchan JE, Stanley JC, Sikes RW, Chronister RB (1980) Convergence of excitatory amygdaloid and hippocampal input in the nucleus accumbens septi. Brain Res 185:183–186

DeLong MR, Georgopoulos AP (1979) Motor functions of the basal ganglia as revealed by studies of single cell activity in the behaving primate. Advances Neurol 24:131–140

Dill RE (1977) Induction and measurement of tremor and other dyskinesias. In: Methods in Psychobiology. Vol III Myers RD (ed) Academic Press New York pp 241–257

Dill RE, Jones DL, Gillin C, Murphy G (1979) Comparison of behavioral effects of systemic L-DOPA and intracranial dopamine in mesolimbic forebrain of nonhuman primates. Pharmacol Biochem Behav 10:711–716

Divac I (1975) Magnocellular nuclei of the basal forebrain project to neocortex, brain stem, and olfactory bulb. Review of some functional correlates. Brain Res 93:385–398

Divac I, Öberg RGE (1979) Current conceptions of neostriatal functions: History and an evaluation. In: The Neostriatum. Divac I, Öberg RGE (eds) Pergamon Press Oxford pp 215–230

Dooley D, Dubach MF, Blake PH, Bowden DM (1981) A chronic, stereotaxic guide-tube platform for intracranial injections in macaques. J Neurosci Meth 3:385–396

Dray A (1980) The physiology and pharmacology of mammalian basal ganglia. Progress Neurobiol 14:221–335

Dubach MF, Bowden DM (1980) Altered behavior of macaques following dopamine injection into caudate n., n. accumbens, and substantia nigra. Society Neurosci Abst 6:721

Fallon JH, Moore RY (1978) Catecholamine innervation of the basal forebrain: IV. Topography of the dopamine projection to the basal forebrain and neostriatum. J Compar Neurol 180:545–580

Féger J (1981) Les ganglions de la base: aspects anatomiques et electrophysiologiques. J Physiol (Paris) 77:7–44

Fog R, Randrup A, Pakkenberg H (1971) Intrastriatal injection of quaternary butyrophenones and oxypertine: neuroleptic effect in rats. Psychopharmacol (Berlin) 19:224–230

Fuxe K, Ungerstedt U (1976) Studies on the cholinergic and dopaminergic innervation of the neostriatum with the help of intraneostriatal injections of drugs. Pharmacol Ther B2:29–36

Glowinski J (1981) In vivo release of transmitters in the cat basal ganglia. Fed Proc 40:135–141

Goldman PS, Nauta WJH (1977) An intricately patterned prefrontocaudate projection in the rhesus monkey. J Compar Neurol 171:369–386

Goldman-Rakic PS (1982) Cytoarchitectonic heterogeneity of the primate neostriatum: subdivision into island and matrix cellular compartments. J Compar Neurol 205:398–413

Goodman M (1975) Protein sequence and immunological specificity: their role in phylogenetic studies of primates. In: Phylogeny of the Primates. Luckett WP, Szalay FS (eds) Plenum Press New York pp 219–248

Grabowska M, Anden N (1976) Apomorphine in the rat nucleus accumbens: effects on the synthesis of 5-hydroxytryptamine and noradrenaline, the motor activity and the body temperature. J Neural Transmission 38:1–8

Graybiel A, Ragsdale W (1979) Fiber connections of the basal ganglia. Prog Brain Res 51:239–283

Groenewegen HF, Arnold DEAT, Lopes da Silva FH (1981) Afferent connections of the nucleus accumbens in the cat with special emphasis on the projections from the hippocampal region: an anatomical and electrophysiological study. In: The Neurobiology of the Nucleus Accumbens. Chronister RB, DeFrance JF (eds) Haer Institute Brunswick Maine pp 41–74

Heimer L, Switzer RD, Van Hoesen GW (1982) Ventral striatum and ventral pallidum: components of the motor system? Trends Neurosci 5:83–87

Heimer L, Van Hoesen GW, Rosene DL (1977) The olfactory pathways and the anterior perforated substance in the primate brain. Inter J Neurol 12:42–52

Heimer L, Wilson RD (1975) The subcortical projections of the allocortex: similarities in the neural associations of the hippocampus, the piriform cortex, and the neocortex. In: Golgi Centennial Symposium Proceedings. Santini M (ed) Raven Press New York pp 177–193

Hemphill M, Holm G, Crutcher M, DeLong M, Hedreen J (1981) Afferent connections of the nucleus accumbens in the monkey. In: The Neurobiology of the Nucleus Accumbens. Chronister RB, DeFrance JF (eds) Haer Institute Brunswick Maine pp 75–81

Hökfelt T, Ljungdahl A, Fuxe K, Johansson O (1974) Dopamine nerve terminals in the rat limbic cortex: aspects of the dopamine hypothesis of schizophrenia. Sci 184:177–179

Hornykiewicz O (1966) Dopamine (3-hydroxytyramine) and brain function. Pharmacol Reviews 18:925–964

Iansek R, Porter R (1980) The monkey globus pallidus: neuronal discharge properties in relation to movement. J Physiol (London) 301:439–455

Iversen LI (1978) The role of dopamine in schizophrenia. In: Chemical Communication Within the Nervous System and Its Disturbance in Disease. Taylor A, Jones MT (eds) Pergamon Press Oxford pp 17–37

Jackson DM, Anden N, Dahlström A (1975) A functional effect of dopamine in the nucleus accumbens and in some other dopamine-rich parts of the rat brain. Psychopharmacol (Berlin) 45:139–149

Jones DL, Berg SL, Dorris RL, Dill RE (1981) Biphasic locomotor response to intra-accumbens dopamine in a non-human primate. Pharmacol Biochem Behav 15:243–246

Jones DL, Dill RE, Dorris RL, Berg SL (1980) Contrasting roles of striatal and accumbens dopamine in the motor activity in squirrel monkeys. Society Neurosci Abst 6:723

Joyce JN, Davis RE, van Hartsveldt C (1981) Behavioral effects of unilateral dopamine into dorsal or ventral striatum. Eur J Pharmacol 72:1–10

Kitai ST (1981) Anatomy and physiology of the neostriatum. Adv Biochem Psychopharmacol 30:1–21

Kokkinidis L, Anisman H (1980) Amphetamine models of paranoid schizophrenia: an overview and elaboration of animal experimentation. Psych Bull 88:551–579

Kozlowski MR, Marshall JF (1980) Rotation induced by intranigral injections of GABA agonists and antagonists: zone-specific effects. Pharmacol Biochem Behav 13:561–567

Krayniak PF, Meibach RC, Siegel A (1981) A projection from the entorhinal cortex to the nucleus accumbens in the rat. Brain Res 209:427–431

Lindvall O, Björklund A (1974) The organization of the ascending catecholamine neuron systems in the rat brain. Acta Physiol Scand Sup 412:1–48

Lindvall O, Björklund A (1978) Anatomy of dopaminergic neuron systems in the rat brain. Adv Biochem Psychopharmacol 19:1–24

Matthysse S (1981) Nucleus accumbens and schizophrenia, 1980. In: The Neurobiology of the Nucleus Accumbens. Chronister RB, DeFrance JF (eds) Haer Institute Brunswick Maine pp 351–359

Mogenson GJ, Jones DL, Yim CY (1980) From motivation to action: functional interface between the limbic system and the motor system. Prog Neurobiol 14:69–97

Nauta HJW, Cole M (1978) Efferent projections of the subthalamic nucleus: an autoradiographic study in the monkey and cat. J Compar Neurol 180:1–16

Neill DB (1981) Discussion. In: The Neurobiology of the Nucleus Accumbens. Chronister RB, DeFrance JF (eds) Haer Institute Brunswick Maine p 362

Newman R, Winans SS (1980) An experimental study of the ventral striatum of the golden hamster. I. Neuronal connections of the nucleus accumbens. J Compar Neurol 191:167–192

Parent A, Gravel S, Olivier A (1979) The extrapyramidal and limbic systems relationship at the globus pallidus level: a comparative histochemical study in the rat, cat, and monkey. Adv Neurol 24:1–11

Pasik P, Pasik T, DeFiglia M (1979) The internal organization of the neostriatum in mammals. In: The Neostriatum. Divac I,Öberg RGE (eds) Pergamon Press Oxford pp 5–36

Pijnenburg AJJ, Honig WMM, van der Heyden JAM, van Rossum JM (1976) Effects of chemical stimulation of the mesolimbic dopamine system upon locomotor activity. Eur J Pharmacol 35:45–58

Pijnenburg AJJ, van Rossum JM (1973) Stimulation of locomotor activity following injection of dopamine into the nucleus accumbens. J Pharm Pharmacol 25:1003–1004

Pilbeam D (1972) The Ascent of Man. MacMillan Co. New York

Randrup A, Munkvad I (1967) Stereotyped activities produced by amphetamine in several animal species and man. Psychopharmacol (Berlin) 11:300–310

Rinvik E (1975) Demonstration of nigrothalamic connections in the cat by retrograde axonal transport of horseradish peroxidase. Brain Res 90:313–318

Rosene DL, Van Hoesen GW (1981) Commissural connections of the hippocampal formation in the rhesus monkey. Society Neurosci Abst 7:257

Seeman P, Titeler M, Tedesco J, Hartley EJ (1978) Anti-schizophrenic drugs: membrane receptor sites of action. In: Proceedings of the VI International Congress on Pharmacology. Boissier JR, Lechat P, Fichelle J (eds) vol 5 Neuropsychopharmacology. Dumont C (ed) Pergamon Press New York pp 3–20

Shantha TR, Manocha Sl, Bourne GH (1968) A stereotaxic atlas of the Java monkey brain. Williams Wilkins Baltimore

Snyder SH (1976) The dopamine hypothesis of schizophrenia: focus on the dopamine receptor. Am J Psychiatr 133:197–202.

Stevens JR (1979) Schizophrenia and dopamine regulation in the mesolimbic system. Trends Neurosci 2:102–105

Swanson LW, Cowan WM (1975) A note on the connections and development of the nucelus accumbens. Brain Res 92:324–330

Swanson LW, Cowan WM (1977) An autoradiographic study of the organization of the efferent connections of the hippocampal formation in the rat. J Compar Neurol 172:49–84

Titeler M, Seeman P (1980) Radioreceptor labeling of pre- and post-synaptic dopamine receptors. Adv Biochem Psychopharmacol 24:159–166

Turillazzi PG, Marchini S, Alessandroni P, Baldo N, Campanella C, Trucchi D (1982) Social grooming in *Macaca fuscata*. In: Anneli Istituto Superiore di Sanita No 2. Rome In press

Van Hoesen GW, Rosene DL, Mesulam MM (1979) Subicular input from temporal cortex in the rhesus monkey. Sci 205:608–610

Van Hoesen GW, Yeterian EH, Lavizzo-Mourey R (1981) Widespread corticostriate projections from temporal cortex of the rhesus monkey. J Compar Neurol 199:205–219

Winer BJ (1971) Statistical Principles in Experimental Design (2nd Edition). McGraw-Hill New York

Yeterian EH, Van Hoesen GW (1978) Corticostriate projections in the rhesus monkey: the organization of certain cortico-caudate connections. Brain Res 139:43–63

Ethopharmacology: Primate Models of Neuropsychiatric Disorders, pages 185–197

Male Dominance, Serotonergic Systems, and the Behavioral and Physiological Effects of Drugs in Vervet Monkeys *(Cercopithecus aethiops sabaeus)*

Michael J. Raleigh, Gary L. Brammer, and Michael T. McGuire

Department of Psychiatry, University of California Los Angeles, School of Medicine, Los Angeles, California 90024 (M.J.R., G.L.B., M.T.M.); Nonhuman Primate Research Laboratory, Veterans Administration Medical Center, Sepulveda, California 91343 (M.J.R., G.L.B., M.T.M.); and Neurobiochemistry Laboratory, Veterans Administration Brentwood Medical Center, Los Angeles, California 90073 (M.J.R., G.L.B.)

INTRODUCTION

We have investigated aspects of the interplay between neural transmitter systems, peripheral biochemical measures, and social and individual behavior in captive, adult male vervet monkeys *(Cercopithecus aethiops sabaeus)*. Two related sets of questions have been of particular interest to us: One concerns the relative role of monoaminergic systems, particularly serotonin, in the mediation of overt behavior. The second deals with the effects of male social dominance on monoaminergic function. Our work does not directly model any particular human psychopathology because we have focused on species-typical, normative behavior. Nevertheless, in our view further specification of the functional relationships between overt behavior, central neurotransmitter systems, and peripheral biochemical profiles in nonhuman primates may provide important insights into understanding and treating human psychiatric disorders.

In this chapter, we will argue that active occupation of the dominant male social position generates a physiological state that is distinct from that of nondominant males. This status-related difference is reflected in the different physiological and behavioral responses to drug interventions and in the different peripheral biochemical profiles exhibited by dominant and other adult males.

We begin the summary of our recent research by reviewing behavioral features of male dominance in captive vervet monkeys. We then report on the interaction between dominant status and the behavioral and physiological effects of drugs enhancing serotonergic activity. Subsequently we describe aspects of the impact of dominant status on peripheral biochemical measures that at least partially reflect central serotonergic activity. We next examine the interplay between dominance, peripheral monoamine oxidase activity, and the behavioral consequences of monoamine oxidase inhibitors. Finally, we discuss the implications of these data for the development of nonhuman primate models designed either to elucidate the behavioral and physiological mechanisms underlying psychopathology or to account for individual differences in response to therapeutic interventions.

BEHAVIORAL FEATURES OF DOMINANCE

Vervets are Old World monkeys that are widespread and not endangered. The animals in our studies are ferally reared on the islands of St. Kitts or Nevis in the East Caribbean and are descendents of West African vervets brought to the Caribbean in the 17th and 18th centuries (McGuire, 1974). In Africa and St. Kitts, free-ranging vervet monkeys have been observed to live in both single and multimale groups (Struhsaker, 1974; Gartlan and Brain, 1968). As in other Old World monkey species, females remain in their natal group and adult males migrate to different groups. Unlike some Old World monkeys, vervets tolerate captivity well, and when housed in large outdoor enclosures the effects of captivity on their behavior appear to be quantitative rather than qualitative (Rowell, 1972). Captivity neither produces novel, pathological behaviors nor distorts the form and relative rates of agonistic and affiliative behaviors (Raleigh et al., 1979; Fairbanks, 1980).

In both free-ranging and captive multimale groups, it is possible to readily distinguish behaviorally one male from all other adult males. This male, the dominant male, is the most successful in intermale dyadic aggression, has the highest control male factor score, and has preferential access to limited resources such as favored sleeping sites (Fairbanks et al., 1979; Raleigh et al., 1983). Unlike East African vervets, the vervets on St. Kitts often do not show clear rank relationships among nondominant males. One nondominant male may rank higher than another nondominant male on success at dyadic aggression but have a lower control male factor score. Rather than constructing a linear dominance hierarchy, we distinguish between the dominant male and all nondominant males in a binary manner. Once dominance relationships are established, a dominant male will typically retain his position for long periods of time (i.e., up to 4 years). Among captive groups with stable dominance hierarchies, there is little aggressing, displaying, or engaging in other dominance-related behaviors between the sexes. After male dominance relationships are established, they persist relatively independently of female dominance interactions. Alterations in female dominance relationships do not seem to exert much impact on male dominance hierarchies or vice versa.

DOMINANCE AND DRUGS ENHANCING SEROTONERGIC ACTIVITY

In our investigations of the behavioral and physiological consequences of drugs enhancing serotonergic activities we used groups containing two or three adult males, two or more adult females, and their immature offspring. These gorups had been together for at least 10 weeks prior to the onset of these studies and each group had an obvious dominant male.

We examined the behavioral effects of three different drugs: tryptophan, fluoxetine, and quipazine. These drugs were selected chiefly because of their predominant effects on central serotonergic systems. In addition to enhancing serotonergic activity, these drugs may alter the functional activity of other transmitter systems. Nevertheless, behavioral commonalities produced by these drugs are most parsimoniously ascribed to their similar impact on central serotonergic systems. The amino acid tryptophan is the natural precursor to serotonin (Yuwiler, 1973); tryptophan administration leads to increases in brain serotonin concentration and turnover (Fernstrom and Wurtman, 1974). Fluoxetine is a fairly specific serotonin reuptake inhibitor (Fuller and Wong, 1977). By inhibiting the reuptake of serotonin, fluoxetine administration increases the amount of serotonin available for binding to serotonin receptors. Quipazine is a serotonin receptor agonist leading to direct stimulation of serotonin receptor sites (Fuller et al., 1976). Thus tryptophan, fluoxetine, and quipazine all increase stimulation of serotonin receptors: tryptophan by enhancing serotinin synthesis resulting in more serotonin available for release, fluoxetine by augmenting the time serotonin is available for the receptors, and quipazine by direct stimulation.

Because of our interest in normative, nonpathological behavior, we have employed low doses of these drugs. In the selected dose ranges animals do not exhibit abnormal or aberrant behaviors or stereotypies. Tryptophan was administered at four dose levels: 10, 20, 40, and 80 mg/kg/day; fluoxetine was given at 0.5, 1.0, 2.0, and 4.0 mg/kg/day; quipazine was given at 0.25, 0.5, and 1.0 mg/kg/day. Only one animal in a given group was treated at any time, and treatment periods lasted 5 days. Each animal received all doses of fluoxetine, tryptophan, and quipazine. For any animal different doses of drug treatment were separated by at least 15 days of saline treatment.

The selected behavioral measures were known on the basis of earlier studies to be serotonergically influenced in vervet monkeys (Raleigh et al.,

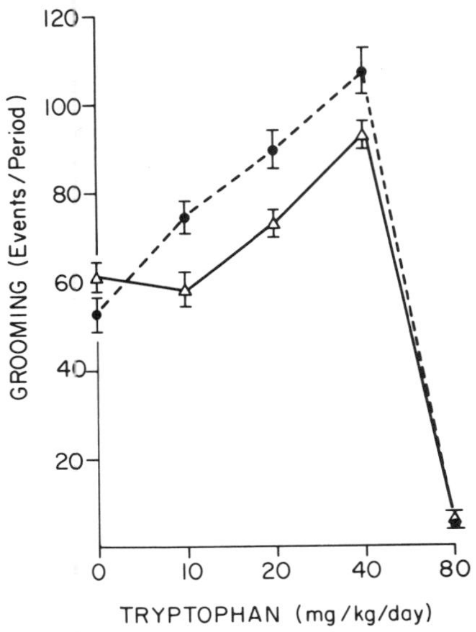

Fig. 1. The effects of tryptophan treatment on social grooming. Four dominant (●) and eight nondominant (△) males were treated with 0, 10, 20, 40, and 80 mg tryptophan/kg/day. Each treatment period lasted five days. Differences between dominant and nondominant males were significant for the 10, 20, and 40 mg tryptophan/kg/day doses. ($P \leqslant .01$ by Scheffe's test.) Data are in $\bar{X} \pm$ SEM. See text for details.

1980). These measures included such social behaviors as "approach," "groom," "avoid," and "be solitary," and such individual behaviors as "rest," "eat," "locomote," and "be vigilant." In these groups, in baseline conditions, there were no significant pairwise correlations among the eight behaviors. Thus, for example, grooming and avoiding were not significantly related. Dominant and nondominant males did not differ in the baseline rates of these behaviors, except for "being vigilant."

Behavioral Drug Effects

The behavioral effects of fluoxetine, tryptophan, and quipazine are depicted in Fig. 1 and Table I. Specifically, Fig. 1 illustrates the effects of tryptophan treatment on grooming. The rate of grooming is increased by tryptophan treatment in both dominant and nondominant males. In baseline conditions the rate of grooming was about 60 events per period. For dominant males treatment with 10, 20, or 40 mg/kg/day of tryptophan augmented grooming to an average of 76, 90, and 106 events per period respectively. For nondominant males 10 mg/kg/day of tryptophan did not alter grooming rates, while 20 and 40 mg/kg/day of tryptophan increased grooming to about 72 and 92 events per period respectively. Thus at 10, 20, and 40 mg/kg/day, the greater effect of tryptophan treatment on the behavior of the dominant animals is readily apparent. The soporific effects of tryptophan obliterated not only the dominant/nondominant difference but also nearly all behavior at the high 80 mg/kg/day dose. Consequently, data on the behavioral effects of the high doses of tryptophan and fluoxetine were excluded from analysis.

Table I qualitatively summarizes the effects of tryptophan, fluoxetine, and quipazine on all eight measured behaviors. The left-hand portion of this table depicts the impact of these drug treatments on the rates of the behavioral endpoints. The right-hand portion indicates whether there were status-related differences in the behavioral effects of these drugs; that is, whether dominant males exhibited larger responses to drug treatment. For example, consider the behavior "approach." The table shows that tryptophan, fluoxetine, and quipazine treatment all produce dose-dependent increases in approach. The table further shows that these increases were significantly greater in dominant males. Each drug treatment increased grooming, approaching, resting, and eating, while locomoting, avoiding, being solitary, and being vigilant decreased. There were significant status–drug treatment interactions for grooming, approaching, being solitary, being vigilant, avoiding, and locomoting; that is, the increases or decreases in these behavioral measures were larger in dominant than in nondominant males. In brief, tryptophan, fluoxetine, and quipazine all produced the same behavioral effects. Furthermore the heightened responsivity of the dominant males to drug treatments was apparent with all three drugs regardless of the direction of the behavioral change.

TABLE I. Drug Dose-Related Behavioral Response

	Direction of effect on rate of behavior			Interaction with status		
	F	T	Q	F	T	Q
Approach	+	+	+	Yes	Yes	Yes
Groom	+	+	+	Yes	Yes	Yes
Be solitary	−	−	−	Yes	Yes	Yes
Locomote	−	−	−	Yes	Yes	Yes
Rest	+	+	+	No	No	No
Eat	+	+	+	No	No	No
Avoid	−	−	−	Yes	Yes	Yes
Be vigilant	−	−	−	Yes	Yes	Yes

F = fluoxetine; T = tryptophan; Q = quipazine. "+" and "−" indicate, respectively, that treatment increases or decreases the frequency of occurrence of the scored behaviors. All effects are significant at $P \leqslant 0.05$.

These status-related differences suggest that there is a difference between dominant and nondominant animals in the responsiveness of their central serotonergic neurotransmitter systems to drug interventions.

Drug Effects on Serotonin in Blood Platelets

Because 20 mg/kg/day of tryptophan produced greater behavioral effects in dominant than in nondominant males, we examined some of the physiological consequences of this dose of tryptophan. In both the central nervous system and peripheral tissue, serotonin biosynthesis is substrate-limited (Fernstrom and Wurtman, 1974). Following tryptophan administration, the elevated brain serotonin concentrations have the same anatomical distribution as endogenous serotonin (Moir and Eccelston, 1968; Kuhar et al., 1972). Tryptophan administration also results in augmented serotonin concentrations in peripheral tissues. An easily measured portion of peripheral serotonin is sequestered in blood platelets (Yuwiler et al., 1981). Consequently in these studies we measured serotonin in whole blood.

Table II shows the effect of an acute dose of 20 mg/kg of tryptophan on whole-blood serotonin concentrations. These investigations were conducted in seven groups containing, in total, seven dominant and nine nondominant males. After a basal blood sample was obtained 20 mg/kg of tryptophan was administered. Sixty minutes later, a time at which the behavioral differences between dominant and nondominant males were pronounced, a second blood sample was obtained. Dominant males differ substantially from nondominant animals in whole-blood serotonin response to tryptophan load. This status-related difference is most clearly apparent in the ratio of the post-tryptophan to basal whole-blood serotonin concentrations. Dominant males exhibit a larger relative rise in whole-blood serotonin than nondominant males in spite of having basal whole-blood serotonin levels approximately twice those of nondominant males. Such a status-related difference in tryptophan conversion to serotonin, should it occur in the central nervous sytem, might explain the greater behavioral change seen in dominant animals treated with tryptophan.

PERIPHERAL MEASURES REFLECTING CENTRAL SEROTONERGIC SYSTEMS

The relationship between social dominance and peripheral biochemical parameters has been investigated in several monkey species. A variety of physiological measures, including but not limited to basal and challenged serum cortisol (Golub et al., 1979; Mendoza et al., 1979), serum testosterone (Rose et al., 1979), plasma dopamine-beta-hydroxylase (Redmond et al.,

TABLE II. Whole-Blood Serotonin Response to Tryptophan Load

	Dominant (N = 7)	Nondominant (N = 9)
Basal level (ng/ml)	1,136 ± 40	668 ± 26
Tryptophan +60 min (20 mg/kg)	2,428 ± 88	1,029 ± 48
Absolute difference	1,292 ± 70	361 ± 36
Relative difference	2.14 ± 0.07	1.54 ± 0.06

Data are mean ± SEM.

1976), platelet and plasma MAO (Redmond et al., 1979), cerebrospinal fluid 5-hydroxyindole acetic acid (CSF 5-HIAA) (Gradwell et al., 1975), and whole-blood serotonin (Raleigh and McGuire, 1980), have been examined. In this section we discuss two peripheral measures that may reflect central serotonergic activity: whole-blood serotonin and CSF 5-HIAA levels.

Three sets of data suggest that blood and brain serotonin are related. Both are similarly affected by several pharmacological treatments (Koe and Weisman, 1966; Yuwiler, 1973); abnormalities in blood serotonin concentration are associated with several psychiatric and behavioral disorders (Ritvo et al., 1970); and aspects of the uptake and storage of serotoninin blood platelets and serotonergic neurons are similar (Stahl and Meltzer, 1978). There is a robust association between active occupation of the dominant male social position and elevated whole-blood serotonin concentrations. In 19 stable multimale captive groups whole-blood serotonin was measured on at least three occasions. Dominant males exhibited whole-blood serotonin concentrations substantially higher than those of nondominant males (960 ± 18 ng/ml (19) vs. 620 ± 20 ng/ml (39); mean ± SEM (n)). Unlike such peripheral measures as testosterone which may exhibit tenfold day-to-day intra-animal fluctuations, whole-blood serotonin concentrations are relatively invariant. When status relationships are stable, it is extremely rare for any animal to have a whole-blood serotonin (WBS) level that deviates more than 15% from the animal's mean concentration. Thus, in contrast to some other peripheral measures, the between-animal differences in WBS concentrations over time correspond closely with the long-term, enduring nature of dominance relationships. Because of its intra-animal stability, robust association with status, and potential relationship to central serotonergic systems, we have been investigating the mechanisms that might underlie the elevated whole-blood serotonin exhibited by dominant males. Such mechansims include elevated tryptophan hydroxylase activity and enhanced platelet uptake and storage of serotonin. The difference between dominant and nondominant males in such a peripheral measure may suggest that a corresponding central nervous system difference might partially account for behavioral differences between dominant and nondominant males.

A second peripheral measure, CSF 5-HIAA, may be more closely related to central serotonergic systems than WBS. We have obtained single samples of cisternal CSF from animals in eight stable social groups. Because metabolite levels in CSF are temporal and spatial integrals of prior neuronal activity, CSF may be regarded as a peripheral measure. Table III shows that the concentration of CSF 5-HIAA in eight dominant males is higher than in 12 nondominant animals. The table also shows that CSF homovanillic acid (HVA), a metabolite of dopamine, is not significantly different between dominant and nondominant males. The observation that HVA concentrations are not higher in dominant than in nondominant males makes it very unlikely that the 5-HIAA difference results from differences in acid transport or some other generalized process. Because CSF 5-HIAA may be an index of total brain serotonergic activity, this difference between dominant and nondominant males may reflect differences in brain function. The CSF 5-HIAA difference is consistent with the dominant males' heightened sensitivity to drugs augmenting central serotonergic activity and with their elevated blood serotonin concentrations.

DOMINANCE, MONOAMINE OXIDASE, AND THE EFFECTS OF MAO INHIBITORS

Platelet monoamine oxidase and plasma amine oxidase are enzymes that catalyze important steps in the degradation of monoamines. Although platelets contain only the "B" isozyme whereas both the "A" and "B" are present in brain, under some basal and experimental conditions the activity of these peripheral enzymes may parallel that of monoamine oxidase in the central nervous system (Tipton et al., 1973; Donnelly and Murphy, 1977; Oreland et al., 1981). Platelet monoamine oxidase acitivity in some patients with

TABLE III. CSF Measures

	Dominant (N = 8)	Nondominant (N = 12)
5-HIAA	109 ± 18*	72 ± 5
HVA	177 ± 8	206 ± 16

*Dominant different from nondominant at $P < 0.05$. Data are mean ± SEM of single samples in ng/ml.

schizophrenia or depression has been reported to be lower than that observed in referent populations (Murphy and Weis, 1972; Murphy and Wyatt, 1972). In addition, the monoamine oxidase inhibitors are an important class of antidepressant drugs. Furthermore, several observations suggest that differences in peripheral monoamine oxidase activity may be associated with different behavioral patterns in humans and monkeys. For example, Buchsbaum et al. (1976) showed that compared to students with high platelet monoamine oxidase activity, those with low MAO activity were more likely to have psychological or psychiatric counseling and problems with the law. Furthermore, relatives of the low MAO proband were more likely to have psychiatric problems than those of the high MAO probands. Similarly, in rhesus monkeys platelet MAO exhibited little intra-animal variation and correlated positively with the incidence of being alone, self-grooming, and resting, and inversely with receiving grooming, social contact, and engaging in dominant agonistic behaviors (Redmond et al., 1979). On the basis of these observations, we were interested in determining whether platelet MAO and plasma AO activities differed between dominant and nondominant males. We also sought to ascertain whether there were status-related differences in the behavioral effects of monoamine oxidase inhibitors.

In these studies the relationship between social status and enzyme activity was investigated in three stable social groups. For each animal monoamine oxidase activity was determined on at least four occasions by the method of Murphy et al. (1976). Table IV shows that there were no significant differences between dominant and nondominant males in either plasma amine oxidase or platelet monoamine oxidase activity. For dominant males, plasma amine oxidase activity was about 23 nmoles/hr/ml blood while it was about 27 nmoles/hr/ml blood for nondominant males. Platelet MAO activity levels were about 223 picomoles/hr/10^6 platelets for both dominant and nondominant males. Both plasma amine oxidase and platelet monoamine oxidase activity exhibited relatively little intra-animal variation between samples.

TABLE IV. Amine Oxidase Measures

	Dominant (N = 3)	Nondominant (N = 4)
Plasma amine oxidase (nmoles/hr/ml blood)	23.4 ± 2.7	27.6 ± 1.9
Platelet monoamine oxidase (pmoles/hr/10E+6 platelet)	224 ± 0.3	232 ± 29

Data are the mean ± SEM of the means of four determinations of each variable per animal.

We examined the behavioral effects of two monoamine oxidase inhibitors: chlorgyline and deprenyl. Chlorgyline preferentially inhibits the A isozyme while deprenyl has its greater affinity for the B isozyme. Chlorgyline was given at a low (10 mg/kg/day) and a high (20 mg/kg/day) dose. Deprenyl was also administered at two dose levels, 7.5 and 15 mg/kg/day. The behavioral effects of the low dose of chlorgyline were examined in three dominant and three nondominant males. The effects of the high dose of chlorgyline and both doses of deprenyl were monitored in six dominant and nine nondominant males. As shown in Table V, the following behavioral measures were taken: groom (GR), approach (AP), rest (RT), eat (ET), locomote (LC), avoid (AV), be solitary (SL), be vigilant (VG), huddle (HD), aggress (AG), be aggressed (BG), and engage in sexual behavior (SX).

Chlorgyline and deprenyl exerted strikingly similar behavioral effects. Both drugs increased grooming, approaching, and being vigilant and decreased being solitary in a dose-dependent fashion. The high dose of both drugs decreased avoiding. The high dose of chlorgyline and both doses of deprenyl increased locomoting. The only behavior that chlorgyline and deprenyl affected differentially was aggressing. This behavior was increased by the high dose of deprenyl but was not altered by the chlorgyline treatments.

Table V also shows that social status was not an important factor influencing the behavioral effects of these drugs. Being vigilant was the only behavior for which there were status-related differences. For this behavior, dominant males were more responsive to deprenyl but not chlorgyline treatment than were nondominant males. The absence of status-related effects was not due to the relatively small number of subjects. Except for "be vigilant," the distribution of the rates at which dominant males engaged in any behavior affected by either dose of either drug overlapped those exhibited by nondominant males. In no case (except for "be vigilant") was the probability of a status-related effect nearly significant ($P \geqslant 0.3$ for all cases). Thus there is a clear concordance between this lack of a social status influence on the behavioral effects of either chlorgyline or deprenyl and the absence of a difference in their platelet MAO and plasma amine oxidase activity levels.

CONCLUSION

Our investigations give credence to the view that a distinct biochemical, physiological, and behavioral state is conferred upon the dominant male. Behavioral studies have shown that there are status-related differences in response to drugs affecting central serotonergic neurotransmission. Biochemical studies have revealed that dominant males differ from other males in

TABLE V. Behavioral Effects of High and Low Doses of Chlorgyline and Deprenyl

	Chlorgyline		Deprenyl		Interaction with status	
	Low	High	Low	High	C	D
GR	143 ± 9*	162 ± 11*	153 ± 11*	173 ± 20*	No	No
AP	133 ± 9*	171 ± 10*	148 ± 13*	168 ± 13*	No	No
RT	104 ± 15	98 ± 14	111 ± 21	97 ± 14	No	No
ET	109 ± 19	113 ± 21	91 ± 10	121 ± 9	No	No
LC	106 ± 15	128 ± 9*	133 ± 10*	149 ± 12*	No	No
AV	79 ± 16	61 ± 10*	84 ± 12	66 ± 10*	No	No
SL	68 ± 6*	63 ± 7*	67 ± 9*	50 ± 6*	No	No
VG	130 ± 8*	148 ± 9*	128 ± 7*	153 ± 11*	No	No
HD	113 ± 17	132 ± 29	96 ± 10	99 ± 10	No	No
AG	131 ± 29	141 ± 20	142 ± 6	163 ± 10*	No	No
BG	113 ± 14	115 ± 7	108 ± 12	116 ± 11	No	No
SX	100 ± 9	108 ± 13	106 ± 9	109 ± 10	No	No

The values are mean ± SEM percentages of baseline values for each behavior and treatment. The behavioral variables and dose levels are indicated in the text. The interaction with status columns indicate whether there were status-related differences in the effects of chlorgyline (C) or deprenyl (D).
$^*P \leqslant 0.05$.

basal whole-blood and CSF metabolite concentrations and in the dynamic serotonin synthesis and sequestering response to a tryptophan load. Investigations of platelet MAO and plasma AO activity and of the behavioral effects of MAO inhibitors indicate that differences between dominant and nondominant males are not ubiquitous. Rather the clear impact of behavioral dominance may be confined to peripheral and central physiological parameters relative to serotonergic function.

The influences of social status on the behavioral effects of drugs and on biochemical profiles has not been specified in humans but may have clear clinical relevance. Among humans differences in social status may be an important factor underlying inter-individual differences in the effects of pharmacological interventions. Moreover, studies in humans analogous to those we have conducted in monkeys may require a more detailed characterization of social status because most individuals simultaneously occupy several dominant and nondominant social positions. Thus, for example, social status–related differences in the effects of drug treatment may be detectable only following distinct changes in social status such as those that may accompany the assumption of a leadership role in a relatively closed group. These possibilities are currently under investigation.

ACKNOWLEDGMENTS

This research was supported in part by HF Guggenheim grant H-80606 and in part by the Research Service of the Sepulveda and Brentwood VA Hospitals. Constructive suggestions were provided by Klaus Miczek, Dana Olsen, and Arthur Yuwiler. Useful technical assistance was provided by Diane Bushberg, David Flannery, Michelle Freier, Mary Harrington, and Brian Vierra.

REFERENCES

Buchsbaum MS, Coursey RD, Murphy DL (1976) The biochemical high-risk paradigm: behavioral and familial correlates of platelet monoamine oxidase activity. Sci 194: 339–341

Donnelly CH, Murphy DL (1977) Substrate- and inhibitor-related characteristics of human platelet monoamine oxidase. Biochem Pharmacol 26: 853–858

Fairbanks LA (1980) Relationships among adult females in captive vervet monkeys: testing a model of rank related attractiveness. Anim Behav 28: 853–859

Fairbanks LA, McGuire MT, Page N (1978) Social roles in captive vervet monkeys *(Cercopithecus aethiops sabaeus)*. Behav Processes 3: 335–352

Fernstrom JD, Wurtman J (1974) Control of brain serotonin levels by the diet. Adv Biochem Psychopharmacol 11: 134–142

Fuller RW, Snoddy HD, Perry KW, Roush BW, Molloy BB, Bymaster FR, Wong DT (1976) The effects of quipazine on serotonin metabolism in rat brain. Life Sci 18: 925–934

Fuller RW, Wong DT (1977) Inhibition of serotonin reuptake. Fed Proc 36: 2154–2158

Gartlan JS, Brain DK (1968) Ecology and social variability in *Cercopithecus aethiops*. In: Jay P (ed) Primates: Studies in Adaptation and Variability. Holt Rinehart Winston, New York, pp 253–292

Golub MS, Sassenrath EN, Goo GP (1979) Plasma cortisol levels and dominance in peer groups of rhesus monkey weanlings. Horm Behav 12: 50–59

Gradwell PB, Everitt BJ, Herbert J (1975) 5-Hydroxytryptamine in the central nervous system and sexual receptivity of female rhesus monkeys. Brain Res 88: 281–293

Koe BK, Weismann A (1966) p-Chlorophenylalanine: a specific depletor of brain serotonin. J Pharmacol Exp Ther 154: 499–516

Kuhar MJ, Aghajanian GK, Roth RH (1972) Tryptophan hydroxylase activity and synaptosomal uptake of serotonin in discrete regions after midbrain raphe lesions: correlation with serotonin levels and histochemical fluorescence. Brain Res 44: 165–176

McGuire MT (1974) The St. Kitts Vervet. Karger, Basel

Mendoza SP, Coe CL, Lowe EL, Levine S (1979) The physiological response to group formation in adult squirrel monkeys. Psychoneuroendocrinol 3: 221–229

Moir ATB, Eccelston D (1968) The effects of precursor loading on the cerebral metabolism of 5-hydroxyindoles. J Neurochem 15: 1093–1108

Murphy DL, Weiss R (1972) Reduced monoamine oxidase activity in blood platelets from bipolar depressed patients. Am J Psychol 128: 1351–1357

Murphy DL, Wright C, Buchsbaum M, Nichols A, Costa JL, Wyatt RJ (1976) Platelet and plasma amine oxidase activity in 680 normals: sex and age differences and stability over time. Biochem Med 16: 254–265

Murphy DL, Wyatt RJ (1972) Reduced MAO activity in blood platelets from schizophrenic patients. Nature 238: 225–226

Oreland L, Wiberg A, Foowler CJ (1981) Monoamine oxidase activity in platelets as related to monoamine oxidase activity and monoaminergic function in the brain. In: Angrist B, Burrows GD, Lader M, Lingjaerde O, Sedvell G, Wheatley D (eds) Recent Advances in Neuropsychopharmacology. Pergamon Press, New York, pp 195–201

Raleigh MJ, Brammer GL, McGuire MT, Yuwiler A, Geller E, Johnson CK (1983) Social status related differences in the behavioral effects of drugs in vervet monkeys *(Cercopithecus aethiops sabaeus)*. In: Steklis HD, Kling AS (eds) Hormones, Drugs, and Primate Social Behavior. Spectrum Press, New York, pp 83–105.

Raleigh MJ, Brammer GL, Yuwiler A, Flannery JW, McGuire MT, Geller E (1980) Serotonergic influences on the social behavior of vervet monkeys *(Cercopithecus aethiops sabaeus)*. Exp Neurol 68: 322–334

Raleigh MJ, Ervin FR, Flannery JW (1979) Sex differences in social behavior among captive juvenile vervet monkeys *(Cercopithecus aethiops sabaeus)*. Behav Neurol Biol 26: 455–465

Raleigh MJ, McGuire MT (1980) Biosocialpharmacology. J McLean Hosp 2: 73–84

Redmond DE, Baulu J, Murphy DK, Loriaux DL, Zeigler MG, Lake CR (1976) The effects of testosterone on plasma and platelet monoamine oxidase (MAO) and plasma dopamine-beta-hydroxylase (DBH) activities in the male rhesus monkey. Psychosom Med 38: 315–326

Redmond DE, Murphy DL, Baulu J (1979) Platelet monoamine oxidase activity correlates with social affiliative and agonistic behaviors in normal rhesus monkeys. Psychosom Med 41: 87–100

Ritvo ER, Yuwiler A, Geller E, Ornitz EM, Saeger K, Plotkin S (1970) Increased blood serotonin and platelets in early infantile autism. Arch Gen Psychiatr 23: 566–577

Rose RM, Bernstein IS, Gordon TP (1975) Consequences of social conflict on plasma testosterone levels in rhesus monkeys. Psychosom Med 37: 50–61

Rowell R (1972) The Social Behavior of Monkeys. Penguin Books, Middlesex England

Stahl SM, Meltzer HY (1978) A kinetic and pharmacological analysis of 5-hydroxytryptamine transport by human platelets and platelet comparison with central serotonergic neurons. J Pharmacol Exp Ther 205: 118–132

Struhsaker TT (1967) Behavior of vervet and other cercopithecines. Sci 156: 1197–1203

Tipton KF, Houslay MD, Garret NJ (1973) Allotopic properties of human brain monoamine oxidase. Nature New Biol (London) 246: 213–214

Yuwiler A (1973) Conversion of d- and l-tryptophan to serotonin and 5-hydroxyindoleacetic acid and to blood serotonin. J Neurochem 20:1099–1109.

Yuwiler A, Brammer GL, Morley JE, Raleigh MJ, Flannery JW, Geller E (1981) Short-term and repetitive administration of oral tryptophan in normal men. Arch Gen Psychiatr 38: 619–626

Ethopharmacology: Primate Models of Neuropsychiatric Disorders,
pages 199–218

Amphetamine Challenge: Effects in Previously Isolated Rhesus Monkeys and Implications for Animal Models of Schizophrenia

Gary W. Kraemer, Michael H. Ebert, C. Raymond Lake, and William T. McKinney

Wisconsin Psychiatric Research Institute and Primate Laboratory (G.W.K.) and Department of Psychiatry (W.T.M.), University of Wisconsin, Madison, Wisconsin 53706; National Institute of Mental Health, Bethesda, Maryland 20014 (M.H.E.); and Uniformed Services University of the Health Sciences, School of Medicine, Bethesda, Maryland 20014 (C.R.L.)

INTRODUCTION

Animal models have contributed greatly to our present understanding of the neurobiological basis of human psychopathology. Hypotheses about the neurochemical substrates of disorders such as depression and schizophrenia derive from studies in animals of the neurochemical effects of pharmacological agents which are either thought to precipitate or exacerbate symptoms of these disorders in humans, or from studies of the neurochemical effects of known therapeutic agents. For instance, the "catecholamine theory of depression" is based in part on the findings that agents that can precipitate depression in some humans, e.g., reserpine, deplete or reduce function in the catecholamine (CA) neurotransmitter systems (norepinephrine [NE] and dopamine [DA]) in animals. Conversely, the mechanism of action of antidepressant agents has long been thought to be their ability to augment CA function, and this hypothesis is based in large measure on studies of the behavioral and neurochemical effects of antidepressant agents in animals. These sorts of findings have been taken as evidence that the neurobiological substrates of depression might involve reductions in the function of the brain CA system (Kraemer and McKinney, 1979). The "dopamine theory of schizophrenia" is based in part on the similarity between amphetamine (AMPH)-induced psychosis and paranoid schizophrenia in humans, and the ability of neuroleptic agents to reverse AMPH-induced psychosis and to serve as therapeutic agents in schizophrenia. Work in animals suggests that many of the effects of AMPH and the antagonism of these effects by phenothiazines and butyrophenones is mediated by actions of these drugs on brain DA receptors (Angrist et al.,

1974; Janowsky and Davis, 1976; Snyder, 1974). This has been taken to suggest that schizophrenia itself is somehow related to disorders in brain DA system function.

Making inferences about the possible substrates of altered brain function in various forms of psychopathology based on studies of drug action on neurochemical systems certainly has its perils. We are only technologically capable of studying a few systems, and biochemical effects central to the pharmacological response may be in systems other than the ones being studied. Interpretation of results is also difficult. The catecholamine theory of depression was based in part on the ability of tricyclic antidepressants to augment CA function by reducing NE and 5HT reuptake at the synapse. However, advances in the study of biogenic amine receptors now suggest that the eventual impact of this may be NE receptor subsensitivity, and a down regulation of NE system function (Sulser et al., 1978). Additionally, most effective antidepressants have effects on a wide variety of neurobiochemical systems, and their central mode of action may not be as specifically related to the NE system function as was once thought. Similarly, the DA theory of schizophrenia has also required significant revision in light of conflicting findings about the sensitivity of schizophrenic patients to psychostimulant drugs. This issue will be addressed at greater length later in the present paper. Therefore, inferences about brain mechanisms based on known biochemical effects of drugs must be reviewed as theoretical constructs that may have to be changed as new information becomes available. Nevertheless, a great deal of empirically useful information about the relationship between changes in brain neurotransmitter systems and changes in behavior has been derived from studies of the neurochemical effects of drugs in animals, and continued work in this area leads to advances in theories about brain mechanisms which are then testable with development of new pharmacological methods and tools.

In the present chapter, we would like to consider the use of pharmacological agents as tools to study the neurobiological substrates of the development of social behavior in primates and the impact of factors which can alter that development. This approach will then be related to theories about some forms of human psychopathology. Extrapolations from rodents to nonhuman primates to humans always generates controversy. The reasons for this are well known and appreciated (McKinney and Moran, 1981). However, in the context of the discussion we will attempt to establish some basis for cross-species comparisons and a rationale for their application.

PHARMACOLOGICAL CHALLENGE

The concept of using a pharmacological agent to reveal some characteristic neurochemical function which is not observable otherwise is not new. Early studies of the effects of reserpine, a drug which depletes brain biogenic amines, revealed that little behavioral change was observed with chronic treatment which depleted brain biogenic amines to 10–20% of control in rodents. Yet, increased dosage of reserpine which produced further depletions affected motor behavior and body posture (Haggendal and Lindqvist, 1964). This suggested that the brain has tremendous reserve homeostatic capacities, and that changes in behavior might only be observable after neurochemical measures had been altered dramatically.

Subsequent work with 6-hydroxydopamine (6OHDA), a neurotoxin thought to be selectively toxic to CA neurons (Breese, 1975), revealed that depletions of brain CA to 10–20% of control had little effect on behavior, but that the deficit could be revealed if CA metabolism were further compromised in subjects previously treated with 6OHDA. It was found in both rodents and nonhuman primates that the CA depleting effects of 6OHDA could be revealed behaviorally, by treating previously lesioned subjects with alpha-methyl-para-tyrosine (AMPT), a drug which inhibits tyrosine hydroxylase and, therefore, the production of CA (Cooper et al., 1972; Kraemer et al., 1981). In this case, AMPT was found to have behavioral depressant effects at much lower doses in subjects that had been previously treated with 6OHDA than in intact controls. These examples support the idea that a previously existing deficit, produced by a pharmacological or neurotoxic treatment, can have little effect on ongoing behavior. However, latent deficits can then be revealed by an additional pharmacological treatment which presumably affects the same underlying systems. On this account, administration of a “challenge” drug, whose mechanism of action has been established to the degree possible in rodents, can tell us something about the function of the neurobiological systems upon which it acts in other species. Thus, in the same way that pharmacological challenge can be viewed as revealing the effects of a prior lesion or pharmacological treatment, inferences can be made about the effects of a variety of experimental treatments on the basis of known neurochemical actions of the challenge drug.

PHARMACOLOGICAL CHALLENGE IN NONHUMAN PRIMATES

One of the central problems in primate research is “individual variability.” In monkeys, as in humans, the sources of variability are probably due to genetic factors which then interact with a variety of environmental inputs over the course of development. Many forms of human psychopathology can be viewed in this way. Systematically specifying the kinds of developmental factors which can have a long-lasting impact on brain function, which is then reflected in behavior, is extremely difficult. However, in nonhuman primates a number of factors can be controlled and investigated experimentally. Nevertheless, there are limitations, both practical and ethical, in the kinds of studies that can be performed on primate species.

Ideally, it would be of value to follow the course of development of brain mechanisms over time in conjunction with a number of experimental manipulations that are hypothesized to have an impact on that development. Direct measures of brain neurotransmitter content, turnover, and receptor binding are possible in rodents but less feasible in primates. For this reason, a greater emphasis has been placed on measures of neurotransmitter metabolism or of neurotransmitters themselves, in cerebrospinal fluid (CSF). Repeated measures of this sort in conjunction with behavioral observations provide the primary basis for inferences about the possible role of changes in neurobiological mechanisms in mediating persistent changes in behavior or responses to experimental manipulations. However, as noted earlier, there is evidence that neurochemical measures may be altered substantially, without apparent changes in behavior. The opposite is also true; behavior can be altered markedly without apparent changes in the brain neurochemical measures that are being taken (Breese et al., 1973). This lack of correspondence between measures at two levels of analysis (behavior-neurochemical) could be due to wide differences in the sensitivity of methods, failure to study the systems central to the behavior, or inappropriate dependent measures. Brain content of neurotransmitter substances may not be as relevant a measure as turnover rate. Turnover rate may not be as important as evaluations of the dynamic characteristics of the system or its homeostatic resilience. Pharmacological challenge provides another route by which inferences about the function of underlying neurochemical systems can be made.

This approach has its limitations: Pharmacological challenge of subjects that have widely differing behavioral repertoires presents an extremely difficult problem in terms of interpreting the differential responses observed. However, in many cases where adequate experimental control of baseline conditions can be achieved, pharmacological challenge can be an effective tool for exploring some parameters of underlying differences that are due to developmental and environmental factors. As with other techniques directed toward the investigation of neurobiological "mechanisms" underlying behavior, including studies of the effects of lesions and the direct measurement of brain neurotransmitter content and receptor binding, interpretations are limited by what can be measured, and the inferences that can be made from these measures about a larger and more complex system are similarly limited. Pharmacological challenge and CSF sampling, as opposed to direct measures of brain tissue, allow repeated measures that can reflect changes over time, and the effects of various treatments.

This is critically important in nonhuman primates for the following reasons: (1) By comparison to research employing rodents, the number of subjects and the techniques that can be used in nonhuman primate studies are greatly limited by practical, ethical, and economic factors. The individual variability of primates necessitates the development of methods to estimate, in advance of experimental treatment, the variance of the measures to be taken. In many cases, if this is done, it is found that the natural variation in the measure exceeds the magnitude of the effect that could conceivably be produced by the experimental treatment. Group composition and adequate baseline data thus become major considerations in evaluating experimental results. (2) Studies in nonhuman primates are time-consuming, expensive, and rarely repeated. Thus, it is necessary to establish methods to determine whether measures that can only be taken once—e.g., brain neurotransmitter content, regional distribution and so forth—are justified and are likely to be central to the mechanisms of interest and therefore affected by the experimental treatment. It is important to take the "right" measures and to have some rational method for deciding when they ought to be taken.

Pharmacological challenge is a method that can be used to minimize or resolve a number of these problems. In conjunction with the use of a variety of other techniques, it can greatly increase the depth and reliability of information that can be obtained about the brain mechanisms that mediate complex behavior in nonhuman primates. While relating indirect measures of neurochemical function to brain mechanisms has its own pitfalls, the methods and data derived from this approach may have empirical validity that could be clinically important before the underlying mechanisms that mediate the effect of interest are elucidated. The present chapter focuses on investigations of some of the behavioral and neurobiological changes that are produced by disrupted social development and can be revealed with pharmacological challenge, and the possible relationship of these changes to similar effects in humans and some forms of human psychopathology.

EFFECTS OF EARLY SOCIAL DEPRIVATION ON RHESUS MONKEYS

The course of nonhuman primate social development has been used as an animal model of similar processes that occur in humans. One experimental method of disrupting social development in rhesus monkeys has been to place them in social isolation during periods of their early life when various kinds of social interaction would otherwise be occurring. The severity of the effect of this treatment varies across primate species (Sackett et al., 1976), and cross-species generalizations must be made with caution. The following background relates predominantly, but not exclusively, to the isolation syndrome as it has been defined in rhesus monkeys.

Mason (1968) summarized the effects of primate social isolation under four headings: (1) abnormal posturing and movements; (2) motivational disturbances, e.g., excessive fearfulness or arousal; (3) poor integration of motor patterns; (4) deficiencies in social communication, such as failure to withdraw after being threatened by a dominant animal. The degree of impairment of social behavior in rhesus monkeys by social isolation initiated at birth depends in part on the amount of time spent in isolation. Monkeys isolated for the first 3 months of life eventually exhibit seemingly normal behavioral development if they are subsequently placed in a nuturing social environment (Griffin and Harlow, 1966). Twelve-month isolates show a devastating loss in social competence which is greater than that seen with 6- or 9-month isolates (Sackett, 1972). Monkeys isolated for the first 6–12 months of life develop patterns of behavior characterized by self-orality, huddling, self-clasping, and stereotypy, and are socially incompetent (Sackett, 1972; Suomi and Harlow, 1971). When placed in social situations, these animals show a persistent absence of appropriate responses and typically withdraw totally from social interaction. In addition to huddling and rocking in the social situation, they may show stereotyped behaviors and engage in self-aggression or inappropriate and unpredictable aggression against infants or large dominant males. Sexual behavior is also inappropriate; males do not mount properly, and females fail to present and make confused and unwilling partners of even experienced feral males. If previously isolated females are impregnated artificially, they are grossly inadequate mothers and may attack and mortally wound their own infants (Arling and Harlow, 1967).

In addition to the duration of isolation, the degree of impairment in social behavior is also related to the age at which animals are isolated. Animals isolated after 3 or 6 months of social experience are not as severely debilitated by this treatment (Clark, 1969), but do show persistent abnormal social and sexual behavior (Sackett, 1972). Monkeys isolated during the second 6 months of life show inordinate levels of conspecific aggression when they are subsequently reintroduced to the social situation (Clark, 1969).

Isolation seems to produce deficits in social behavior or tasks related to social perception without affecting acquisition or performance of abstract problem-solving (Harlow, 1969). This finding must be accepted with the provision that isolation rearing does produce major changes in the response to experimental environments and contingencies, and in the approach to problem-solving, which may complicate interpretation of learning studies (Sackett, 1972; Mason, 1978). However, the perception of social cues does appear to be impaired on a long-term basis. Isolates have been found to be ineffective in perceiving and sending facial expressions that form a discriminative stimulus enabling an isolate or a socially competent partner to perform an active avoidance task. They also did not respond physiologically to cues of imminent shock as provided by the facial expression of the other subject (Mirsky, 1968).

SOCIAL REHABILITATION

The effects of early social deprivation can persist into adulthood, and at one time it was thought that these effects were irreversible (Sackett, 1972). However, it has been demonstrated that providing social experience with younger, socially developing monkeys—"monkey therapists"—can eliminate most of the bizarre behavior patterns of isolated monkeys (Novak and Harlow, 1975; Suomi et al., 1974; Suomi and Harlow, 1972). Over long periods of group housing social behavior develops, and by 3–4 years of age previously isolated monkeys are indistinguishable on a daily basis from their chronically socially reared counterparts. However, these subjects show latent deficits when challenged with socially stressful situations that require complex social discriminations (Anderson and Mason, 1978). In these instances, inappropriate social behavior (withdrawal or aggression) and increased stereotypic behaviour surfaces. This suggestion of a latent and extremely persistent effect of early social deprivation represents one case in which pharmacological challenge is a useful technique in revealing possible underlying neurochemical changes that are attributable to social deprivation.

Deprivation of early sensory experience may produce changes in CNS neurochemical systems which are later translated into altered behavior in challenge situations or in response to treatment with drugs that act through neurochemical pathways. Very few studies have examined the neurobiological effects of isolation in primates. Neuroanatomical studies have shown a reduction in prefrontal cortical dendritic branching in previously isolated monkeys (Struble and Riesen, 1978). However, in rodents, isolation alters the turnover rate of brain biogenic amines (Modigh, 1973; Segal et al., 1973; Stolk et al., 1974) and the nature and magnitude of stress-related cortical neurochemical changes in later tests (Blanc et al., 1980).

Catecholamines have been shown to play a significant role in the regulation of cortical plasticity. Treatment of developing kittens with 6OHDA prevented visual experience from exerting its normal effects on cortical development (Kasamatsu and Pettigrew, 1976). Conversely, infusions of NE can maintain cortical plasticity (Pettigrew and Kasamatsu, 1978), and environmental variables may have an impact on the maintenance and recovery from CA system lesions. Thus, enriched environments can contribute to behavioral and physiological recovery from the effects of neonatal treatment with 6OHDA (Pearson et al., 1980). These data suggest a relationship between CA mechanisms, sensory input, and CNS development. Sensory deprivation may result in inadequate cortical CA innervation, and this may be manifested by an inability to alter responses to specific features of subsequent stimuli (Kasamatsu and Pettigrew, 1976; Pettigrew and Kasamatsu, 1978). The overall effect, in terms of brain CA content, would be difficult to detect since these cortical systems represent only a small proportion of total brain content. Nevertheless, differences in cortical CA systems could be manifested by differences in behavioral and biochemical response to CA agonists and antagonists.

By extrapolation from extensive work in rodents, it appears that if there are long-standing changes in brain neurotransmitter mechanisms induced by early social deprivation, then one way to reveal these changes would be to challenge apparently normal, but previously isolated (rehabilitated) monkeys with drugs that act primarily through brain CA systems. We will present and discuss the results of some of our studies using AMPH in this capacity. In another report (Kraemer et al., in press), we have related these AMPH challenge data to inferences about primate development. In the present discussion, we would like to consider the implications of these findings for animal models of psychostimulant-induced psychosis and their relationship to human schizophrenia.

EFFECT OF EARLY SOCIAL DEPRIVATION ON THE SOCIAL BEHAVIORAL RESPONSE TO AMPH

Two control groups (N = 8) were reared in social housing conditions, and two experimental groups (N = 8) were isolated for different periods in the first year of life, and then housed in social groups until 30 months of age with no further treatment. This was followed by AMPH challenge. The group composition was as follows: Four (3 male, 1 female) control monkeys were reared in single cages with their mothers until 6 months of age, when they were separated from their mothers and placed in a social group. The other four (male) control monkeys were separated from their mothers at birth, reared for 1 month in the laboratory nursery, and then placed in a social group. Four (male) experimental subjects were reared with their mothers until 6 months of age, when they were separated from their mothers and placed in social isolation chambers for 1 month and then placed in a social group. Another four (male) experimental subjects were separated from their mothers at birth, reared for 1 month in the laboratory nursery, and then housed for 11 months in social isolation; at approximately 1 year of age, they were placed in a social group. Beginning at the time of social grouping until 30 months of age, all groups were housed in the same room and received identical animal care and experimental treatment. The long intervening period of social housing was instituted so that, over time, levels of social behavior in the isolates would recover and later effects of AMPH could be evaluated in terms of comparable levels of social behavior between groups.

AMPH challenge was administered to all of the groups between 30 and 36 months of age. Throughout this phase of the study, the monkeys were intubated daily at 8:00 and 16:00 with placebo (tap water) or d-amphetamine sulfate (0.5, 1.0, 2.0, and 3.0 mg/kg/day, dose expressed as weight of the free base). Five-day drug treatment conditions at each dose were intercalated with 2 weeks of placebo administration. Social behavioral data were collected between 8:00–11:00 and 13:00–15:00, using a previously described 20-category scoring system (Kraemer et al., 1976).

The most prominent effects of AMPH were revealed by the behaviors of Contact Cling and Submit. These particular behaviors represent two ends of the spectrum of individual reactions. Contact Cling is highly affiliative and involves close body contact (hugging); Submit (fear grimace, screeching, oriented withdrawal) is a response usually emitted in response to displays of hostility (facial threats, barking, approach) or aggression.

The baseline data in Table I show that constant peer group housing over long time periods in the controlled laboratory setting is a great "equalizer." No baseline differences in social behavior occurred in any of the groups despite the wide range of early experience, and despite the potential for group-specific behaviors to develop. Thus, by 30 to 36 months of age, early experience with mother-rearing or isolation did not produce behavior different from that of constant peer housing over the same time. This uniformity was shattered by AMPH challenge. Comparisons were made between behavior during the preceding placebo treatment period and on each dose of AMPH that all of the groups would tolerate (0.5 and 1.0 mg/kg/day). In groups without early isolation, AMPH reduced Contact Cling and increased the proportion of time spent in nonsocial behaviors, particularly intensive stereotypic environmental exploration. The socially reared groups continued to interact socially on 0.5 mg/kg/day with increased levels of Submit. At 1.0 mg/kg/day, Submit returned to baseline values, and the animals spent most

TABLE I. Mean Duration of Contact Cling (max 300 sec ± SD) and Mean Frequency of Submit in 300 (± SD) in Four Social Groups (N = 4 each) With Different Rearing Conditions

	Amphetamine dose (mg/kg/day)					
	Placebo		0.5		1.0	
Rearing condition	Contact cling	Submit	Contact cling	Submit	Contact cling	Submit
Mother-peer	154.2 ± 24.5	5.2 ± 5.0	7.0* ± 6.2	25.0* ± 4.2	15.3* ± 23.0	4.5 ± 3.5
Peer-peer	126.7 ± 27.3	3.4 ± 1.4	79.1* ± 17.6	0.3* ± 0.5	1.5* ± 1.9	4.6 ± 2.0
Mother-isolate-peer (1 month)	132.4 ± 10.7	5.8 ± 2.1	127.3 ± 40.8	17.5*[a] ± 0.7	73.7 ± 45.0	22.0*[b] ± 7.0
Isolate-peer (1 year)	158.3 ± 43.8	3.6 ± 1.2	147.3 ± 47.3	15.0*[b] ± 2.8	52.0* ± 45.3	23.0*[c] ± 8.4

*=P < .05 versus placebo.

Wounding during amphetamine treatment weeks. [a]Lacerations and abrasions; [b]lacerations, abrasions, and lethargy; [c]features of a + b plus loss of body weight, dehydration—required intervention by experiment.

of their time intensively exploring the environment. Increasing doses up to 3.0 mg/kg/day induced progressively more stereotypic behavior in these groups, and social interactions were greatly reduced.

The response of the previously isolated animals to AMPH was distinctly different from the nonsocially deprived animals. Submit frequencies increased dramatically at 0.5 mg/kg/day with no concurrent decreases in Contact Cling, and some wounding occurred. At 1.0 mg/kg/day, Contact Cling was only slighlty reduced, Submit increased even further, and wounding was severe enough to require separation of the animals and termination of AMPH administration. The level of wounding for each dose is shown in Table I. The displacement of social behavior to environmental stereotypies did not occur in socially deprived animals.

To summarize, AMPH produced a wide variety of changes in motor behavior in all subjects. In chronically socially housed groups, there was a rapid reduction in social contact. In these subjects stereotypic behavior patterns were not manifested in social interactions. Rather, they appeared to redirect their altered behavior toward the inanimate environment in the form of prolonged bouts of manual and oral exploration of the home cage. In previously isolated subjects, altered behavior was not adaptively redirected to the environment. Instead, these monkeys maintained high levels of affiliative contact concurrently with high levels of Submit. The increase in Submit behavior was not paired with increased Threat displays but actually occurred in the context of close social contact. It did not appear to be a response to any other behavior that the human observers could detect. This highly unstable situation was punctuated with bouts of severe aggression and wounding.

EFFECT OF SOCIAL DEPRIVATION ON NONSOCIAL BEHAVIORAL AND NEUROCHEMICAL RESPONSES TO AMPH

Five of eight previously isolated monkeys showed toxic reactions to AMPH at doses of 1.0 mg/kg and above. This was characterized by postural collapse and convulsions. These monkeys were not used in subsequent AMPH trials because of the danger to the subjects and the obvious difficulty in interpreting data collected from subjects in this condition. The following dose-response study was conducted 1 month after the social study. Six control monkeys and three 1-month isolates were available for further study.

Each monkey received a single dose (1.0, 2.0, 3.0 mg/kg/day) at 8:00, and CSF and plasma were collected at 9:00 and 13:00 to correspond to the times of the prior behavioral testing sessions. The order of presentation of dosage level and time of sampling were counterbalanced across animals. Each animal was sampled at each time and dose level. An observer who was blind to the treatment protocol recorded the relative duration out of 10 minutes of stereotypic behavior at 8:50, 10:50, and 12:50 on a ten-point scale (0 = not present, 10 = always present) on days when CSF samples were taken at 13:00. Stereotypy was defined as motor movement in a stable pattern occurring without deviation for three or more cycles.

NE in CSF was analyzed using a radioenzymatic assay to convert endogenous NE to tritiated epinephrine with phenylethanolamine-N-methyl transferase and tritiated S-adenosylmethionine (Lake et al., 1976). CSF homovanillic acid (HVA) was analyzed using gas chromatography and mass spectrometry (GC-MS) with a trifluoroacetic anhydride derivative and a deuterated internal standard (Gordon et al., 1974). CSF 5-hydroxyindoleacetic acid (5HIAA) was analyzed using GC-MS with a trifluoroacetic anhydride derivative and a deuterated internal standard (Godfe et al., 1977).

The only significant behavioral difference between groups was in stereotypy. Table II shows the relative duration (± SEM) out of 10 minutes for each group at each dose level.

The data suggest that acute treatment with AMPH increases stereotypy in socially deprived monkeys but not in chronically socially reared monkeys. AMPH may actually reduce stereotypy in chronically socially reared monkeys.

These behavioral differences in the response to AMPH between groups were paired with significant neurochemical differences. Table III shows the concentration of CSF NE at 13:00 following placebo or a single dose of either 1.0, 2.0, or 3.0 mg/kg of AMPH given at 8:00 to individually housed members of the socially reared groups as compared to those of the 1-month isolation-reared group. Comparisons of NE values on placebo versus AMPH

TABLE II. Relative Duration of Stereotypy out of 10 Mintues (± SEM)

	Amphetamine dose (mg/kg)			
Rearing condition	0	1.0	2.0	3.0
Chronic social (N = 6)	1.8 ± 1.1	1.5 ± 0.7	0.6 ± 0.4	0.4 ± 0.4
One-month isolate (N = 3)	0.7 ± 0.4	2.2 ± 0.8[a]	6.9 ± 2.3[a,b]	3.6 ± 2.6

Harmonic mean ANOVA groups F = 6.86, df = 1/7, P < .05; Dose F = 4.37, df = 3/21, P < .025.
Fisher Least Significant Difference: [a] = P < .05 versus base line.; [b] = P < .05 between groups.

(1.0 mg/kg/day, the dose at which behavioral data were collected) show that the previously isolated monkeys had CSF NE values that were significantly higher than their own baseline ($P < .01$ Fisher Least Significant Difference [LSD]), and higher than the control monkeys at the same dose ($P < .05$ Fisher LSD). These differences were reduced at higher dose levels. There were no significant differences in CSF 5HIAA, HVA, or plasma AMPH levels between groups at any dose.

SUMMARY AND DISCUSSION

We have found that socially "rehabilitated" rhesus monkeys are hypersensitive to AMPH in terms of behavioral responses, toxicity, and changes in measures of brain neurochemical function. Furthermore, this effect can be demonstrated years after the social deprivation experience when the animals have apparently recovered, which suggests a long-term impact of developmental factors on later behavior and drug responses. In rodents, the effects of isolation are short-lived and there do not appear to be long-lasting neurobiological effects (Brain, 1975). In monkeys, it appears that the opposite is true. Monkeys isolated for periods in excess of 3 months in the first 6 months of life show behavioral abnormalities that, if left untreated, persist into adulthood (Sackett, 1972). Our pharmacological challenge data indicate that even short periods of deprivation may have a lasting impact on neurobiological mechanisms even in monkeys that have been socially rehabilitated.

It is well known that repeated or high doses of AMPH induce or increase motor stereotypies (rapid side-to-side head and eye movements [checking], intensive and repetitive manual or oral exploration of the inanimate environment, self-grooming, pacing), and disrupt social behavior in macaques, vervets, and marmosets (Machiyama et al., 1970; Kjellberg et al., 1973; Schiorring and Hecht, 1979; Schiorring, 1977; Garver et al., 1975; Haber et

TABLE III. Cerebrospinal Fluid Norepinephrine Concentration (ng/ml ± SEM)

Rearing condition	Amphetamine dose (mg/kg) 0	1.0	2.0	3.0
Chronic social (N = 6)	422 ± 123	693 ± 118	625 ± 112	909[a] ± 74
One-month isolate (N = 3)	543 ± 20	1,005[a,b] ± 120	1,201[a,b] ± 240	1,311[a] ± 107

Harmonic mean ANOVA groups $F = 10.97$, $df = 1/7$, $P < .025$; dose $F = 8.98$, $df = 3/21$, $P < .001$.

Fisher Least Significant Difference: [a] = $P < .01$ versus base line; [b] = $P < .05$ between groups at same dose.

al., 1981). Several investigators have suggested that these behavioral effects in nonhuman primates, including increased agonistic behavior, are comparable to the symptoms of paranoid schizophrenia that can be produced by AMPH in humans (Garver et al., 1975; Haber et al., 1981). These findings complement the much more extensive work that has been conducted using psychostimulant models of schizophrenia in rodents (Segal and Janowsky, 1978). They suggest that to the degree that it can be accepted that psychostimulant psychosis resembles some forms of schizophrenia in humans, then the motor patterns and abnormal behaviors induced in animals are analogs of the human disorder. However, this is not the only context in which the behavior of monkeys has been likened to that of schizophrenic patients.

The striking behavioral similarities between the bizarre stereotypic and cataleptic-like behaviors of the isolation syndrome in rhesus monkeys and of some forms of schizophrenia, together with the long-term persistence of these behaviors and of inappropriate social and sexual behavior and aggression, at one time suggested that the isolation syndrome could be used as a primate model of schizophrenia (Sackett, 1972). Also, treatment with the antipsychotic agent chlorpromazine reduces abnormal behavior in rhesus monkey isolates (Moran and McKinney, 1975). Thus, the variety of abnormal individual and social behaviors produced, and the reduction of these behaviors following neuroleptic treatment, seemed to be isomorphic with the behavior and drug responses of some human schizophrenics. However, it was also found that social learning paradigms (using monkey therapists) can almost totally reverse the behavioral effects of isolation (Novak and Harlow, 1975). The fact that the isolation syndrome is reversible, whereas schizophrenia generally is not, suggested that despite the similarities in behavior and drug response, human schizophrenia and the isolation syndrome are probably mediated by different underlying mechanisms. Nevertheless, early investigators, many with clinical experience, did remark upon the potent behavioral similarities between schizophrenic patients and isolated monkeys. Are the similarities adventitious, or is there some basis for cross species comparisons?

The primate social deprivation-rehabilitation syndrome adds a new dimension to our understanding of how these similarities might arise, and how the isolation syndrome, while not identical to schizophrenia, may be an important component of what is clinically labeled as schizophrenia. Three basic comparisons can be drawn.

(1) Previously socially deprived monkeys living in social groups interact socially but they do not respond to many social cues and are less sophisticated in using social coping strategies to deal with stressful situations (Anderson and Mason, 1978). When stressed, their bizarre stereotypic behavior and

inappropriate social behavior in the form of withdrawal or aggression surfaces. This propensity is evident in 4- to 5-year-old monkeys deprived of social contact for brief periods in infancy, and is probably permanent.

Social deprivation is a variable but salient factor in human development. It is well known that social deprivation alone does not produce schizophrenia. However, social developmental theories of schizophrenia have long emphasized the role of social deprivation, fragmented or disordered family communication patterns, seclusiveness, and parental rejection as contributing factors that can interact with genetic predisposition and precipitate the disorder (Neal and Oltmans, 1980). Also, primary psychopathology in individuals or families can lead to social deprivation as a derivative phenomenon (Neal and Oltmans, 1980). Thus, while the cause and effect relationship between schizophrenia and social deprivation may be difficult to unravel in the context of studies in humans, there is a wealth of evidence that the problems are often paired.

(2) The bizarre behavior of socially deprived monkeys, until recently, has not been associated with physiological changes that can be measured peripherally (Meyer and Bowman, 1972), but it is well known that early social deprivation produces brain neuroanatomical changes (Struble and Riesen, 1978). Our preliminary data indicate that socially deprived monkeys have normal levels of CSF biogenic amine metabolites but tend to have increased CSF NE.

This parallels the human situation in that reliable differences in measures of peripheral physiological function, or of DA metabolites in CSF between schizophrenic patients and controls have not been found (van Kammen, 1979; Bowers, 1974; Post et al., 1975; van Praag, 1977). Elevations of CSF NE have been found in paranoid schizophrenic patients (Lake et al., 1980). It is not clear how this finding fits with the DA hypothesis, or why reduction in CSF NE should be associated with clinical improvement following treatment with the DA receptor blocker pimozide (Sternberg et al., 1981).

(3) AMPH increases stereotypic and inappropriate social behavior and CSF NE in previously isolated monkeys at dose levels that have no effect in controls.

It has been suggested that schizophrenia may be caused by hyperactive brain DA systems. The foundations of this hypothesis relate to the ability of AMPH 1) to exacerbate the symptoms of schizophrenic patients at low doses (Janowsky and Davis, 1976; Snyder 1974); 2) to induce symptoms of paranoid schizophrenia in normal subjects at higher doses or with prolonged administration (Angrist et al., 1974; Snyder, 1974); and 3) to induce abnormal behavior in animals (McKinney and Moran, 1981; Haber et al., 1981).

The foundations of this hypothesis also relate to the fact that these effects can be reversed with drugs that block DA receptors and are also useful in the treatment of schizophrenia (Angrist et al., 1974; Snyder, 1974).

However, there are several established findings that are inconsistent with this hypothesis: 1) AMPH administration does not always exacerbate symptoms in well-diagnosed schizophrenic patients, and there are reports of acute improvement. This is also true of treatment with L-dopa; 2) some schizophrenic patients are not helped by neuroleptic treatment and some may show improvement during withdrawal; 3) psychotic behavior can be induced with psychostimulants (AMPH, methylphenidate) even while patients are on long-term treatment with neuroleptics; and 4) combined treatment with psychostimulants and antipsychotic agents sometimes results in no change or a slight improvement in schizophrenic symptoms (Post et al., 1975; Meltzer 1979; Crow, 1980; van Kammen et al., 1982).

Results of this sort have led clinical investigators to suggest that there are two types of schizophrenia, DA-sensitive (type 1) and DA-insensitive (type 2) (Crow, 1980; Angrist et al., 1980), or that patients are differentially sensitive to AMPH challenge depending on state-related factors at the time of challenge (van Kammen et al., 1982). The state versus trait issue, and more global hypotheses about how the presence or lack of AMPH sensitivity relates to the neurobiological substrates of schizophrenia, would be a lot easier to sort out if there were more information about the etiology of such differences, and if changes in brain neurochemical mechanisms could be related to more specific changes than those produced by AMPH.

The studies reported herein, using AMPH as a pharmacological challenge of previously isolated monkeys, are directed, in part, toward this goal. One of the most parsimonious interpretations of the data is that AMPH-induced psychosis in humans and abnormal behavior in animals are likely to be a pharmacological model of the isolation syndrome (withdrawal, aggression, and stereotypy) rather than human schizophrenia. The sensitivity of some schizophrenic patients to AMPH has been assumed to reflect an underlying difference in brain DA system function which produces the disorder. The etiology of these changes is not known, and they have been presumed to be irreversible although DA blocking agents provide symptomatic relief. One etiological factor for increased sensitivity to AMPH in monkeys is early social deprivation, and this sensitivity is marked by increases in behaviors which a number of investigators have likened to those of paranoid schizophrenic patients. Increased CSF NE has also been associated with paranoid schizophrenia in humans, and increased CSF NE also appears to discriminate previously isolated monkeys from controls following AMPH challenge. It may be that AMPH challenge exacerbates the symptoms of the isolation syndrome in humans, and that this has been confused with the effects of a more basic brain dysfunction which is centrally involved in producing the cognitive and perceptual symptoms of schizophrenia. The more primary dysfunction may lead to social deprivation, whether imposed by the individual or the society, and this may lead to the kinds of neurochemical and resultant drug sensitivity changes seen in some schizophrenic patients but not others. The data reported herein do not "prove" that social deprivation, as opposed to some other underlying disease state, is the basis for differential AMPH sensitivity in schizophrenic patients. Rather, they suggest that this is one factor worth attending to, and one which deserves further investigation in humans and animal models. The primate isolation syndrome could be a component of what is clinically labeled as schizophrenia.

ACKNOWLEDGMENTS

The research reported herein was supported by grants MH21892 (NIMH) and HD10570 (NICHD). D-amphetamine was kindly provided by Smith, Kline and French Laboratories.

REFERENCES

Anderson CO, Mason WA (1978) Competitive social strategies in groups of deprived and experienced rhesus monkeys. Develop Psychobiol 11(4): 289–299.

Angrist B, Rotrosen J, Gershon S (1980) Responses to apomorphine, amphetamine, and neuroleptics in schizophrenic subjects. Psychopharmacol 67: 31–38.

Angrist B, Sathananthan G, Wilk S, Gershon SJ (1974) Amphetamine psychosis: Behavioral and biochemical aspects. J Psychiatr Res 11:13–23.

Arling GL, Harlow HF (1967) Effects of social deprivation on maternal behavior of rhesus monkeys. J Compar Physiol Psychol 64(3): 371–377.

Blanc G, Herve D, Simon H, Lisoprawaki A, Glowinski J, Tassin JP (1980) Response to stress of mesocortical-frontal dopaminergic neurons in rats after long term isolation. Nature 284: 265–266.

Bowers MB (1974) Central DA turnover in schizophrenia syndromes. Arch Gen Psychiatr 31:50–54.

Brain PF (1975) What does individual housing mean to a mouse? Life Sci 16: 187–200.

Breese GR (1975) Chemical and immunochemical lesions by specific neurotoxic substances and antisera. In: Handbook of Psychopharmacology, Vol. I. Iversen LL, Iversen SD, Snyder SH (eds) Plenum Press, New York, pp 137–174.

Breese GR, Smith RD, Mueller RA, Howard JL, Prange AJ Jr, Lipton MA, Young LD, McKinney WT, Lewis JK (1973) Induction of adrenal catecholamine synthesizing enzymes following mother-infant separation. Nature New Biol 246(151): 94–96.

Clark DL (1969) Immediate and delayed effects of early, intermediate, and late social isolation in the rhesus monkey. (Doctoral Dissert Univer Wisconsin 1968) Dissert Abs 29: 4862B.

Cooper BR, Breese GR, Howard JL, Grant LD (1972) Enhanced behavioral depressant effects of reserpine and alpha-methylparatyrosine after 6-hydroxydopamine treatment. Psychopharmacol 27: 99–110.

Crow TJ (1980) Molecular pathology of schizophrenia: More than one disease process? Brit Med J 280: 66–68.

Garver DL, Schlemmer RF, Maas JW, Davis JM (1975) A schizophreniform behavioral psychosis mediated by dopamine. Am J Psychiatr 132(1): 33–38.

Godfe DD, Warsh JJ, Stanser HC (1977) Analysis of acetic monoamine by GC-MS. Anal Chem 49(7): 917–918.

Gordon EK, Oliver J, Black K, Kopin IJ (1974) Simultaneous assay by mass fragmentography of vanillylmandelic acid, homovanillic acid, and 3-methoxy-4-hydroxy-phenylethylene glycol in cerebrospinal fluid and urine. Biochem Med 11: 32–40.

Griffin GA, Harlow HF (1966) Effects of three months of total social deprivation on social adjustment and learning in the rhesus monkey. Child Develop 37(3): 535–547.

Haber S, Barchas P, Barchas JD (1981) A primate analogue of amphetamine-induced behaviors in humans. Biol Psychiatr 16(2): 181–195.

Haggendal J, Lindqvist M (1964) Brain monoamine levels and behavior during long-term administration of reserpine. In J Neuropharmacol 3: 59–64.

Harlow HF, Schiltz KA, Harlow KK (1969) Effects of social isolation on learning performance in rhesus monkeys. In: Proceedings of the Second International Congress of Primatology I: Behavior. Carpenter CP (ed) Basel: Karger, pp 178–185.

Janowsky DS, Davis JM (1976) Methylphenidate, dextroamphetamine, and levamphetamine effects on schizophrenic patients. Arch Gen Psychiatr 33: 304–308.

Kasamatsu T, Pettigrew JD (1976) Depletion of brain catecholamines: Failure of ocular dominance shift after molecular occlusion in kittens. Sci 194: 206–209.

Kjellberg B, Randrup A (1973) Disruption of social behavior of vervet monkeys *(Cercopithecus)* by low doses of amphetamines. Pharmakopsychiatr 6: 287–293.

Kraemer GW, Breese GR, Prange AJ, Moran EC, Lewis JK, Kemnitz JW, Bushnell PJ, Howard JL, McKinney WT (1981) Use of 6-hydroxydopamine to deplete brain catecholamines in the rhesus monkey: Effects on urinary catecholamine metabolites and behavior. Psychopharmacol 73: 1–11.

Kraemer GW, Ebert MH, Lake CR, McKinney WT (in press) Early social deprivation: A possible etiology for long-lasting hypersensitivity to d-amphetamine in rhesus monkeys. Psychopharmacology

Kraemer GW, McKinney WT (1979) Interactions of pharmacological agents which alter biogenic amine metabolism and depression: An analysis of contributing factors within a primate model of depression. J Affective Disorders 1: 33–54.

Kraemer GW, McKinney WT, Prange AJ, Breese GR, McMurray TM, Kemnitz J (1976) Isoniazid: Behavioral and biochemical effects in rhesus monkeys. Life Sci 19: 49–60.

Lake CR, Sternberg DE, van Kammen DP, Balenger JC, Ziegler MG, Post RM, Kopin IJ, Bunney WE (1980) Schizophrenia: Elevated cerebrospinal fluid norepinephrine. Sci 207: 331–333.

Lake CR, Ziegler MG, Kopin IJ (1976) Use of plasma NE for evaluation of sympathetic neurone function in man. Life Sci 18: 1313–1326.

Machiayama Y, Utena H, Kikuchi M (1970) Behavioral disorders in Japanese monkeys produced by the long-term administration of methamphetamine. Proc Japan Acad 46(7): 738–743.

Mason WA (1968) Early social deprivation in the nonhuman primates: Implications for human behavior. In: Glass DC (ed) Environmental Influences. New York, Rockefeller University Press and Russell Sage Foundation, pp 70–100.

Mason WA (1978) Social experience and primate cognitive development. In: Burghardt GM, Bekoff M (eds) The Development of Behavior: Comparative and Evolutionary Aspects. Garland Press, New York, pp 233–251.

McKinney WT, Moran EC (1981) Animal models of schizophrenia. Am J Psychiatr 138: 478–483.

Meltzer HY (1979) Biology of schizophrenia subtypes: A review and proposal for method of study. Schiz Bull 5(3): 460–479.

Meyer JS, Bowman RE (1972) Rearing experience, stress and adrenocortico-steroids in the rhesus monkey. Physiol Behav 8: 339–343.

Mirsky IA (1968) Communication of affects in monkeys. In: Glass DC (ed) Environmental Influences. Rockefeller University Press and Russell Sage Foundation, New York, pp 129–137.

Modigh K (1973) Effects of isolation and fighting in mice on the rate of synthesis of noradrenaline, dopamine, and 5-hydroxytryptamine in the brain. Psychopharmacol 33: 1–17.

Moran EC, McKinney WT (1975) Effects of chloropromazine on the vertical chamber syndrome in rhesus monkeys. Arch Gen Psychiatr 32:1409–1413.

Neal JM, Oltmans TF (1980) Schizophrenia. John Wiley and Sons, New York, pp 288–387.

Novak MA, Harlow HF (1975) Social recovery of monkeys isolated for the first year of life: 1. Rehabilitation and therapy. Develop Psychol 11(4): 453–465.

Pearson DE, Teicher MH, Shaywitz BA, Cohen DJ, Young JG, Anderson GM (1980) Environmental influences on body weight and behavior in developing rats after neonatal 6-hydroxydopamine. Sci 209: 715–717.

Pettigrew JD, Kasamatsu T (1978) Local perfusion of noradrenaline maintains visual cortical plasticity. Nature 271: 761–763.

Post RM, Fink E, Carpenter WT, Goodwin FK (1975) Cerebrospinal fluid amine metabolites in acute schizophrenia. Arch Gen Psychiatr 32:1063–1069.

Sackett GP (1972) Isolation rearing in monkeys: Diffuse and specific effects on later behavior. Colloques Internationaux du CNRS, No. 198, Models Animaux Du Comportement Humain. Editions Du Centre National De La Recherche Scientifique 15, Quai Anatole-France, Paris VIIe, pp 61–110.

Sackett GP, Holm RA, Ruppenthal GC (1976) Social isolation rearing: Species differences in behavior of macaque monkeys. Develop Psychol 12(4): 283–288.

Schiorring E (1977) Changes in individual and social behavior induced by amphetamine and related compounds in monkeys and man. In: Ellinwood EH, Kilbey MM (eds) Cocaine and Other Stimulants. Plenum Press, New York, pp 481–522.

Schiorring E, Hecht A (1979) Behavioral effects of low, acute doses of d-amphetamine on the dyadic interaction between mother and infant vervet monkeys *(Cercopithecus aethiops)* during the first six postnatal months. Psychopharmacol 64: 219–224.

Segal DS, Janowsky DS (1978) Psychostimulant-induced behavioral effects: Possible models of schizophrenia. In: Psychopharmacology: A Generation of Progress. Lipton MA, DiMascio A, Killam KF (eds) Plenum Press, New York, 1113–1123.

Segal DS, Knapp S, Kuczenski RT, Mandell AJ (1973) The effects of environmental isolation on behavior and regional rat brain tyrosine hydroxylase and tryptophan hydroxylase activities. Behav Biol 8: 47–53.

Snyder SH (1974) Catecholamines as mediators of drug effects in schizophrenia. In: Schmitt FO, Worden FG (eds) The Neurosciences Third Study Program. MIT Press, pp 721–732.

Sternberg DE, van Kammen DP, Lake CR, Ballenger JC, Marder SR, Bunney WE Jr (1981) The effect of pimozide on CSF norepinephrine in schizophrenia. Am J Psychiatr 138(8): 1045–1051.

Stolk JM, Conner RL, Barchas JD (1974) Social environment and brain biogenic amine metabolism in rats. J Compar Physiol Psychol 87:203–207.

Struble RG, Riesen AH (1978) Changes in cortical dendritic branching subsequent to partial social isolations in stumptailed monkeys. Develop Psychobiol 11(5): 479–486.

Sulser F, Vetulani J, Mobley PL (1978) Commentary: Mode of action of antidepressant drugs. Biochem Pharamcol 27: 257–261.

Suomi SJ, Harlow HF (1971) Abnormal social behavior in young monkeys. In: Hellmuth J (ed) The Exceptional Infant, Vol. II. Bruner-Mazel, New York, pp 483–529.

Suomi SJ, Harlow HF (1972) Social rehabilitation of isolate-reared monkeys. Develop Psychol 6(3): 487–496.

Suomi SJ, Harlow HF, Novak MA (1974) Reversal of social deficits produced by isolation rearing in monkeys. J Human Evolution 3: 527–534.

van Kammen DP (1979) The dopamine hypothesis of schizophrenia revisited. Psychoneuroendocrinology 4: 37–46.

van Kammen DP, Docherty JP, Marder SR, Rayner JN, Bunney WE (1982) Long-term pimozide pretreatment differentially affects behavioral responses to dextroamphetamine in schizophrenia. Arch Gen Psychiatr 39: 275–281.

van Praag HM (1977) The significance of dopamine for the mode of action of neuroleptics and the pathogenesis of schizophrenia. Brit J Psychiatr 130: 463.

Ethopharmacology: Primate Models of Neuropsychiatric Disorders,
pages 219–253

Maternal Separation Studies: Rationale and Methodological Considerations

Martin Reite and Robert Short

Department of Psychiatry, University of Colorado School of Medicine, Denver, Colorado 80262

INTRODUCTION

This chapter examines maternal separation research in nonhuman primates from the following viewpoints: (1) why separation research is important, (2) what some of the advantages and disadvantages of maternal separation paradigms are, (3) how such research is done from a methodological standpoint in our laboratory, and (4) what has been learned to date from such research.

RATIONALE FOR SEPARATION RESEARCH

In psychiatry, separation and loss have long been thought to lead to more serious affective disorders. Richard Burton's "Anatomy of Melancholia," written in 1621, described losses as a central causative factor in affective disorders and extended the concept of loss to include persons, objects, propitious surroundings, and life circumstances (Brink, 1979). In Freud's classic 1917 paper "Mourning and Melancholia," attention was directed at the role of loss in subsequent affective disorders (Freud, 1959). A variety of additional reports have generally supported the relationship between separations and losses and subsequent psychiatric disturbances, most frequently affective disorders (Sethi, 1964; Cadoret et al., 1972; Heinicke, 1973; McKnew and Cytryn, 1973; Stenback, 1965; Paykel et al., 1969).

Clayton, studying psychological reactions to loss, found that 35% of recent widows and widowers met criteria for depression at 1 month, 25% at 4 months, and 17% at 1 year. All in all, a total of 45% of the bereaved met the criteria for a major affective disorder during the first year of bereavement (Clayton, personal communication).

A number of studies have shown that there is a significant increase in morbidity and mortality among the recently bereaved. This work, especially the more recent, embodies the research traditions and techniques of epidemiology, including somewhat better control and improved statistical analysis.

It also tends to be more empirical, deemphasizing particular theoretical explanatory viewpoints. Reviews of this area may be found in Parkes (1972), Jacobs and Ostfeld (1977), and Epstein et al. (1975). Explanations for this observed relationship vary, but include the notion that there may be an as of yet poorly understood set of physiological changes activated by loss or separation.

There is also a large literature linking separation and loss to the onset of a variety of nonpsychiatric medical illnesses. Table I lists medical disorders that at one time or another have been thought to have been precipitated and/or aggravated by separation or loss. This list is not meant to be comprehensive, but rather to indicate the broad scope of disorders thought by various investigators over the past half century to be related in some way to separation or loss. Much of this literature, especially the older literature, comes from the tradition of early psychoanalytically oriented psychosomatic medicine, depends upon anecdotal case reports, and suffers from lack of controls. Some of the more recent studies include appropriate control groups, however, and improved experimental designs. While the prospective controlled studies necessary to substantiate an etiologically significant relationship between separation and loss and the onset of medical disorders have yet to be performed, the existing evidence is certainly suggestive of such a relationship.

Thus separation and loss may rank among the most potent of pathogens with very significant public health implications, yet we know very little about the physiological mechanisms that underlie such pathogenicity. It is for this reason that basic research on the biology of separation and loss is so important.

HISTORICAL PERSPECTIVE OF MATERNAL SEPARATION: RESEARCH IN PRIMATES

The first formal mother-infant separation study in monkeys was reported by Seay et al. (1962). This experiment, in which 4 mother-infant rhesus macaque *(M. mulatta)* pairs were separated from each other for a 3-week period, was designed to determine whether the protest-despair-detachment reaction described by Bowlby (1960, 1961) in human children would similarly be seen in monkey infants. Harlow's group stated that "if the mechanisms producing Bowlby's separation syndrome are as biologically basic as the activation of basic component instinctual responses, a similar syndrome should be produced in infant monkeys following maternal separation." Such was indeed the case, as the rhesus infants responded with initial violent protest followed by a period "appropriately described as despair." Evidence

TABLE I. Review of the Literature of the Past Several Decades in Which Separations and/or Losses Are Implicated as Etiologically Significant Antecedents of a Variety of Medical Illnesses[a]

Disease	Authors	Year	Comment
Asthma	French	1934	Asthma attacks precipitated by temptation which threatens to estrange the patient from a mother figure. No controls. Anecdotal.
Cancer	Evans	1926	Anecdotal case reports of cancer onset frequently following losses of various types.
	Bacon et al.	1952	Anecdotal. No control. Losses and separations precede some cases of cancer.
	Peller	1952	". . . widows have higher cancer incidence than other women of the same age."
	Greene	1954	Separations and losses important antecedents of leukemia and lymphoma in 17 of 20 men and boys.
	Kowal	1955	Review of 18th and 19th century literature found relationship between despair and hopelessness on onset of cancer.
	Greene et al.	1956	Losses and separations precede onset of lymphoma and leukemia in adults. No controls.
	Greene and Miller	1958	Separation from a significant object often precedes development of leukemia in children. No controls.
	LeShan	1959	Review article. "The most consistently reported relevant psychological factor has been the loss of a major emotional relationship prior to the first-noted symptoms of the neoplasm."
	Bahnson and Bahnson	1966	". . . loss and depression may be significant antecedents to the onset of clinical cancer. . ."
	Jacobs and Charles	1980	25 children, retrospective, matched control group.
Congestive failure	Chambus and Reiser	1953	Stress considered generally, some separations and losses. Analytic, retrospective, no controls.
	Perlman et al.	1971	105 patients, 50 controls. Separation an important event antedating hospitalization.
Diabetes mellitus	Hinkle and Wolf	1952	Real or fantasized loss related to ketosis; retrospective, not controlled.

(continued)

TABLE I. Review of the Literature of the Past Several Decades in Which Separations and/or Losses Are Implicated as Etiologically Significant Antecedents of a Variety of Medical Illnesses[a] (continued)

Disease	Authors	Year	Comment
	Slawson et al.	1963	25 new adult diabetics; 14 had history of definite object loss; retrospective, no controls.
	Stein and Charles	1971	Adolescents with diabetes had higher incidence of loss and severe family disturbance than matched nondiabetic chronically ill adolescents.
	Leaverton et al.	1980	37 children with matched controls showed parent loss significantly higher in children who later developed diabetes.
Functional uterine bleeding	Heiman	1956	Experience of loss preceding bleeding in significant number of cases. Retrospective, no controls.
Hypertension	Mammen	1979	Adult uncontrolled retrospective case report.
Hyperthyroidism	Mittelmann	1933	Onset of Graves disease may follow loss. Retrospective. Anecdotal.
	Conrad	1934	Relationship between fear or loss and symptom onset. Retrospective, no controls.
	Litz	1949	Separation or loss anecdotally related to onset in many cases. Retrospective, no controls.
	Kleinschmidt et al.	1956	Loss or separation may precede thyrotoxicosis. Retrospective, anecdotal, no controls.
	Morillo and Gardner	1979	4 case reports in children; retrospective, anecdotal, no controls.
Infectious hepatitis	Papper and Handy	1956	12 of 25 patients had threatened or actual separation or loss.
Lupus erythematosus	McClary et al.	1955	Loss of significant personal relationship preceded exacerbation of complaints. Case reports, retrospective, anecdotal.
Obesity	Hamburger	1951	Some cases related to separation and/or feared or fantasized loss. Retrospective, no controls.
Peptic ulcer	Christodoulou et al.	1977	25 children; retrospective, matched control group.
	Ackerman et al.	1981	24 children; retrospective, matched control group.

(continued)

TABLE I. Review of the Literature of the Past Several Decades in Which Separations and/or Losses Are Implicated as Etiologically Significant Antecedents of a Variety of Medical Illnesses[a] (continued)

Disease	Authors	Year	Comment
Porphyria	Fedders	1972	Attacks of AIP apparently triggered by loss and subsequent mourning. Case report. Retrospective. No controls.
Reynaud's disease	Millet et al.	1953	Vasospasm attacks brought on by conflict activated by fear of loss. No controls.
Rheumatoid arthritis	Cobb et al.	1939	Mentions grief as antecedent.
	Ludwig	1952	Onset and subsequent exacerbations related to events implying loss of security. Retrospective; no controls.
	Henoch et al.	1978	88 children; matched control group, retrospective.
Streptococcal infection	Meyer and Haggerty	1962	Losses are among the significant stresses that precede onset of streptococcal infections in children. Retrospective, no controls.
Tuberculosis	Wittkower	1949	Separations important antecedents in some cases. Retrospective, no controls.
	Kissen	1956	Emotional factors found to precede onset of TB significantly more frequently than in control group—mainly real or threatened separations or losses. Retrospective.
	Kissen	1957	Real and/or threatened separations or losses frequent antecedents to relapse in pulmonary tuberculosis. Retrospective.
Ulcerative colitis	Lindemann	1945	History showed various forms of bereavement as the most important precipitating factor in 45 patients. No controls, retrospective.
	Engel	1955	Review article. Losses or separations as antecedents of helplessness or despair, thought to be etiologically significant.

[a]Most of this literature is of a retrospective, anecdotal, case report type, as the proper prospective controlled studies are virtually impossible to perform in man.

of detachment, following reunion, was apparent in only one of the four infants, however. These authors interpreted their findings as "being generally in accord with Bowlby's theory of primary separation anxiety as an explanation principle for the basic primate separation mechanisms."

In a second study reported by Seay and Harlow in 1965, eight rhesus mother-infant pairs were separated from each other for a 2-week period. Olfactory, auditory, and visual contact, present in the first study, were denied in this experiment. Once again a two-stage protest-despair like reaction was noted in the separated infants.

The first of a series of studies of maternal separation in rhesus infants was reported by Hinde et al. in 1966. This report described an initial period of distress followed by behavioral "depression" during a 6-day period of separation during which the four separated infants (aged 30–32 weeks) remained in their social groups. Again, no evidence of detachment was noted on reunion. A subsequent study in Hinde's laboratory demonstrated that infants separated from their mother for 13 days exhibited a greater degree of depression of locomotor and play behavior following reunion with the mother than did those separated for 6 days. Further, some of the effects of 6-day separations were still evident up to 6 to 24 months later, suggesting early maternal separation experiences might have long-term effects on behavioral development (Hinde and Spencer-Booth, 1971).

During the same time period, Kaufman and Rosenblum were examining the effects of maternal separation on pigtail *(M. nemestrina)* and bonnet *(M. radiata)* monkey infants. In a study of four group-living pigtailed infants whose mothers were removed for 4 weeks, three of the infants became profoundly depressed behaviorally for a period of about a week, exhibiting a reaction phenomenologically similar to the "anaclitic depression" described by Spitz in 1946 (Kaufman and Rosenblum, 1967). Kaufman and Rosenblum interpreted the depressed behavior in the separated pigtail infants as a manifestation of Engel's theory of conservation withdrawal (Engel, 1962). In contrast, similar maternal separation experiments in group-living bonnet infants disclosed that the separated infants exhibited an initial period of behavioral agitation, but no clear-cut evidence of behavioral depression (Rosenblum and Kaufman, 1968). These apparent species differences in the response to maternal separation were attributed to differences in bonnet and pigtail social group behavior patterns which permitted separated bonnet infants to approach and be adopted by other adults, an uncommon occurrence in pigtail social groups (Kaufman and Rosenblum, 1969a).

A more recent seminal experiment by Kaufman and Stynes (1978), in which a bonnet infant was separated not only from its mother, but from all conspecifics as well, and was left with the adult pigtail members of a mixed-species group, demonstrated that under these conditions, a bonnet infant might exhibit as severe a behavioral depression as is characteristic of a separated pigtail infant.

Maternal separation experiments have been performed as well in several other species of monkeys, including *Erythrocebus patas* (Preston et al., 1970), squirrel monkey *(Saimiri sciureus)* (Jones and Clark, 1973; Kaplan 1970), java monkey *(Macaca irus)* (Schlottmann and Seay, 1972), *M. fascicularis* (Hrdina and van Kulmiz, 1978), and langur monkey *(Presbytis entellus)* (Dolhinow, 1980). All species studied to date have demonstrated considerable similarity in the initial, or protest, response to separation. The subsequent period of behavioral depression or despair has been shown to be quite variable in form and degree from one study to another, likely owing in part to both species differences and differences in experimental design.

A number of different separation paradigms have been used, including variations on the mother-infant separation paradigm (Chappel and Meier, 1975; Hinde and McGinnes, 1975; Suomi et al., 1976), and varying age peer separations (Suomi et al., 1970), nuclear family separations (Suomi et al., 1975), mixed-species paradigms (Kaufman and Stynes, 1978; Reite and Snyder, 1982), and, in adult pigtailed monkeys, separation from important social companions (Rasmussen and Reite, 1982). Variables such as age, sex, maternal dominance, social group composition, and the like have also been studied (Hinde and Spencer-Booth, 1971; Hinde and McGinnes, 1977). This large body of work has recently been reviewed by Mineka and Suomi (1978).

The behavioral response to separation has been viewed from several theoretical perspectives, including Bowlby's (1960a, 1961) theory of primary separation anxiety (Seay et al., 1962), Spitz's (1946) anaclitic depression (Harlow et al., 1972), Engel's (1962) conservation withdrawal (Kaufman and Rosenblum, 1967), Seligman's (1975) theory of learned helplessness (Kaufman, 1977), and Solomon and Corbett's (1974) opponent process theory of motivation (Mineka and Suomi, 1978). The two-stage agitation-depression or protest-despair behavioral response to maternal separation has been thought by several investigators to represent a valuable animal model of certain human loss-related depressive disorders, and much of the research on maternal separation has proceeded with this goal in mind (McKinney and Bunney, 1979; Reite, 1977).

We and others have suggested that the organismic reaction to maternal separation may be homologous in monkeys and humans (Bowlby, 1973; Reite, 1977) and that this may be due to the high probability that attachment systems generally may be homologous among high primates, all of which share a significant common evolutionary history. Thus, we believe that what we learn from studying attachment systems and the response to separation and loss in one species (e.g., an Old World monkey) may have general relevance to improved understanding of similar phenomena in other species, including humans. We are by no means suggesting equivalence across species, but only a high likelihood of homology of significant heuristic import.

Consideration of the historical origin of separation research is not complete without considering two additional factors. First, most of the early research began with mother-infant separation paradigms, but for a variety of reasons a number of other experimental paradigms arose from this beginning. Among these reasons for developing new designs are that the mother-infant separations are intrinsically more expensive than the type of repeated separations possible with peer-raised animals. Also, the elaboration of similarities and differences among the various separation paradigms (e.g., mother from infant, infant from surrogate, peer from peer, adult from nuclear family) is both interesting and conceptually important.

Secondly, the rationale for separation research has evolved with time. Original studies were designed primarily to evaluate certain seemingly fundamental psychological principles using an animal model. For example, some of Harlow's early work was designed to evaluate what aspects of the mother-infant relationship were most important, this being partly in response to some of Freud's early psychoanalytic theories, especially as concerns orality. Similarly, some of Hinde's work was designed to evaluate Bowlby's theories of separation anxiety, and Kaufman's early work was designed to examine the concept of object loss. It was not long after the beginning of this research that it was seen as being relevant to the area of clinical depression, with separation in nonhuman primates serving as a model for certain aspects of human loss-related depression (McKinney and Bunney, 1969; Reite, 1977). More recently, the broader issue of the role of separation and loss as etiologically significant pathogenic factors in human health generally has become an important rationale for continued research in this area.

As the rationale for this work has seen its emphasis shift with time, scientists involved in this research have seen the nature of the questions change in terms of what data are of most relevance. The work began with simple descriptive behavioral changes, with the emphasis shifting during the last decade to understanding the physiological changes accompanying such behavioral changes and, more recently, to understanding the mechanisms underlying what is clearly a very complex psychobiological reaction. This shift in emphasis with time has been due in part to improvements in our technological capability to monitor physiological variables, stemming from recent advances in microelectronic and to improvements in instrumentation for measuring biochemical and pharmacological correlates of behavioral change.

ADVANTAGES AND DISADVANTAGES OF MOTHER-INFANT SEPARATION PARADIGMS

As mentioned, a number of different types of separation paradigms have been used in nonhuman primate research to study the behavioral and, in some more recent studies, physiological correlates of separation and loss. Each paradigm, whether it is mother-infant, peer-peer, infant-surrogate, or nuclear family separations, has specific advantages and disadvantages. The paradigm to be chosen depends to a large extent on the emphasis of the study, including its theoretical basis as well as a number of practical considerations. In this section, some of the advantages and disadvantages specific to mother-infant paradigms will be examined.

When viewing separation from the standpoint of attachment theory, i.e., the disruption of attachment bonds, the mother-infant separation paradigm is important in that the mother-infant bond is likely the strongest attachment bond the infant will ever experience. Its nature may certainly be influenced to some extent by the nature of the mother-infant relationship, and the as yet poorly understood individual differences in the abilities of both mother and infant to form attachments, but by limiting oneself to considering separations of infants from mothers, one is hopefully examining "attachment" in as close to an unadulterated form as possible.

Additionally, the mother-infant attachment bond is likely to be prototype of subsequent attachments to be formed by the infant, including peer bonds, nuclear family bonds, and, as appropriate (which is true at least in the case of man), more derivative attachment relationships to broader aspects of culture, including material objects and theoretical constructs such as self-image. Thus, experimental manipulation of the early mother-infant bond allows one to address empirically the issue to what extent such manipulations may alter, skew, or interfere with the development of subsequent attachment relationships, or, perhaps more broadly, the general area of object relations.

Finally, there would appear to be a high likelihood of homology between mother-infant attachment and infant-from-mother separation, in both human and at least some nonhuman primates. When dealing with the very young organism of either group, we avoid the complexities that accompany subsequent development, especially in the case of man, including such entities as psychic mechanisms, highly developed cognitive structures and processes, and complex social influences. But also the nonhuman primate model offers direct applicability to separated human infant reactions to temporary or permanent separations from the primary care giver. The elucidation of the physiological reactions are especially important in understanding the problems children may experience after loss.

There are as well, however, disadvantages to mother-infant separation paradigms. First, it is likely that more contributes to the response to separation, both behaviorally and physiologically in the case of the infant, than the disruption of an attachment bond. The mother plays several important roles in the relationship including such things as being a source of nutrition, providing a buffer between the infant and other individuals, soothing the infant in times of distress, and in general serving as an important regulator of the timing and rhythmicity of behavioral and biological rhythms. It is difficult to separate these factors from attachment as each may be an important component of the overall construct. Indeed, emerging evidence suggests that alteration of nutritional status or some closely related factors may be involved in modulating and shaping the response to separation from mother in young monkeys.

Second, rapid developmental changes occurring in young infants may serve to increase the variability in the model, especially if repeated separations are performed. Infants change rapidly with time in a number of important domains; thus age at separation, as it may relate to the specific developmental status and rate of development for a particular infant, may be a significant confounding influence on outcome. The interactions of development with the social and physical environment are not yet well understood.

Finally, as mentioned earlier, mother-infant separation paradigms in nonhuman primates are intrinsically expensive, generally more so than either peer separation paradigms or nuclear family separation paradigms. There is only a limited time period over which separations can be performed, and keeping infants and mothers together means that the mothers are not available for continued breeding. Separations performed before approximately 4 months of age are unnecessarily confounded by the concurrent withdrawal of mother's nutritional support. After approximately 10–12 months of age, the mother-infant separation experiments are confounded by the infant's moving into the transition to adolescence. The time constraint restricts the number of repeated separations possible, and hence more subjects are required to detect the subtleties of the response.

The aforementioned disadvantages can also be seen, however, as typical areas of central importance to our improved understanding of the complexities of early human development. Thus research that helps define these, at present somewhat unclear, areas and interactions should prove to have considerable clinical relevance for proper assessment and management of disturbances in early development.

METHODOLOGICAL CONSIDERATIONS

The behavioral and physiological data we have collected to date during various separation experiments has spanned over a decade. While we have constantly been striving toward a goal of computer based behavioral scoring and on-line processing of physiological information, the technology (hardware and software) available to do so has changed rapidly during this time period. We began by scoring behavior on mechanical keyboard clock counters, then moved to dictating observed behavior onto audio tape and later playing it back and scoring it on a computer keyboard, to the present time when remote terminals are used on line for all behavior observations. With physiological data we began by hand-scoring physiological variables from the paper polygraph record, to computer analysis of prerecorded physiological data from FM analog tape, to the present time when all physiological variables (except nocturnal sleep patterns) can be processed on line in real time. In this section, we will describe the current status of the behavior and physiology data collection and processing systems as they are used at present in our laboratory.

The System for Behavioral Data Collection and Analyses

Behavioral samples are obtained using a continuous real-time measuring technique (cf. Sackett, 1978). For a predetermined period of time (software variable anywhere from 1 to 30 minutes), an observer watches a single "focal" animal through a one-way window and records behavioral events as they occur on a computer terminal using the BEIN software (software, discussed later, is summarized in Fig. 1). The taxonomy in use was originally derived from the behavioral taxonomy for pigtail and bonnet monkeys by Kaufman and Rosenblum (1966), with additions and alterations as appropriate for particular experimental designs and questions. Our current taxonomy is composed of over 100 possible behavioral events which are coded by unique alphanumeric keystrokes, each of which can be modified with additional symbols, indicating the initiator and recipient of interactions if appropriate. Some behaviors are "duration" items, having discrete start and stop times and finite durations; others are "frequency" items which are considered to be momentary events which have but a single time of occurrence. Software provides continuous visual feedback on the observer's terminal as to which

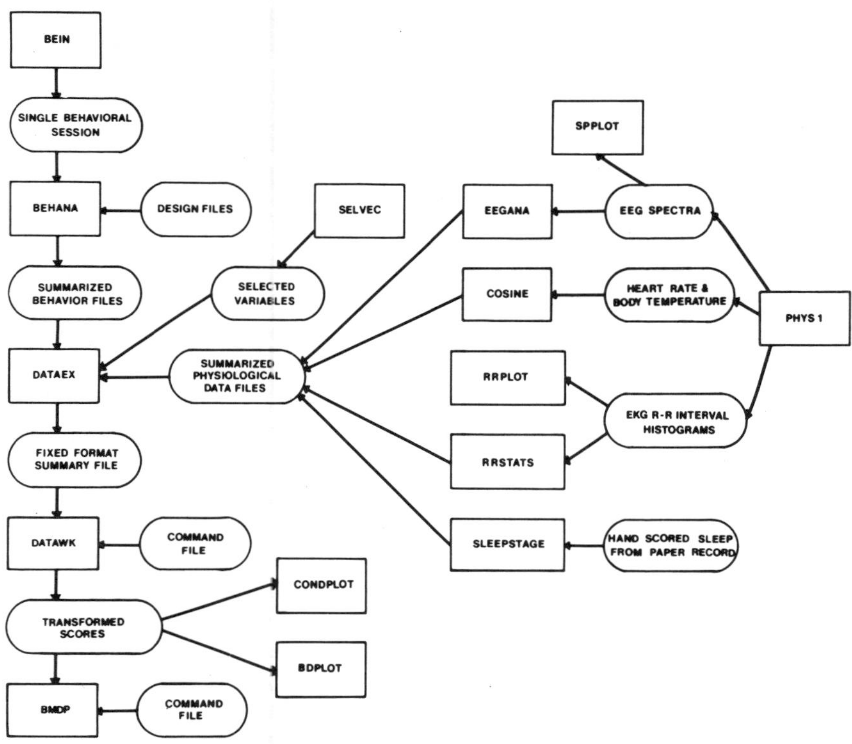

Fig. 1. A summary of the interactive software developed for managing the behavioral and physiological data base. Rectangles represent software systems; ovals represent command and data files. Behavioral data originates with keyboard entry of ongoing behavior via BEIN. Physiological data are collected and partially processed via PHYS1.

events are currently ongoing. Experienced observers rarely look at the terminal, using a "touch-type" method of keyboard entry and keeping their eyes on the animal. The visual display is very useful for beginning observers, however, who may need to be reminded to end certain behaviors, and which and how many behaviors are simultaneously ongoing. An editing mode is available at the end of a session which allows the addition, deletion, and/or modification of individual entries and the inclusion of a narrative comment if desired. Sessions are stored on a computer disk file retaining the subject identification, start time, observer, condition, and date, plus the absolute start and stop times with temporal sequence for each recorded behavioral event.

Our present computer system used for behavioral data collection and analysis is presented as a block diagram in Fig. 2. The system is composed

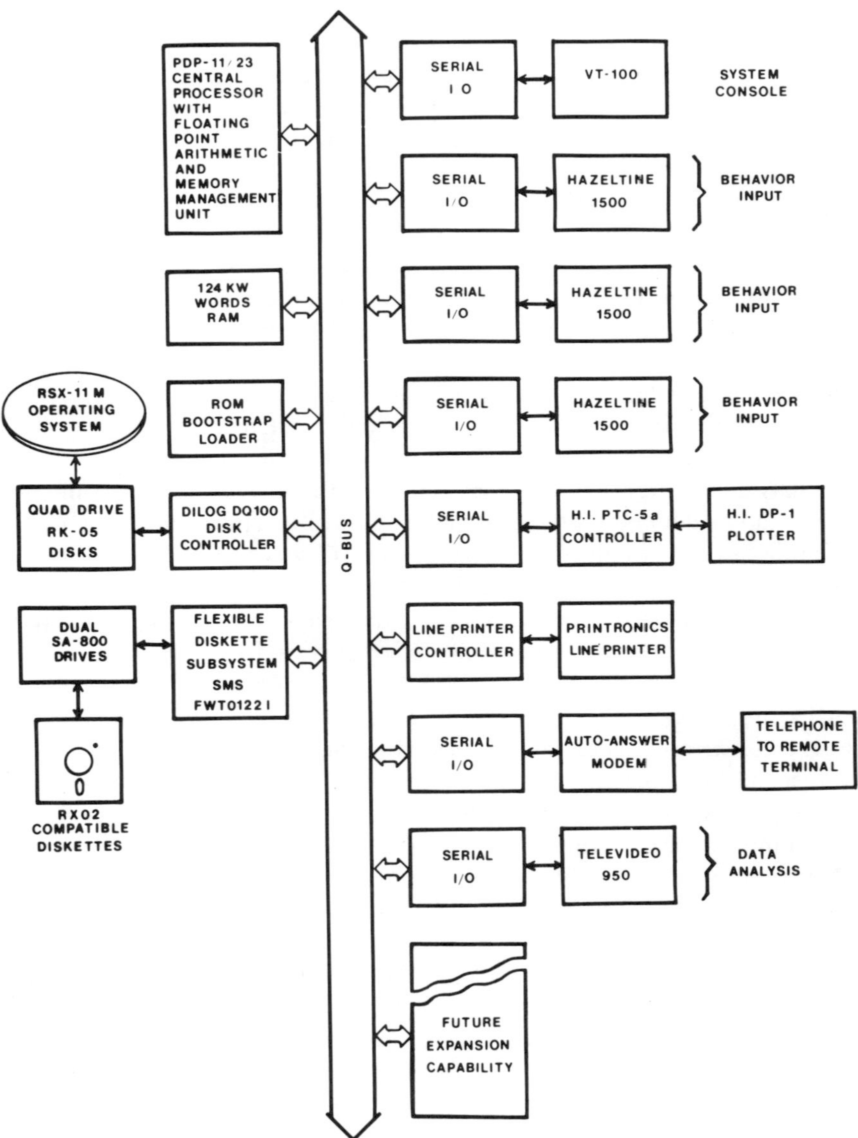

Fig. 2. Block diagram of our current PDP-11/23 processor-based computer system.

of a PDP-11/23 central processor, running under the RSX-11M operating system, with seven input/output (I/O) ports, a line printer, 4 RKO5 disk drives, a dual floppy disk system, and 120 K words of memory. RSX is a time-sharing system, and thereby permits several observers to collect behavioral data simultaneously. Generally only three terminals are used for behavior data collection, and the other I/O lines support CRT terminals used primarily for software design, system maintenance, and interactive data analysis. Also, an incremental digital plotter fills a port for plotting of physiological and behavioral data.

Our approach for summarizing behavioral data to date has been to calculate the durations and frequencies for all behavioral categories across a number of sessions. Scores are normalized by computing the percent of total time observed, in the case of the duration items, and frequency per 1,000 seconds for the frequency items. The period of time over which sessions are summarized in this manner depends on the experimental design, but up to approximately 9 hours of observation time can currently be analyzed to obtain a single summary score for each taxonomic item.

The software, developed in house, for summarizing and managing data is summarized in Fig. 1. Depending on the experimental design, summary scores can be automatically computed by animal or observation time period using the proper design file as input to the BEHANA controlling software. Generally a summary file is retained at this step containing scores for all variables summarized over the particular time period or treatment condition. Behavioral variables of interest may be selected using the SELVEC routine and, when desired, merged with physiological information using the DATAEX program, which organizes the scores into a fixed format summary matrix in which the columns correspond to the selected variables and rows correspond to the cases. DATAWK optionally linearly combines, rescores, rearranges, deletes, and/or transforms scores either interactively or by use of a command file. Variables may also be added to the summary file from other similar summary files. A number of graphic routines (BDPPLOT, CONDPLOT in Fig. 1) have been written to plot summary statistics across time or to create profiles of individuals. Alternatively, scores can easily be entered into canned statistical packages; we currently use the BMDP system (Dixon et al., 1981), which is supported by the RSK-11M operating system.

In addition to focal animal observation, "scan" type observations, in which an entire social group is watched continuously for occurrence of relatively low frequency behaviors (e.g., aggressive or dominance altercations, sexual behaviors, and complex social interactions involving several animals simultaneously), can be recorded on line as well.

The Physiological Data Collection System

The physiological data collection system consists of three major components: (1) the implantable biotelemetry system, (2) the receiving/demodulating system, and (3) the physiology data collection, storage, and processing system.

The implantable biotelemetry systems transmit seven channels of data using a pulse-amplitude modulated 1.7 KHz subcarrier and an FM carrier in the VHF band (for details, see Pauley and Reite, 1981). The system consists of two packages, an interconnecting cable, and cables to record sites of interest. One package contains the amplifier and signal conditioning circuitry, multiplexer, temperature-sensing thermistors, and RF circuitry; the second package contains a 3.7 V, 1/2 AA lithium cell, and a magnetically activated bistable latching reed switch. The first (electronics) package measures 19 × 19 × 6 mm prior to implantation. The entire system, complete with battery, weighs approximately 25 grams when fully encapsulated prior to implantation. Physiological information transmitted includes the electrocardiogram (EKG), body temperature (BT), eye movement (EOG), muscle activity (EMG), and three channels of electroencephalographic (EEG) activity. The transmission range is nominally 10 m in a noisy environment, with a battery life of about 1,000 hours.

All surgical procedures are performed under general (pentobarbital) anesthesia. The two biotelemetry packages are implanted extraperitoneally, beneath abdominal wall musculature. Electrode cables are routed subcutaneously to recording sites of interest. Details of the surgical procedure have been published previously (Reite et al., 1973; Reite and Pauley, 1976).

The implanted infants and their mothers are usually housed apart from the group just prior to and during recovery from surgery for the administration of prophylactic antibiotics. Sutures are removed 10 days after surgery and the mother and infant are returned to the social group. Once the telemetry systems are turned on, physiological data transmission is normally continuous (24 hours a day) for the duration of the experiment.

The telemetered RF signal is received on one of several tuned dipole antennas, the antenna with the best signal being selected automatically (Pauley and Reite, 1977). The signal is then routed to an FM receiver, demodulated, and amplified and conditioned by a Grass model 78 polygraph with 7P511 amplifiers. A continuous paper record is obtained at night during the lights-out period (2000–0700 hours); during the day generally only short samples of paper recording are obtained. An example of the polygraph output is illustrated in Fig. 3.

A block diagram of the physiology data collection system is illustrated in Fig. 4. Three channels of physiological data are continuously monitored by

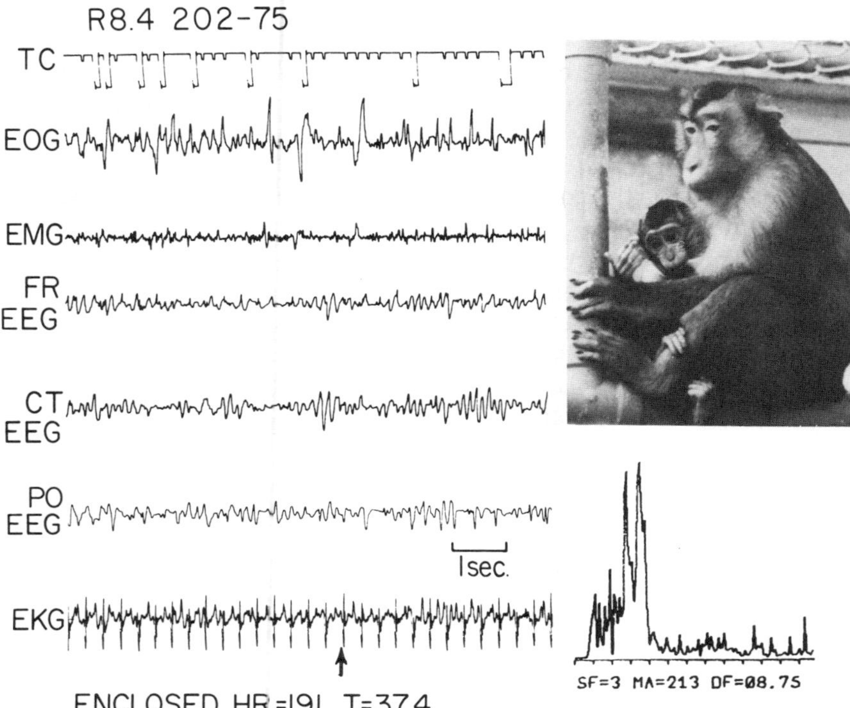

Fig. 3. Infant number R8.4 enclosed by her mother. The simultaneously transmitted physiological data are illustrated on the left. Abbreviations are as follows: TC = time code, EOG = electro-oculogram, EMG = electro-myogram, FR EEG = frontal electroencephalogram, CT EEG = central temporal EEG, PO EEG = parietal-ocipital EEG, EKG = electrocardiogram. Photo was taken at the time indicated by the arrow. The infant's heart rate was 191 beats per minute and her body temperature was 37.4°C. In the lower right-hand corner is the power spectrum of the illustrated epoch of CT EEG.

a dedicated LSI 11/03 based computer system, providing on-line collection, processing, and floppy disk storage. For each 1-minute period we obtain numerical values for heart rate (HR), body temperature (BT), 64 components of the EEG power spectrum, providing a possible 1,440 such samples per 24 hour day. The program controlling the acquisition of physiological data is labeled PHYS1 in Fig. 1. Typically, at the beginning of each 1 minute (determined by the system clock), body temperature (encoded on a temperature sensitive, frequency-modulated square wave) is sampled for 1 second, converted, and stored, then EEG and EKG are alternately sampled for the remainder of the 1-minute period. A total of approximately 20 seconds of EKG is sampled during each 1-minute period.

A pattern recognition algorithm written by R.T. Mast (unpublished manuscript) is used to separate true QRS complexes from noise, as noise introduced at various points in the overall system precludes the use of a Schmitt trigger or other simple threshold-detecting techniques. The algorithm computes the first difference between points sampled at the rate of 500 samples/sec to obtain the velocity of the EKG signal. The resultant velocity is plotted against the amplitude to obtain a loop (see Fig. 5). The clockwise trajectory of any QRS complex follows, within certain limits, the same path each time; spurious noise spikes tend to follow a different trajectory. By employing a dynamic learning set within the algorithm, which simply keeps track of a subset of coordinates for the last five accepted QRS complexes, a window can be defined. Candidate QRS complex trajectories pass through the window whereas noise spikes have random paths. When the incoming signal trajectory meets certain criteria, the spike is either discarded or identified as a QRS complex, and the selected coordinates from its trajectory are used to update the learning set. The time of each detected QRS complex is stored and used in computing heart rate inbeats per minute and the resulting value included in the R-R interval histogram.

HR and BT values can be processed by a variety of routines. Normally our processing includes obtaining a 24-hour (from 0900 to 0900) plot of HR and BT each day and estimates of a number of circadian parameters. A hard copy printout of such a plot and the estimated parameters are illustrated in Fig. 6.

Additionally, sequentially stacked R-R interval histograms with hidden line suppression may be plotted as a function of time. The two 4½-hour sequentially stacked R-R interval histograms, illustrated in Fig. 7, were obtained from a normative baseline condition (top trace) and the first night of maternal separation (bottom trace). Each vertical line represents a single histogram of the R-R intervals for 1 minute of data. Each line represents, therefore, about 20 seconds of actual EKG, and provides an estimate of the mode and variabiltiy of R-R intervals within that time sample. Such a display technique gives an indication of the variability of heart rate across time, the prominence of ultradian rhythms, and shows, when compared with EEG spectra plots and sleep-stage plots, the correspondence of HR and rhythm with EEG and sleep-stage patterns. The existence of cardiac arrhythmias is suggested by bimodal or multimodal peaks on each R-R interval histogram; skipped beats, for example, would be indicated by a second (smaller) peak at a rate of one-half the modal rate. In Fig. 7, the top trace shows the type of

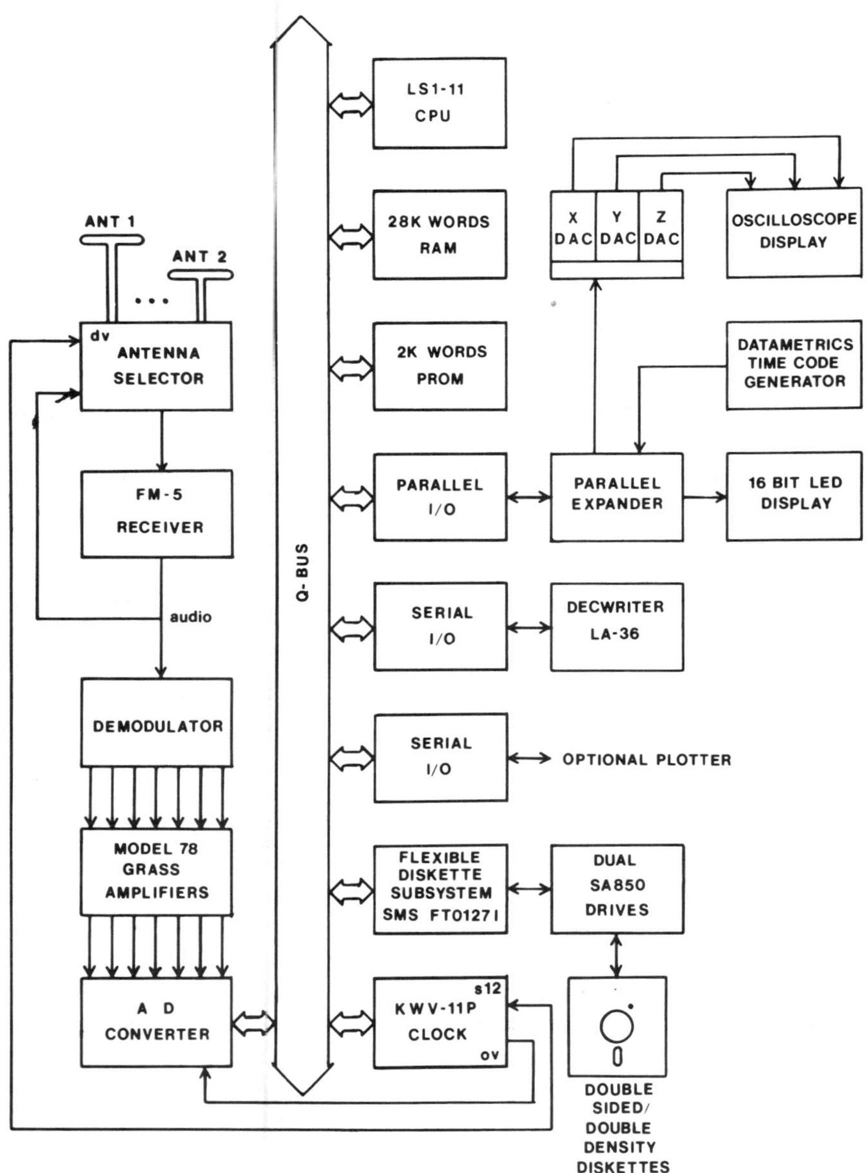

Fig. 4. Block diagram of our current LSI-11 processor-based physiological data acquisition system, including the antenna selector, FM receiver, demodulator, and Grass amplifiers. Processed data are stored on floppy diskettes.

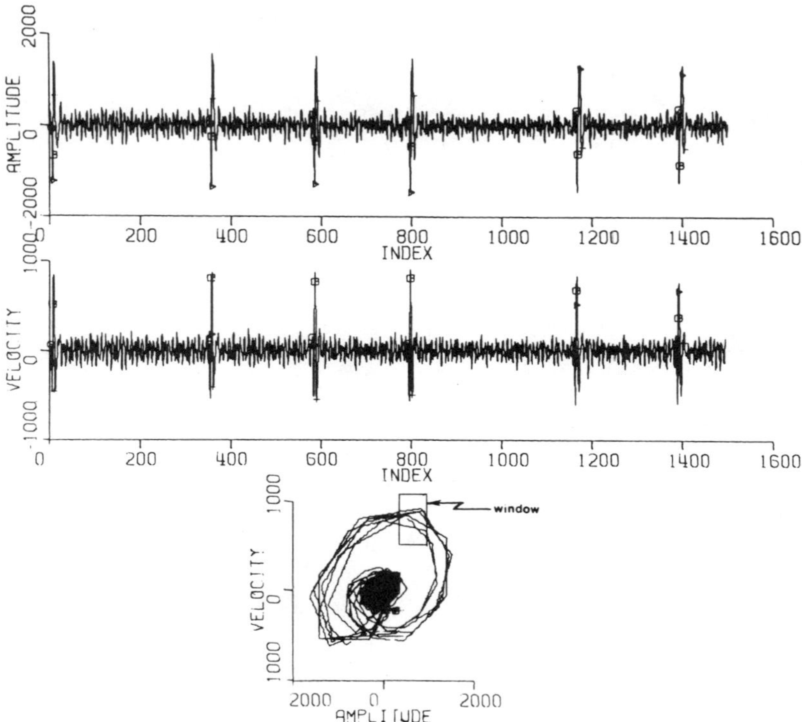

Fig. 5. The top plot is the EKG data sampled at 500/sec plotted as a function of time. The middle plot represents the lag one difference or velocity as a function of time. The bottom plot is the velocity plotted as a function of amplitude.

variability seen in heart rate during sleep in a typical baseline night, from about 2130 hours to after 0200 hours. Contrast this record with that obtained from a first night of separation directly below. The baseline night trace (top) shows a mean rate of approximately 130–140 bpm, with considerable variability of the peak rate as a function of time, as well as a comparatively tight modal distribution of R-R intervals. By comparison, the separation night stacked histogram (bottom) shows a mean rate of less than 120 bpm, loss of minute-to-minute variability of the maximum, and a considerable skewness of the distribution in the downward direction indicative of arrhythmias.

The analog EEG signal is sampled for a total of about 20 seconds during each minute at a rate of 128 samples per second. Fast fourier transforms are

FI1:P492.193

```
COSIN3 : COSINE ANALYSIS FOR DATA IN "PHYS1A" FORMAT

ENTER INPUT DIRECTORY FILE SPECIFICATION : FI1:P492.193

HEART RATE---
LEVEL =   160.08      A =      8.48       B =     52.23
CENTERED LEVEL =   162.16       AMPLITUDE =     52.92         PHASE =       5.38
MSE=469.15   F=338.83     NN=215    MEAN D=199.84    MEAN N=112.31

BODY TEMP---
LEVEL =     37.69      A =      0.09       B =      1.76
CENTERED LEVEL =    37.80       AMPLITUDE =      1.76         PHASE =       5.80
MSE=   0.18   F=945.00     NN=209    MEAN D= 39.07    MEAN N= 36.33

NUMBER OF TIME POINTS PER DATA POINT =        6
```

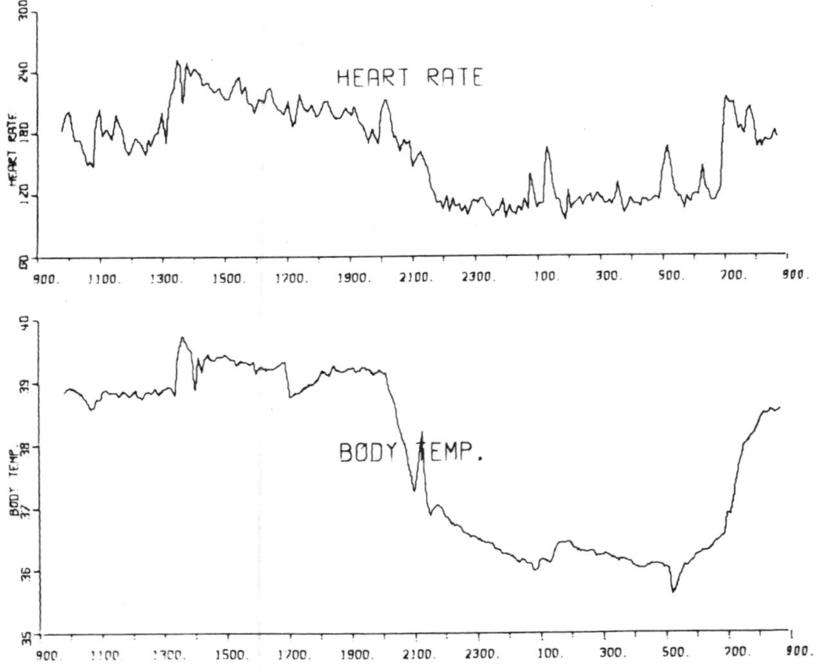

Fig. 6. Plots of 24-hour HR and BT samples collected by the dedicated LSI-11 microprocessor and circadian parameters from the COSINE program. Each point is an average of approximately 6 minutes of data. Least-squares cosine functions are fit to the data yielding estimates of level, amplitude, and phase for both HR and BT. Also computed are the mean day and mean night HR and BT. The statistical fit of the fitted cosine is assessed with the F ratio with 2 and NN degrees of freedom.

computed on two second samples, and the resulting ten power spectra averaged to provide a single mean spectrum for each minute. Each averaged spectra has ½ Hz resolution from ½ to 31½ Hz. Stored EEG power spectra can be processed as desired. Normally we plot a stacked spectral display with hidden line suppression for each 24-hour period, using spectra obtained for each 1-minute epoch, as well as plots representing the absolute amount of power in any selectable EEG frequency band during the same time period (SPPLOT in Fig. 1). Alternatively, ratios of power in one band to power in another can be examined.

The all-night paper polygraph record is visually scored by hand for sleep stage on a computer terminal by entering a keyboard character for each page (20 second) of paper record; this sleep file is then processed by the SLEEP-STAGE program (see Fig. 1) to provide an all-night sleep-stage plot and numerical values for each of 15 different sleep variables.

Fig. 8 illustrates a plot of stacked EEG power spectra recorded from the central-temporal cortical region for a 4-hour period from 2000 hours to 0000 hours (midnight) during a baseline night, as well as a portion of the all-night sleep-stage plot. Also included are plots of the EEG power in the delta band (1–4 Hz), and the percent of total power in the EEG for each of four bands (see legend). Note these bands are somewhat different from conventional human EEG frequency bands. The occurrence of deep sleep (stages 3 and 4) is accompanied by an increase in absolute power of the delta band. Also note the redistribution in power across the four bands preceding sleep onset and the onset of the illustrated REM period.

Overall then, this behavioral and physiological data collection/analysis system provides for on-line collection of both behavioral and physiological data, a good bit of real-time processing of physiological data, and rapid turnaround for the preliminary analysis of the remainder of the data. The ability to record continuous physiological data enhances the opportunity to detect alterations in biological rhythmicity of various frequencies, and diminishes the likelihood of errors introduced by sampling bias. Similarly, the ability to perform detailed correlations of physiology with behavior is limited only by how much behavior one wishes to collect (behavioral observations being very labor intensive).

PHYSIOLOGICAL CORRELATES OF SEPARATION

Since the beginning of our laboratory's research efforts studying the physiology of separation in monkeys, we have studied over 60 pigtailed and bonnet macaque infants in a variety of separation paradigms. Most of these

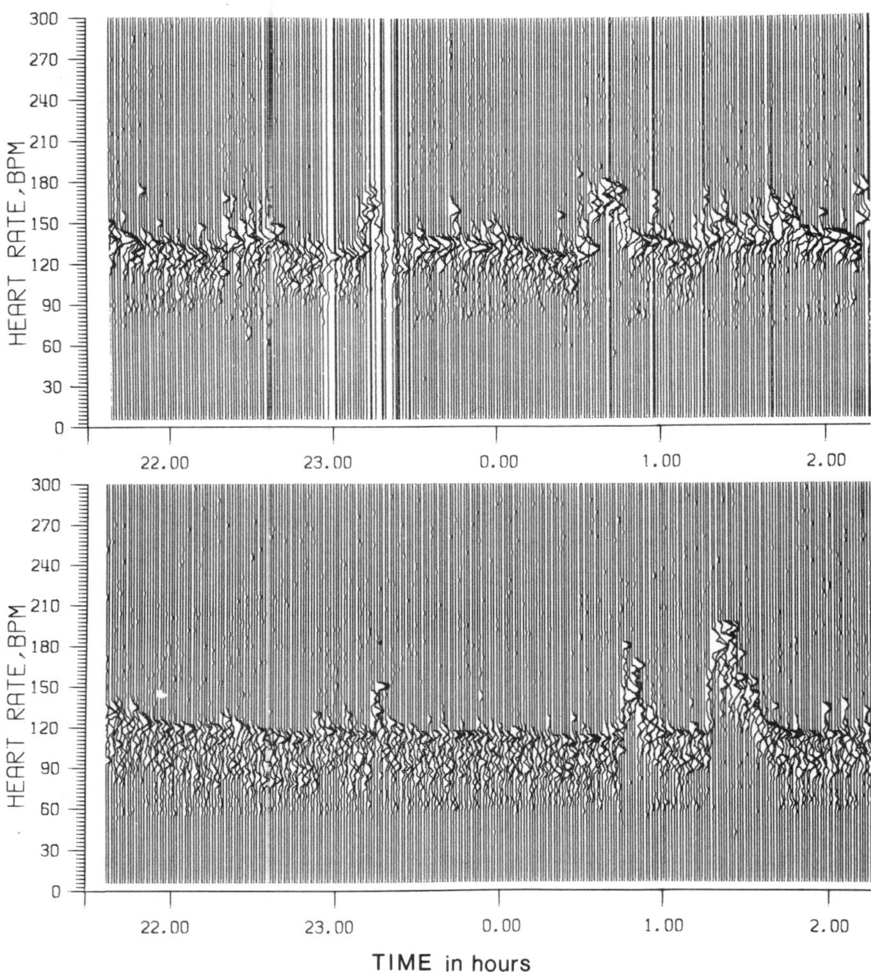

Fig. 7. Sections from a 24-hour plot of R-R internal histograms from the RRPLOT software. Each vertical trace represents a 1-minute histogram, and the histograms are plotted with hidden line suppression as a function of time. The top trace is from the baseline condition and the bottom trace from the night following maternal separation.

studies have involved maternal separation paradigms, although limited work has been done as well with peer-separation and infant-surrogate separation. In this section, we will summarize briefly our findings to date on the physiological correlates of separation in mother-infant and other paradigms, as well as some relevant data from other laboratories.

It is our goal to summarize briefly major findings that have potential clinical relevance in terms of addressing those issues presented earlier in this chapter. We should also point out that the comprehensive behavioral and physiological data collection/analytic system described in the preceding section was not available when most of the data described in this section were collected. Many of the questions that can now be answered with currently available methods could not be addressed with older methodologies.

In a typical mother-infant separation paradigm, infants are born and raised by their mothers in social groups in the laboratory. When the infants are about 4 months of age, they are surgically implanted with multichannel biotelemetry systems similar to those previously described. Following recovery from surgery, the infants and their mothers are returned to the social groups, where behavioral observations (which began at birth) continue. Shortly thereafter the telemetry systems are turned on and 24-hour-a-day physiological data transmission begins. This period of simultaneous behavioral and physiological data collection (prior to separation or other manipulation) is termed a "baseline" period; we have used this time period as a measure of normal behavior and physiology in young monkeys and for the construction of a "biobehavioral developmental profile" (BDP) for the pigtailed infant (Reite and Short, 1980). Following the collection of sufficient baseline data, the mothers are separated from the infants (who remain in the social groups in which they were raised). The ensuing agitation/depression behavioral reaction is accompanied by collection of both behavioral and physiological data. Following 10 days of maternal separation, the mothers are returned to the social groups and "reunion" data collection continues for another 4–5 (or more) days. Peer separation and infant-surrogate separation protocols follow generally similar patterns although timing may vary depending upon experimental demands.

Heart Rate

In pigtail infants, immediately following separation, and accompanying the "agitation" behavioral reaction, heart rate (HR) increases markedly. The increase in heart rate usually does not persist beyond sleep onset the first night of separation. During the first night of separation, mean night heart rate often drops lower than any preceding baseline night and, during 10-day separations, reaches its lowest mean during the first third of separation. A gradual recovery toward baseline value accompanies the remainder of separation (Reite et al., 1981b).

Individual variability in the response to separation is marked, and long-term changes in heart rate extending through and beyond the period of reunion have been found in a number of infants to date, suggesting that

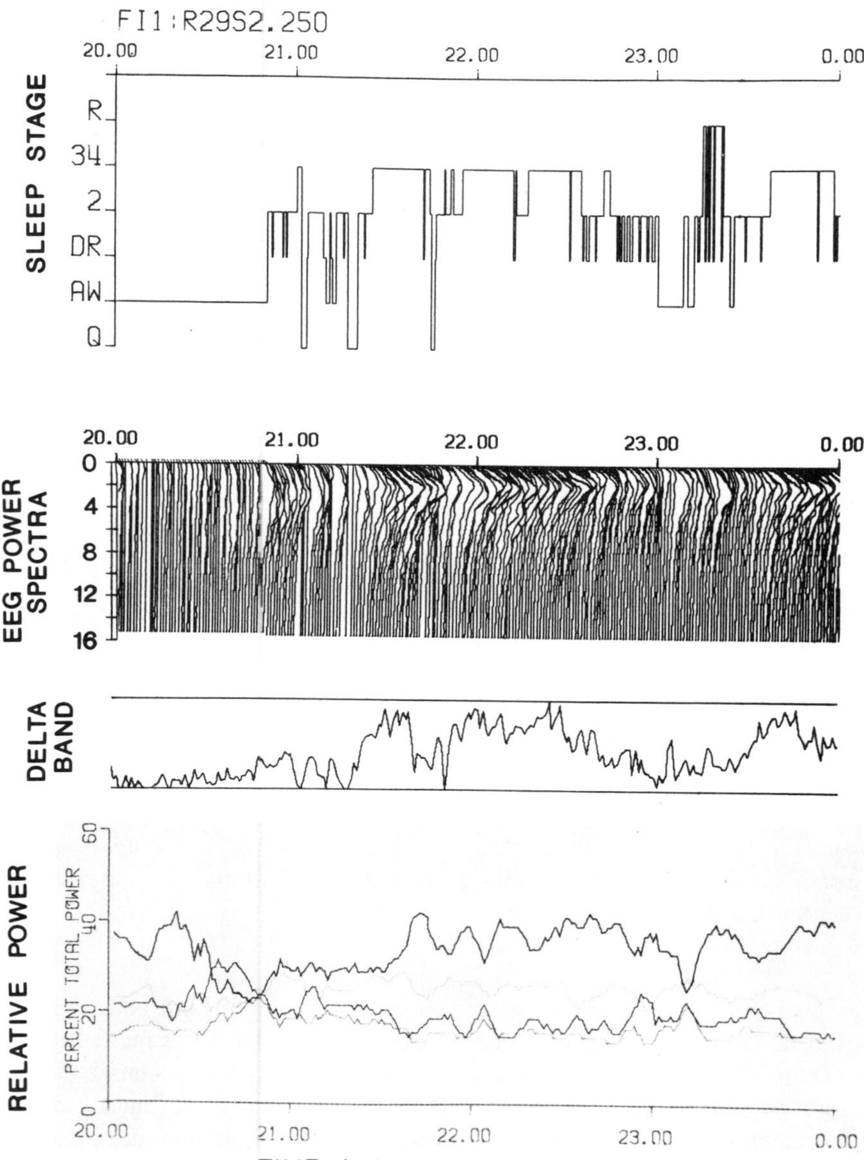

Fig. 8. Sleep stage, EEG power spectra, power in delta band, and percent of total EEG power plotted on the same time scale with the SPPLOT software. Ordinate of sleep stage plots as follows: AW = awake, R = REM, 34 = stages 3 and 4 sleep combined, 2 = stage 2 sleep, DR = drowsy sleep, Q = questionable (noisy). Ordinate of stacked spectra is in Hertz. Ordinate of the delta band plot is an arbitrary index directly proportional to the absolute power in the EEG between 0.5 and 2.5 Hz. The bottom plot is the percent of total power in each frequency band. Band widths are as follows: delta: 0.5–2.5 Hz; theta: 3.0–5.5 Hz; alpha: 6.0–10.0 Hz; beta: 10.5–15.5 Hz. These frequency bands are slightly different from conventional human EEG bands. Going from the top to the bottom trace, the bands are delta, theta, beta, and alpha.

sustained alterations in heart rate regulation may well exceed the duration of separation. It is, of course, not uncommon for a response to stress to persist long after the termination or resolution of the stressful event, but most often (in man), psychic defenses have been used as explanatory mechanisms (Horowitz, 1976).

Normal (i.e., unseparated) pigtail infants exhibit cardiac arrhythmias to a varying degree. Generally, most arrhythmias are seen when the infants are asleep at night, and animals with slow heart rates also tend to have more arrhythmias. The incidence of cardiac arrhythmias often increases dramatically during the depressive behavioral reaction following separation (Seiler et al., 1979). We believe that most of the cardiac arrhythmias that we have observed to date have been atrial in origin, although isolated apparent ventricular arrhythmias have also been observed.

Body Temperature

Body temperature increases dramatically immediately following separation and during behavioral agitation. It is striking to observe a recently separated infant sitting on a bar or bench in a social group, perhaps running about from door to window on occasion (but not as physically active as during vigorous play) with his body temperature quickly climbing over several minutes to higher readings than those observed during baseline. The first night of separation mean night body temperature often decreases to a value lower than any preceding baseline night; mean night body temperature values remain lower than baseline throughout a 10-day period of separation, although the time course of body temperature change is quite variable between individuals. Following reunion, most infants have body temperature values returning to or slightly above normal baseline values (Reite et al., 1981b).

Circadian Rhythms

HR and BT circadian rhythms both show changes after maternal separation. Halberg's cosinor type of analysis (Halberg et al., 1972) was applied to all HR and BT samples collected over a 24-hour period (best-fit least-squares method), providing estimates for cosine level, amplitude (similar to the maximum day/night or peak/trough difference), and time of acrophase (cosine peak). Using this technique we have shown decreases in HR and BT level to accompany separation, as well as increases in BT amplitude. Both HR and BT exhibit a phase lag of about 1 hour during separation (Reite et al., 1982).

Especially interesting is the fact that we have observed a phase shift in circadian rhythms, even though the circadian synchronizers such as light/

dark cycle, time of feeding, and social activity patterns (of the other group members) were not altered. Our findings support the view that disturbance in the rhythmic regulation or control of circadian systems is a prominent component of the reaction to loss or separation, and emphasizes the pervasive nature of the physiological changes induced by the disruption of an attachment bond and/or related maternal regulatory influences.

Sleep Patterns

Nocturnal sleep patterns in separated pigtail infants demonstrate a generalized disruption, consisting predominantly of increases in sleep latency, more frequent arousals during the night, a marked increase in REM latency, a decrease in percent REM, increase in time spent awake during the night, and fragmentation and shifting of stage 3, 4 sleep from early in the night to later in the night. Absolute amounts of slow-wave sleep do not appear to be significantly altered, and sleep latency tends to return toward baseline levels later in separation, whereas time awake and number of arousals both remain increased throughout separation. REM percent and REM in total minutes does not return to baseline levels, even after 10 days of separation (Reite and Short, 1978; Reite et al., 1981b). Infant monkeys normally sleep in contact with or enclosed by the mother; the absence of the mother at night is therefore a unique experience for the infants and represents a marked alteration in its normal sleep environment. Data from another experiment, however, mitigate against this being a sole explanation of our findings. In that study, we separated three infant pigtail monkeys from their mothers at birth and raised them on cloth surrogates. When, at a later date, their cloth surrogate mothers were removed from the cages, markedly and suddenly altering the infants' sleep environment, the infants exhibited disturbances in sleep patterns similar to those reported in this study except that the disturbances were not as pronounced nor as long-lasting. We believe that the infant surrogate attachment bond is considerably less intense (or more fundamentally different) than the infant-mother attachment bond, and that the sleep pattern changes accompanying its disruption are more likely related to the altered sleep environment per se than to the loss of the mother as an important object with the disruption of the more significant attachment bond (Reite et al., 1978).

EEG Changes

Evidence of episodic slowing of certain daytime EEG patterns as well as alterations in EEG alpha activity (just before sleep onset) have been found in many separated infants (Reite et al., 1981b; Short et al., 1977), although the significance of these alterations remains unclear.

Studies in Bonnet Infants

Changes in HR, BT, and sleep patterns qualitatively identical to those observed in pigtail infants have also been found in several bonnet *(M. radiata)* infants during 10-day maternal separations, using both mixed-species social group (Reite and Snyder, 1982) and bonnet social group paradigms (unpublished data). Such physiological changes are therefore clearly not species-specific.

Cortisol Changes With Maternal Separation

Studies in other laboratories have shown that, in rhesus infants separated from their mothers, there may be relatively short-lived increases in circulating plasma cortisol when samples are obtained in the midafternoon (Gunnar et al., 1981). If samples are obtained earlier in the day, however, there is evidence of a plasma cortisol rise throughout at least several days of separation (Levine, personal communication), suggestive of a possible phase lag in time of maximal cortisol secretion.

Immunological Correlates of Separation

In a pilot peer separation study, a pair of young pigtail monkeys that had been raised together since shortly after birth were separated from each other for a 10-day period, during which time lymphocyte response to mitogen stimulation (PHA and Con A) was evaluated. Both infants exhibited an impaired lymphoproliferative response to mitogen stimulation during and shortly after the separation, suggesting a possible separation-induced alteration in immunoregulation (Reite et al., 1981b). A subsequent experiment examined lymphoproliferative response to mitogen stimulation in both members of two bonnet mother-infant pairs and found evidence of similar disturbances—i.e., an impairment in the lymphoproliferative response to the mitogens PHA and Con A mitogen stimulation during the separation in both the mothers and infants (Laudenslager et al., 1982). These two studies suggest a commonality in the maternal and peer separation paradigms, at least in regard to these measures, and are consistent with Bartrop and colleagues' (1977) earlier descriptions of impaired lymphoproliferative responses to mitogenic stimulation in recently bereaved human adults. Together, these data support the hypothesis that altered immune system function is one aspect of the physiology of separation.

Responses to Psychoactive Drugs

Based upon the possible relationships between the response to separation and depression, several studies have been reported at other laboratories involving the use of antidepressants in monkey separation paradigms. Suomi et al. (1978) administered imipramine, 10 mg/kg, to infant rhesus monkeys in a peer separation paradigm and found that chronic imipramine-treated infants showed less passive and self-directed behaviors and more interest in the environment than placebo-treated infants. These data were interpreted as evidence that imipramine treatment resulted in behavioral improvement with a time course similar to that seen in man. Similarly, Hrdina et al. (1979) administered desmethylimipramine (DMI), 5 mg/kg, to young *M. fascicularis* infants in a modified mother-infant (no social group) separation paradigm and found that during maternal separation, DMI-treated subjects exhibited less change in play, less behavioral distress and less self-directed behavior than non-DMI-treated infants.

Other investigators have reported that administration of the catecholamine-depleting agent alpha-methyl-para-tyrosine (AMPT) potentiated the behavioral despair response to peer separation in rhesus monkeys, although the selected depletion of norepinephrine (and possible slight increase in dopamine) produced by dopamine beta-hydroxylase inhibition with fusaric acid resulted in less despair behavior (Morrison et al., 1976; Kraemer et al., 1977; see also Kraemer and McKinney, 1979). Decreased serotonin synthesis produced by para-chlorophenyl-alanine (PCPA) did not appear to affect the behavioral response to peer separation (Kraemer and McKinney, 1979). The results of these studies suggest that certain of the drugs which influence amine metabolism also modify the behavioral response to peer separation in young monkeys. By implication, therefore, such amine systems may be involved in the response to separation.

Cerebral Spinal Fluid Amine Studies

Recently Kraemer et al. (in press) have reported that rhesus monkeys that have relatively low CSF levels of norepinephrine (NE) are more likely to show a severe despair response to social separation than those with higher NE levels, and animals with lower CSF NE levels may also be more sensitive to the catecholamine-depleting effects of AMPT and exhibit greater evidence of behavioral depression resulting from administration of the latter drug. These authors suggest that low CSF norepinephrine may be a trait-related predisposing factor to severe responses to separation, again implicating brain amine systems in the response to separation.

Overview of Physiological Studies

Comparison of the studies involving physiological and endocrinological changes seen in maternal separation paradigms in rhesus, pigtail, and bonnet infants, with modulation of the despair response seen in peer-separated rhesus infants with various drugs, is complicated by the fact that as of this date, no comprehensive physiological studies of the response to peer separation have been performed in rhesus monkeys, and responses of mother-infant separation to various drug treatments have yet to be reported in pigtail infants. Thus the question of comparability across paradigms and species remains an issue subject to investigation.

The sum total of the various physiological responses to maternal separations seen in macaque monkey infants including alterations in the regulation of heart rate and rhythm, body temperature, disturbances in the regulation of circadian rhythms, and alterations in immunological function suggest a generalized impairment of autonomic/homeostatic regulation compatible with a functional disturbance at a hypothalamic level (Reite et al., 1981b). There are, of course, prominent limbic influences on hypothalamic function (Dreifuss et al., 1968), and there is evidence that limbic regions may subserve attachment and affiliative behaviors (Kling and Steklis, 1976). Thus, it seems not unreasonable to postulate that the disruption of an attachment bond may alter limbic activity which in turn could alter hypothalamic function. Direct evidence for such mechanisms is not yet available, but it represents a testable hypothesis.

We should mention at this point a possible caveat, for there are recent data implicating other factors as possibly important in the physiological response to maternal separation. It has been previously postulated that the physiological correlates of separation might include autonomic imbalance with a relative parasympathetic dominance and/or a decrease of central adrenergic output (Reite et al., 1981b). Short-term fasting has been shown to decrease centrally mediated sympathetic activity in the rat (Young and Landsberg, 1977). In pilot studies we have shown that short-term fasting also produces a prominent bradycardia in young monkeys, a physiological response not dissimilar to the separation response. Similarly, if a nursing infant is deprived of the ability to nurse by putting a leather vest on the mother, physiological changes similar to those seen during separation can be produced (Reite et al., unpublished data). In the latter case, it is not clear whether the observed changes are due to alteration in the infant's nutritional status or to an alteration in the mother-infant relationship due to the vest. Clearly, further work in these areas is indicated to further define which aspects of the physiological response to maternal separation may be related to factors other than the disruption of the attachment bonds, including the multiple roles of the mother as a regulator of the infant's psychobiological state, as well as a source of food. It is, of course, unlikely that such mechanisms would account for changes observed to accompany other separation paradigms.

In summary, separation research addresses issues of broad clinical relevance. Work conducted to date in several laboratories has outlined major organismic changes accompanying the reaction to separation, and has provided the information necessary to begin now to develop a specific hypothesis as to underlying mechanisms. As improved methodologies and techniques become available and are applied in this area of research, we will be able to directly address fundamental issues such as neurophysiological and neurochemical mechanisms underlying the observed changes. At that point, we will be in a position to answer questions of major clinical concern including prediction (who is vulnerable and how are they vulnerable), intervention (can or should the physiological changes be treated), and prevention.

ACKNOWLEDGMENTS

Supported by USPHS Grant No. MH19514. Dr. Reite is supported by an NIMH Research Scientist Award No. 5 K02 MH46335.

REFERENCES

Bacon CL, Renneker R, Cutler M (1952) A psychosomatic survey of cancer of the breast. Psychosom Med 14: 453–460

Bahnson CB, Bahnson MB (1966) Role of the ego defenses: Denial and repression in the etiology of malignant neoplasm. Ann New York Acad Sci 125: 827–845

Bartrop RW, Lazarus L, Luckhurst E, Kiloh LG (1977) Depressed lymphocyte function after bereavement. Lancet 1(8016): 834–836

Bowlby J (1960a) Separation anxiety. In J Psychoanal 41: 89–113

Bowlby J (1960) Grief and mourning in infancy and early childhood. Psychoanal Stud Child 15: 9–52 (Discussion pp 53–94)

Bowlby J (1961) Separation anxiety: A critical review of the literature. J Child Psychol Psychiatr 1: 251–269

Bowlby J (1973) Attachment and Loss. Vol. 2. Separation. Basic Books, New York, pp 444

Brink A (1979) Depression and loss, a theme in Robert Burton's Anatomy of Melancholy (1621). Can J Psychiatr 24: 767–772

Cadoret RJ, Winokur G, Dorzab J, Baker M (1972) Depressive disease: Life events and onset of illness. Arch Gen Psychiatr 24: 767–772

Chambers W, Reiser M (1953) Emotional stress in the precipitation of congestive heart failure. Psychosom Med 15: 38–60

Chappel PF, Meier GW (1975) Modification of the responses to separation in the infant rhesus macaque through manipulation of the environment. Biol Psychiatr 10: 643–657

Christodoulou GN, Gargoulas A, Paploukas A, Marinopoulou A, Sideris E (1977) Primary peptic ulcer in childhood: Psychosocial, psychological and psychiatric aspects. Acta Psychiatr Scand 56: 215–222

Cobb S, Bavber W, Whiting I (1939) Environmental factors in rheumatoid arthritis. J Am Med Assoc 113: 668–670

Conrad A (1934) The psychiatric study of hyperthyroid patients. J Nerv Ment Dis 79: 505–529

Dixon WJ et al. (chief ed) (1981) BMDP Statistical Software. Berkeley Univ Calif Press

Dolhinow P (1980) An experimental study of mother loss in the Indian langur monkey *(Presbytis entellus).* Folia Primatol 33: 77–128

Dreifuss JJ, Murphy JT, Gloor P (1968) Contrasting effects of two identified amygdaloid efferent pathways on single hypothalamic neurons. J Neurophysiol 31: 237–248

Engel GL (1955) Studies of ulcerative colitis. Am J Med 19: 231–256

Engel GL (1962) Anxiety and depression-withdrawal: The primary effects of unpleasure. In J Psychoanal 43: 89–97

Epstein G, Weitz L, Roback H, McKee E (1975) Research on bereavement: A selective and critical review. Comp Psych 16(6): 537–546

Evans E (1926) A psychology study of cancer. Dodd-Mead, New York

French TM (1939) Psychogenic factors in asthma. Am J Psychiatr 96: 87–101

Freud S (1917) Mourning and Melancholia. In: Jones E (ed.) (1959) Sigmund Freud. Collected Papers. Vol. 4. New York, Basic Books

Greene WA (1954) Psychological factors and reticuloendothelial disease: I. Preliminary observations on a group of males with lymphomas and leukemias. Psychosom Med 16: 220–230

Greene WA (1966) The psychosocial setting of the development of leukemia and lymphoma. Ann New York Acad Sci 125: 794–801

Greene WA, Miller G (1958) Psychological factors and reticuloendothelial disease: IV. Observations on a group of children and adolescents with leukemia: An interpretation of disease development in terms of the mother child unit. Psychosom Med 20: 124–144

Greene WA, Young LE, Swisher SN (1956) Psychological factors and reticuloendothelial disease: II. Observations on a group of women with lymphomas and leukemias. Psychosom Med 18: 284–303

Gunnar MR, Gonzalez CA, Goodlin BL, Levine S (1981) Behavioral and pituitary-adrenal responses during a prolonged separation period in infant rhesus macaques. Psychoneuroendocrinology 6:66–75

Halberg F, Johnson E, Nelson W, Runge W, Sothern R (1972) Autorhythmometry procedures for physiologic self-measurements and their analysis. Phys Teacher 1: 11

Hamburger WW (1956) Emotional aspects of obesity. Med Cl N Am 35: 483–499

Harlow HF, Gluck JP, Suomi SJ (1972) Generalization of behavioral data between nonhuman and human animals. Am Psychologist 27: 709–716

Heiman M (1956) The role of stress situations and psychological factors in functional uterine bleeding. J Mt Sinai Hosp 23: 775–781

Heinicke C (1973) Parental deprivation in early childhood. In: Scott J, Senay E (eds) Separation and Depression: Clinical and Research Aspects. Wash DC: AAAS

Henoch MJ, Batson JW, Baum J (1978) Psychosocial factors in juvenile rheumatoid arthritis. Arthritis Rheumatism 21(2): 229–233

Hinde RA, McGinnis L (1977) Some factors influencing the effects of temporary mother-infant separation: Some experiments with rhesus monkeys. Psychol Med 7: 197–212

Hinde RA, Spencer-Booth Y (1971) Effects of brief separation from mother on rhesus monkeys. Sci 173: 111–118

Hinde RA, Spencer-Booth Y (1971) Towards understanding individual differences in rhesus mother-infant interaction. Anim Behav 19: 165–173

Hinde RA, Spencer-Booth Y, Bruce M (1966) Effects of 6-day maternal deprivation on rhesus monkey infants. Nature 210: 1021

Hinkel LE, Wolf S (1952) A summary of experimental evidence relating life stress in diabetes mellitus. J Mt Sinai Hosp 19: 537–570

Horowitz MJ (1976) Stress Response Syndromes. Aronson, New York

Hrdina PD, von Kulmiz P (1978) Separation-induced behavioral disorder in infra-human primates: An animal model of depression. In: Garattine S (ed) Depressive Disorders. Stuttgart Schattauer

Hrdina PD, von Kulmiz P, Stretch R (1979) Pharmacological modification of experimental depression in infant macaques. Psychopharmacol 64: 89–93

Jacobs S, Ostfeld A (1977) An epidemiological review of the mortality of bereavement. Psychosom Med 39(5): 344–357

Jacbos TJ, Charles E (1980) Life events and the occurrence of cancer in children. Psychosom Med 42: 11–24

Jones BC, Clark DL (1973) Mother-infant separation in squirrel monkeys living in a group. Dev Psychobiol 6: 259–269

Kaplan J (1970) The effects of separation and reunion on the behavior of mother and infant squirrel monkeys. Dev Psychobiol 3: 43–52

Kaufman IC (1977) Developmental considerations of anxiety and depression: Psychobiological studies of monkeys. In: Shapiro T (ed): Psychoanalysis and Contemporary Science. Vol. 5. International Univ. Press, New York, pp 317–363

Kaufman IC, Rosenblum LA (1966) A behavioral taxonomy for *Macaca nemestrina* and *Macaca radiata:* Based on longitudinal observation of family groups in the laboratory. Primates 7: 206–258

Kaufman IC, Rosenblum LA (1967) The reaction to separation in infant monkeys: Anaclitic depression and conservation-withdrawal. Psychosom Med 29: 649–675

Kaufman IC, Rosenblum LA (1969a) Effects of separation from mother on the emotional behavior of infant monkeys. Ann NY Acad Sci 159: 681–695

Kaufman IC, Rosenblum LA (1969b) The waning of the mother-infant bond in two species of macaque. In: Foss BM (ed) Determinants of Infant Behavior. Methuen, London, pp 41–59

Kaufman IC, Stynes AJ (1978) Depression can be induced in a bonnet macaque infant. Psychosom Med 40: 71–75

Kissen DM (1957) The relapse in pulmonary tuberculosis due to specific psychological causes. Health Bulletin 15. Issued by the Chief Medical Officer of the Dept of Health, Scotland

Kleinschmidt HJ, Waxenberg SE, Cuker R (1956) Psychophysiology and psychiatric management of thyrotoxicosis: A two year follow-up study. J Mt Sinai Hosp 23: 131–153

Kling A, Steklis HD (1976) A neural substrate for affiliative behavior in nonhuman primates. Brain Behav Evol 13: 216–238

Kowal SJ (1955) Emotions as a cause of cancer, 18th and 19th century contributions. Psychoanaly Rev 42: 217–227

Kraemer GW, Ebert MH, McKinney WT (in press) Separation models and depression. In: Angst J (ed) The Origins of Depression: Current Concepts and Approaches. Dahlem Konferenzen, Berlin Heidelberg New York, Springer-Verlag

Kraemer GW, Klopf FH, Suomi SJ, McKinney WT (1977) Effects of alterations in biogenic amine metabolism on the protest-despair response to peer separation in rhesus monkeys. Soc Neurosci Abst 3: 443

Kraemer GW, McKinney WT (1979) Interactions of pharmacological agents which alter biogenic amine metabolism and depression. J Affect Disorders 1: 33–45

Laudenslager ML, Reite M, Harbeck R (1982) Suppresed immune response in infant monkeys associated with maternal separation. Behav Neural Biol 36:40–48

Leaverton DR, White CA, McCormick CR, Smith P, Sheikholislam B (1980) Parental loss antecedent to childhood diabetes mellitus. J Am Acad Child Psych 19: 678–689

LeShan L (1959) Psychological states as factors in the development of malignant disease: A critical review. J Natl Cancer Inst 22: 1–18

Lindeman E (1945) Psychiatric problems in conservative treatment of ulcerative colitis. Arch Neurol Psychiatr 53: 322–324

Litz T (1949) Emotional factors in the etiology of hyperthyroidism. Psychosom Med 11: 2–8

Ludwig AG (1952) Psychogenic factors in rheumatoid arthritis. Bull Rheumatic Dis 2: 33–34

Mammen S (1979) Grief and its manifestation as a psychosomatic disease— hypertension. Nursing J India 70: 299–301

McClary AR, Meyer E, Weitzman E (1955) Observations on the role of the mechanism of depression in some patients with disseminated lupus erythematosus. Psychosom Med 17: 311–321

McKinney WT, Bunney WE (1969) Animal model of depression. Arch Gen Psychiatr 21: 240–248

McKnew DH, Cytryn L (1973) Historical background in children with affective disorders. Am J Psychiatr 130: 1278–1280

Meier GW (1975) Introductory comments to Symposium on Environmental Contingencies in Early Primate Development. Biol Psychiatr 10(6): 605–607

Meyer RJ, Haggerty ZJ (1962) Streptococcal infections in families: Factors altering individual susceptibility. Pediatrics 29: 539–549

Millet J, Lief H, MiHelmann B (1953) Raynaud's disease: Psychogenic factors and psychotherapy. Psychosom Med 15: 61–65

Mineka S, Suomi SJ (1978) Social separation in monkeys. Psychol Bull 85(6): 1376–1400

Mittelman B (1933) Psychogenic factors and psychotherapy in hyperthyreosis and rapid heart imbalance. J Nerv Ment Dis 77: 465–488

Morillo E, Gardner L (1979) Bereavement as an antecedent factor in thyrotoxicosis of childhood: Four case studies with survey of possible metabolic pathways. Psychosom Med 41: 545–555

Morrison HL, Kraemer GW, McKinney WT (1976) Protest-despair response to peer separation in rhesus monkeys and its potentiation by alteration of catecholamine metabolism. Psychosom Med 38: 66

Papper S, Handy J (1956) Observations in a "control" group of patients in psychosomatic investigation. N E J Med 255: 1067–1071.

Parkes CM (1972) Bereavement. International Univ Press, New York

Pauley JD, Reite M (1977) Automatic antenna selector for use in biotelemetry applications. Physiol Behav 18: 169–170

Pauley JD, Reite M (1981) A microminiature hybrid multichannel implantable biotelemetry system. Biotelemetr Patient Monitor 8: 163–172

Paykel ES, Myers JK, Dienelt MN, Klerman GL, Lindenthal JJ, Pepper MR (1969) Life events and depression. Arch Gen Psychol 21: 753–760

Peller S (1952) Cancer in Man. International University Press, New York, p 556

Perlman LV, Ferguson S, Bergum K, Isenberg EL, Hammarsten JF (1975) Precipitation of congestive heart failure: Social and emotional factors. Ann Intern Med 75: 1–7

Poland RE, Rubin RT (1982) Saliva cortisol levels following dexamethasone administration in endogenously depressed patients. Life Sci 30: 177–181

Preston DG, Bakeer RP, Seay B (1970) Mother-infant separation in the patas monkey. Dev Psychol 3:298–306

Rasmussen KLR, Reite M (1982) Loss-induced depression in an adult macaque monkey. Am J Psychiatr 139:679–681

Reite M (1977) Maternal separation in monkey infants: A model of depression. In: Hanin I, Usdin E (eds) Animal Models in Psychiatry and Neurology. Pergamon Press, Oxford New York, pp 127–139

Reite M, Harbeck R, Hoffman A (1981a) Altered cellular immune response following peer separation. Life Sci 29: 1133–1136

Reite M, Pauley JD (1976) Multichannel implantable biotelemetry: Problems, pitfalls, and rewards. In: Fryer TB, Miller HA, Sandler A (eds.) Biotelemetry III. Academic Press, New York, pp 59–62

Reite M, Seiler C, Crowley TJ, Hydinger-Macdonald M, Short R (1982) Circadian rhythm changes following maternal separation in monkeys. Chronobiologia 9: 1–11

Reite M, Seiler C, Short R (1978) Loss of your mother is more than loss of a father. Am J Psychiatr 135: 370–371

Reite M, Short R (1978) Nocturnal sleep in separated monkey infants. Arch Gen Psychiatr 35:1247–1253

Reite M, Short R (1980) A biobehavioral developmental profile (BDP) for the pigtailed monkey. Dev Psychobiol 13(3): 243–285

Reite M, Short R, Seiler C (1978) Physiological correlates of separation in surrogate reared infants: A study in altered attachment bonds. Dev Psychobiol 11: 427–435.

Reite M, Short R, Seiler C, Pauley JD (1981b) Attachment, loss, and depression. J Child Psychol Psychiatr 22: 141–169

Reite M, Snyder D (1982) Physiology of maternal separation in a bonnet macaque infant. Am J Primatol 2: 115–120

Reite M, Walker SD, Pauley JD (1973) Implantation surgery in infant monkeys. Lab Primate Newslet 4: 1–6

Rosenblum L, Kaufman IC (1967) Laboratory observations of early mother-infant relations in pigtail and bonnet macaques. In: Altmann SA (ed) Social Communication Among Primates. Chicago Univ Chicago Press

Rosenblum L, Kaufman IC (1968) Variations in infant development and response to mother loss in monkeys. Am J Orthopsychiatr 38: 418–426

Rosenblum L, Kaufman IC, Stynes AJ (1966) Some characteristics of adult social and autogrooming patterns in two species of macaque. Folia Primatol 4: 438–451

Sackett GP (ed) (1978) Observing Behavior. Vol 2. Data Collection and Analysis Methods. Baltimore Univ Park Press

Schlottmann R, Seay B (1972) Mother-infant separation in the Java monkey *(Macaca irus).* J Comp Physiol Psychol 79: 334–340

Seay BM, Hansen EW, Harlow HF (1962) Mother-infant separation in monkeys. J Chil Psychol Psychiatr 3: 123–132

Seay BM, Harlow HF (1965) Maternal separation in the rhesus monkey. J Nerv Ment Dis 140: 434–441

Seiler C, Cullen JS, Zimmerman J, Reite M (1979) Cardiac arrhythmias in infant pigtail monkeys following maternal separation. Psychophysiology 16: 130–135

Seligman MEP (1968) Chronic fear produced by unpredictable electric shock. J Comp Physiol Psychol 66: 402–411

Seligman MEP (1975) Helplessness. WH Freeman Co, San Francisco

Sethi BB (1964) Relationship of separation to depression. Arch Gen Psychiatr 10:486–496

Short R, Iwata S, Reite M (1977) EEG changes during the depressive reaction following maternal separation. Psychophysiology 14: 120

Slawson PF, Flynn WR, Kollar EF (1963) Psychological factors associated with the onset of diabetes mellitus. J Am Med Assoc 185: 166–170

Solomon RL, Corbit JD (1974) An opponent-process theory of motivation: I. Temporal dynamics of affect. Psychol Review 81: 119–145

Spitz RA (1946) Anaclitic depression. Psycholanal Stud Child 2: 313–342

Stein SP, Charles E (1971) Emotional factors in juvenile diabetes mellitus: A study of early life experience of adolescent diabetes. Am J Psychiatr 128: 700–704

Stenback A (1965) Object loss and depression. Arch Gen Psychiatr 12:144–151

Suomi SJ, Collins ML, Harlow HF (1976) Effects of maternal and peer separations on young monkeys. J Child Psychol Psychiatr 17: 101–112

Suomi SJ, Eisele CD, Grady SA, Harlow HF (1975) Depressive behavior in adult monkeys following separation from family environment. J Ab Psychol 84: 576–578

Suomi SJ, Harlow HF, Domek EJ (1970) Effect of repetitive infant-infant separation of young monkeys. J Ab Psychol 76: 161–172

Suomi SJ, Seaman SF, Lewis JK, DeLizio RD, McKinney WT (1978) Effects of imipramine treatment of separation-induced social disorders in rhesus monkeys. Arch Gen Psychiatr 35: 321–325

Wittkower E (1949) A Psychiatrist Looks at Tuberculosis. National Assoc Prevention Tuberculosis. Tavistock Sq, London, p 152

Young JB, Landsberg L (1977) Suppression of sympathetic nervous system during fasting. Sci 196: 1473–1475

Ethopharmacology: Primate Models of Neuropsychiatric Disorders,
pages 255–275

Substance Abuse Research in Monkey Social Groups

Thomas J. Crowley

Department of Psychiatry, University of Colorado School of Medicine, Denver, Colorado 80262

INTRODUCTION

What is the relevance of animal studies in problems of human drug abuse? Many studies now have shown that animals, when given the means to do so, self-administer most of the same drugs abused by human beings (e.g., Deneau et al., 1969; Goldberg et al., 1971; Hoffmeister and Schlichting, 1972; Balster et al., 1973; Woods and Winger, 1974; Thompson and Pickens, 1975; Harringan and Downs, 1978). These studies demonstrate that particular kinds of psychopathology, poverty, racism, or other peculiarly human stressors are not required for drug abuse to occur; indeed, drugs reinforce their own self-administration even in species lacking those complexities of human psychology and sociology. Such observations forced a renewed interest in reinforcement of self-administration as a pharmacologic property of certain drugs, in addition to earlier emphasis on individual psychopathology and personality deficits among human drug abusers (Knight, 1937; Wieder and Kaplan, 1969).

To examine the reinforcing properties of drugs, the above studies used individually housed animals to reduce complicating social influences on self-administration. But important social influences do affect drug use by human drug abusers (Crowley and Rhine, 1981; Crowley 1972a). Some balance of social reinforcement and social punishment (Crowley, 1983; Anker and Crowley, 1982) may be very important in determining the frequency of drug use. In addition, other social behaviors such as playing on sport teams appear to compete with and diminish drug-use behaviors in some patients. Conversely, repeated drug intoxications may severely impair certain social behaviors of the user, blocking the user's access to important social reinforcers; for example, repeated episodes of drunkenness may render the alcoholic unemployable. Moreover, medications used in the treatment of drug abuse, such as methadone or disulfiram (Antabuse), could adversely alter social behavior of patients.

Examples of social influences on drug use, and drug influences upon the user's social behavior, are familiar to most clinicians. While these very important issues are difficult to study in the natural human social situation, they may be examined in three ways. The first, clinical observation, is notoriously uncontrolled. Second, more controlled research in these matters may be accomplished on research wards (e.g., Mello and Mendelson, 1970, 1971; Meyer and Mirin, 1979), but these very expensive studies are ethically limited to subjects who already abuse drugs; such studies cannot examine social influences upon the initiation of drug abuse. In a third method, studies are conducted in animal social groups; they are amenable to environmental control, and the initiation of drug-abuse behavior can be examined in these settings. Of course, generalizations to human problems from animal studies may be made only with great caution. But with a combination of clinical observations, studies in clinical research wards, and examinations of animal social groups, we gradually are accumulating an understanding of drug effects upon social behavior, and of social influences on drug self-administration. Each technique has its own limitations, but together the three techniques have been quite instructive.

This paper reviews our studies of drugs in primate social groups.

MATERIALS AND METHODS

Setting and Animals

The Primate Research Laboratory of our Department of Psychiatry includes 13 pens for the study of social behavior in primate groups. Each pen is tile-walled and has wire mesh ceilings for brachiation and a sawdust-covered floor. There are bars and shelves for climbing and resting. Artificial lighting is electrically timed. Automatic equipment provides continual access to water. One-way glass windows permit an observer to watch the animals without disturbing them. The pens, measuring about 3 × 3 × 3 m, permit far more locomotion than do cage facilities, although recent work makes it clear that even in such relatively commodious quarters, social interactions may be different than in larger outdoor areas (Wallen, 1982).

In these pens, we study groups of two to 35 individuals, including newborn to very aged animals of both sexes. We study *Macaca nemestrina* (pigtail macaques) and *Macaca radiata* (bonnet macaques) because of their availability; they were introduced into our laboratory by Dr. Charles Kaufman many years ago and have bred readily there. Fortunately, other laboratories have examined drug self-administration by *M. nemestrina* (Young and Woods, 1980; Bowden and Jones, 1980; Elton et al., 1976).

Behavioral Taxonomy

Monkeys in social groups emit chains of discrete behaviors. Each of these behaviors can be observed, objectively described, and counted. When a sufficiently large number of such behaviors have been catalogued, a well-trained observer can name and record the duration of nearly all of the discrete activities of an animal. Our "catalogue," or taxonomy, now includes about 100 different behaviors, closely following but slightly expanded from taxonomies of Kaufman and Rosenblum (1966) and Maxim (1978). Behaviors fall into such general categories as hierarchical (dominance and subordinance) behaviors, sexual behaviors, resting behaviors, social contact behaviors, nutritive behaviors, mother-infant behaviors, behaviors of environmental exploration, and drug-induced behaviors (which occur only during intoxication with various drugs). Within each of these general categories are specific, objectively described behaviors, partially listed in Table I.

We recently assessed inter-rater reliability for bahaviors in our taxonomy. Each member of a group of *M. nemestrina* was videotaped for at least 5 min, producing a total tape of about 2.5 hr duration. Twenty-five sections of about 5 min duration on the tape were demarcated with the words "Start" and "Stop." Two experienced observers then recorded each behavior which they saw in each 5-min observation period. They recorded the frequency of instantaneous behaviors (such as "Bite") and the duration of more prolonged behaviors (such as "Upright Rest"). Across the 25 observation sessions, we then correlated between observers the frequency or duration of observation of the 44 behaviors observed at least once by either observer (Table II). The majority of correlations exceed 0.75, and only eight infrequently observed behaviors had correlations below 0.47. Clearly, the objectivity of our descriptions, coupled with the experience of our observers, yields quite acceptable inter-rater reliability for most behaviors.

Motility Measurement

The seemingly interesting observation that a dose of some drug reduces sexual behavior turns out to be trivial if the drug simply renders animals comatose. Clearly, it is important to distinguish general motor sedation or stimulation from drug effects upon specific social behaviors. To help with this distinction, the subjects in most of our studies wear individually tailored leather vests. A small FM radio transmitter, connected to a mercury switch motion transducer and encased in a hard plastic box, is attached to the back of the vest; our current version of this unit weighs about 360 grams. The device continually transmits information about movements of the animal to a

TABLE I. Descriptions of Selected Behaviors From 100-Item Behavioral Taxonomy

I. Hierarchical behaviors
   A. Dominance behaviors
      1. Bite. Common usage.
      2. Manual attacks. The use of one or both hands for grabbing and pulling the fur, striking, pushing, and/or restraining the motion of another animal, rarely causing serious injury.
      3. Pursuit. Vigorous chasing of another animal while showing repeated threats and invariable attacks on the opponent upon capture. Pursuit is sometimes abruptly terminated as soon as the other animal flees. May occur concurrently with bite and manual attacks.
      4. Threat. Rapid movements including any or all of the following: opening of the mouth with exposure of teeth, thrusting the head forward, flattening the ears against the head and retracting the brow; the body is held still and upright and is thrust forward.
      5. Stare. Intense visual fixation of another animal, frequently catching its gaze for several seconds. The head is generally held slightly forward and the brow protruded.
      6. Brow movement. Slow or rapid retraction of the scalp and brow, often with accompanying ear movement.
      7. Threat shake. Usually an act of the alpha male who abruptly jerks his body up and down on the bars or the shelf. In the wild, this movement shakes tree limbs.
      8. Initiate proper mount. Climbing upon the partner with feet clasping the calves and hands grasping the loins, and with pelvic thrusting beginning as the position is attained. (This pattern does not include intromission; it is performed by either sex on either sex, but is invariably part of copulation.) Counted as a hierarchical dominance behavior (rather than sexual behavior) when performed by members of the same sex.
   B. Subordinance behaviors
      1. Defensive aggression. Hesitant and tentative retaliatory attacks by an animal under attack. Unlike full fighting, the head is withdrawn from (rather than extended toward) the opponent.
      2. Withdrawal. A movement of at least 12 inches, in a deliberate manner, away from a partner in response to the latter's initiation of some social act.
      3. Flight. Rapid, agitated withdrawal from another animal, accompanied by squealing vocalization.
      4. Present. Assumption of a posture in which the hindquarters are raised and oriented toward the partner, and the front legs are generally rigid or only slightly flexed, though occasionally the forelegs may be completely bent and the chest pressed to the floor. Counted as an hierarchical subordinance behavior when performed by same-sex partners.
      5. Grimace. A facial expression directed toward partner; lips retracted and teeth sometimes tightly clenched, resembling a smile.
      6. Lip smacking. Rapid opening and closing of the pursed lips, producing a soft clicking sound, similar to the "tsk-tsk" sound produced by humans.
      7. Crouch. "Frozen" posture with ventral surface lowered toward floor but head raised and alert.

II. Associative behaviors
   A. Grooming solicitation. A presentation of the head, throat, chest, or side to another animal lasting 2 sec or longer.

(continued)

TABLE I. Descriptions of Selected Behaviors From 100-Item Behavioral Taxonomy (continued)

- B. Give groom. Animal picks through, and/or brushes aside, the fur of another with one or both forepaws. The material that is picked out, such as small hairs and flakes of skin, may be placed in the mouth.
- C. Receive groom. Animal accepts the picking through and/or slow brushing aside of the fur by forepaws of one or more animals.
- D. Proximity. Passive standing or sitting within 12 inches of another animal without making contact or engaging in any additional categorized social behavior.
- E. Passive contact or clasp. Remaining in physical contact with another for at least 15 sec without engaging the other in any additional categorized social behavior while quietly at rest.

III. Sexual behaviors

- A. Autosexual behaviors; masturbation. Manipulating the animal's own genitals, accompanied by evidence of sexual excitement, i.e., erection in the male during self-manipulation of the penis, or pelvic thrusting in the female when the labia are repetitively rubbed by pulling the tail between the legs.
- B. Homosexual behaviors; present-present. A proper present in response to the proper present of a partner, the two subjects backing toward one another until the anogenital regions make contact. They then reach back through their legs and manipulate the genitals of the partner.
- C. Heterosexual behaviors
    1. Present. Assumption of a posture in which the hindquarters are raised and oriented toward the partner, and the front legs are generally rigid or only slightly flexed, though occasionally the forelegs may be completely bent and the chest pressed to the floor. Counted as a sexual behavior when a female presents to a male.
    2. Inadequate present. A properly oriented present posture in which the hindquarters are not raised and the hind legs are not properly extended to allow proper mount.
    3. Disoriented present. A present which is not appropriately directed to the partner.
    4. Initiate proper mount. Climbing upon the partner with feet clasping the calves and hands grasping the loins, and with pelvic thrusting beginning as the position is attained. (This pattern does not include intromission; it is performed by either sex on either sex, but is invariably part of copulation.) Counted as sexual behavior when performed by a male upon a female, and as a dominance behavior when performed by one member of one sex upon a same-sex partner.
    5. Inadequate mount. A properly oriented mount where the mounting animal may not have a good grasp on the calves or loin of the mounted animal or where no thrusting occurs.
    6. Disoriented mount. A mount which is not appropriately directed to the partner (mounting the wrong area).
    7. Anogenital exploration. Sniffing at, engaging in close visual inspection (within 12 inches) of, or manual or oral contact with, the perineum of the partner.
    8. Clonic jaw. A complex behavior involving the following: rhythmic to-and-fro movements of the head and shoulders, rhythmic contraction of the brow and scalp, retraction of the lips and exposure of the teeth while the jaws rapidly and rhythmically open and close, providing audible clicking sound. Used by males to summon females for copulation, and performed by males during copulation.

(continued)

TABLE I. Descriptions of Selected Behaviors From 100-Item Behavioral Taxonomy (continued)

9. Intromission. Penis enters vagina.
10. Ejaculation. Common usage—generally indicated by a pause in rhythmic thrusting followed by staccato thrust and body stiffening.

IV. Resting behaviors

1. Upright rest. Sitting motionless with eyes open without accompanying involvement in any more complex activity.
2. Upright sleep. Sitting with shoulders hunched over and eyes closed.
3. Recumbent rest. Lying on either side or back for brief periods with eyes open and limbs partially outstretched, without accompanying involvement in any more complex activity.

V. Drug-related behaviors

1. Nodding. Sitting in an upright position, the monkey's head bobs (chin to chest); eyes partly closed. Common with opiates.
2. Stereotypic pacing. The monkey repeatedly and immediately retraces a route at least three times, sometimes characterized with a stereotyped twist in his walk. Common with amphetamines.
3. Stereotypic other. Other repeated frequent, fragmentary and non-goal-directed behavior; includes excessively frequent normal behaviors—i.e., blinking, licking, chewing. Common with amphetamines.
4. Ataxia. Any clumsy movement. Common with alcohol, sedatives.

receiver located outside the pen, providing 24-hour records of animal motility. These motility counts, integrated over a few minutes, may be printed out on paper tape (Crowley et al., 1974) for later keypunching and analysis, or they may be directly entered into a computer (Mast et al., 1982).

Such motility measurements enhance data like those in Fig. 1, which records the combined frequency of occurrence of several sexual behaviors in *M. nemestrina* males following various doses of morphine. The figure shows that these morphine doses clearly suppressed sexual activity, but motility records showed that those doses did not alter spontaneous motility. Thus, we could conclude that in doses which were not generally sedating, morphine specifically reduced sexual behavior in primates (Crowley et al., 1974); clinicians have long suspected that opioid drugs suppressed sexual activity, but this may be the clearest demonstration of that suppression in a primate (including human) species.

We also studied pentobarbital and methamphetamine in male *M. nemestrina*. The drugs affected the relative frequency of occurrence of dominance and subordinance behaviors; pentobarbital increased the dominance/subordinance ratio while methamphetamine decreased that ratio. In other words, the animals behaved in a relatively more dominant manner after receiving the

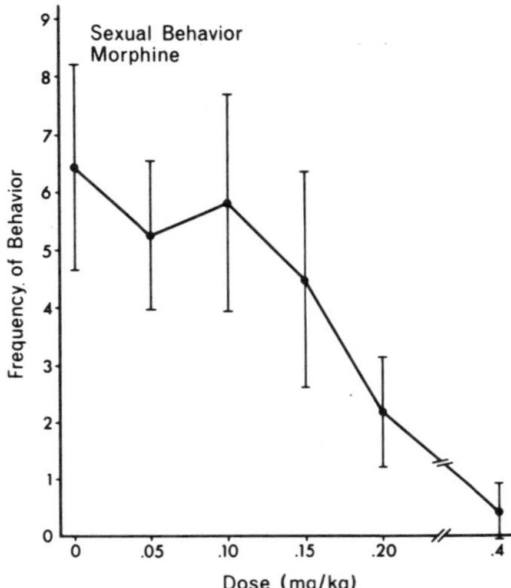

Fig. 1. Frequency of sexual behaviors among male *M. nemestrina* following various doses of morphine. (Reprinted with permission from Arch Gen Psychiatr 31:829–838, 1974.)

barbiturate and in a relatively more subordinate manner after receiving the amphetamine. While changing this ratio, methamphetamine also produced motor stimulation, but pentobarbital changed the dominance/subordinance ratio in doses which did not affect spontaneous motility (Fig. 2). Again, the conjoint recording of social and motor behavior permitted more precise conclusions about specific social effects of the drugs.

Round-the-clock monitoring also permits assessment of effects upon circadian rhythms of motility by relatively long-acting drugs. For example, methadone, which replaces heroin for heroin addicts, has a half-life in man of about 24 hours. We found that when the drug was given chronically, once daily to monkeys, it significantly changed the circadian rhythm of motility in the animals (Crowley et al., 1975, 1977). In comparison to baseline drug-free observations, the drug produced significant motor stimulation among the animals for several hours after its daily oral administration, and it suppressed night-time motility (Fig. 3). As a result, the average 24-hour level of motility increased, the amplitude of the circadian rhythm increased, and the phase of the circadian rhythm advanced about 84 min during methadone administration. Thus, we identified a potentially important drug side effect by recording drug effects upon motor behavior of group-living monkeys.

Data Management

In a typical recent study by our group, an observer recorded the frequency or duration of social behaviors (as described above) from five animals, in

TABLE II. Inter-Rater Reliability for Counting of Social Behaviors

Behavior	Duration (D) as percent of total observation time, or Frequency (F) per 1,000 sec observation time			Inter-rater correlation coefficient, 25 tape sections
	Observer A	D or F	Observer B	
Drinking	0.64	D	0.63	1.00
Give groom	1.60	D	1.50	1.00
Food play	0.37	D	0.03	1.00
Chew food	2.60	D	2.65	1.00
Food foraging	6.18	D	6.61	1.00
Body shake	0.52	F	0.52	1.00
Vaginal self-inspection	0.25	D	0.21	0.99
Vest manipulation	0.33	D	0.51	0.99
Self-manipulation	4.36	D	3.99	0.98
Recumbent rest	1.21	D	1.08	0.98
Upright rest	51.40	D	51.60	0.98
Lick wall	2.11	D	2.02	0.96
Tree shake	3.41	F	2.62	0.96
Anogenital exploration	0.60	D	0.37	0.95
Manual attack	0.92	F	1.31	0.92
Locomotion	20.99	D	26.01	0.92
Object manipulation	1.29	D	1.30	0.91
Receive groom	1.50	D	2.00	0.91
Contact	5.84	D	7.23	0.91
Autogroom	0.71	D	0.51	0.89
Window looking	2.15	D	1.44	0.79
Threat	1.84	F	1.44	0.78
Proximity	24.39	D	16.88	0.76
Lip smack	0.31	D	0.23	0.76
Brow jerk	0.66	F	1.31	0.71
Scratch self	2.66	D	1.94	0.70
Yawn	0.26	F	0.13	0.69
Withdraw	1.05	F	0.39	0.61
Vocalize	0.66	F	0.66	0.58
Ceiling hang	0.03	D	0.14	0.57
Present	0.39	F	0.13	0.55
Flee	0.39	F	0.13	0.55
Stereotyped pacing	3.54	D	0.18	0.49
Solicit groom	0.42	D	0.30	0.49
Stand still	2.51	D	1.74	0.48
Nuzzle	1.05	F	0.26	0.47
Displace	0.53	F	0.39	0.10
Positioning	0.00	F	0.52	0.00
Bite	0.26	F	0.00	0.00
Grimace	0.00	F	0.66	0.00
Play-fight	0.00	D	0.13	0.00
Other stereotypies	0.05	D	0.00	0.00
Present-present	0.00	F	0.26	0.00
Raise tail	0.26	F	0.13	−0.06

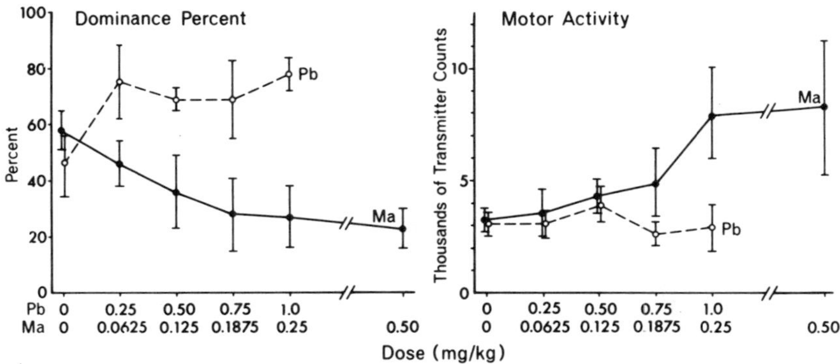

Fig. 2. Left, dominance ratio [Dom/(Dom + Subm)] after pentobarbital (Pb) or methamphetamine (Ma). Right, motor activity counts from backpack transmitter after pentobarbital or methamphetamine. (Reprinted with permission from Arch Gen Psychiatr 31:829–838, 1974.)

four sessions (each of which lasted a total of 20 min), 4 days per week. We also recorded spontaneous motility continually from the same animals. We integrated motility counts for 6 min from one animal, then automatically switched to the transmitter of another animal and recorded motility counts for 6 min, then automatically switched to another for 6 min, etc. These observations continued as we administered a placebo for 6 weeks, an active drug for 13 weeks, and a placebo for another 3 weeks. Obviously, such a study accumulates enormous quantities of data. Our techniques for recording, storing, and retrieving data have beeen modified from those of our colleagues (Walker and Reite, 1975), and are reported in Mast et al. (1982). Briefly, an observer enters social behavior records directly into a DEC LSI-11 computer; the observer, seated at the one-way glass window, punches into a computer terminal a code for each behavior as it occurs. When the behavior ends, the observer enters the code for the next behavior which occurs. This results in a string of behavioral entries, and the computer determines the duration and exact time of occurrence of each entered behavior. Meanwhile, the output from the FM receiver, representing decoded motility information, also is entered directly into the computer; at selected intervals, the computer tunes the receiver from one animal's transmitter to the transmitter of the next animal. In a pre-selected rotation the computer thus receives motility data from each animal in turn, collecting such data around the clock. Programs for data retrieval permit us to examine the frequency or duration of each

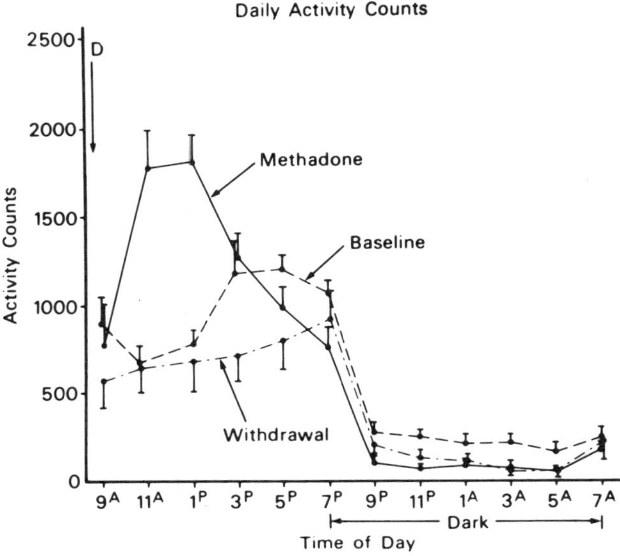

Fig. 3. Mean daily activity counts (± s.e.m.) from five monkeys during 6 baseline weeks of daily placebo administration, 10 weeks of daily methadone administration, and 3 withdrawal weeks of daily placebo administration. Arrow indicates time of dosing. (Reprinted with permission from Psychopharmacol (Berl) 43:135–144, 1975.)

behavior during different treatment conditions, or on different days, or from different animals. Plotting programs permit the graphing of motility data, and programs for cosinor analyses (Halberg et al., 1972) allow circadian analyses of the motility data.

HIGHLIGHTS OF PREVIOUS RESEARCH

Our work began with demonstrations that classical pharmacologic factors such as dose, duration of administration, and type of drug determine drug effects upon social behavior. While the importance of these matters may seem obvious to a pharmacologist, public policy often is predicated upon the simple notion that "drug abuse" produces some unidimensional impairment of social function, with little consideration of dose, duration of administration, or of which drug is involved.

In preliminary studies with rats we showed that shock-induced fighting between two rats increased with modest doses of the stimulant, methamphetamine, or of the sedative, phenobarbital. Higher doses of either drug suppressed fighting below baseline levels (Crowley, 1972b), but the apparent reasons for the changes in fighting were different. High doses of phenobarbital sedated the animals and slowed their fighting behavior. High doses of methamphetamine stimulated the animals, resulting in excessive motor activity; the animals seemed unable to organize a fighting response after a high dose of methamphetamine. Thus, we demonstrated that for two commonly abused drugs, dose was very important in determining the amount of a subsequent social behavior.

Next, we showed that when rats were treated chronically with either methamphetamine or phenobarbital in doses which suppressed body weight, shock-induced fighting times also were markedly depressed. Moreover, animals withdrawn from prior treatment with these drugs slowly increased their tendency to fight, eventually fighting far more than animals that continued to receive the drugs. The results suggested that prolonged duration of administration might alter social behavior far more than acute administration (Crowley and Rutledge, 1974).

Building on those original studies, we next reported drug effects on monkey social behavior (Crowley et al, 1974). We administered ethanol, methamphetamine, pentobarbital, and morphine to each of five sub-dominant male *M. nemestrina* living in a troop of about 30 animals. With a wide range of doses of each drug given to each animal, we determined dose-response curves for a large number of social behaviors, examining how the drugs differed in their capacity to alter primate social behavior.

The drugs did produce decidedly different effects. For example, alcohol induced playful fighting, a behavior almost never seen among adult male *M. nemestrina* in our laboratory. The sexual behavior of these sub-dominant males was mainly autosexual and rarely involved any contact with females, who consorted only with the dominant male; but with increasing doses of alcohol there was a dramatic, almost linear increase in the ratio of heterosexual to autosexual behaviors among these males (Fig. 4). Surprisingly, alcohol had almost no effect on dominance or subordinance behaviors, contrary to its reputation as an "aggressogen."

Pentobarbital did not alter sexual behavior or induce playful fighting, but it did reduce the number of subordinance behaviors, increasing the ratio of dominance behaviors to total hierarchical behaviors (Fig. 2). This dose-related increase in aggressiveness agrees with the findings of Tinklenberg et al. (1974) regarding barbiturate effects upon human aggression.

Contrary to the familiar slogan, "Speed kills," methamphetamine did not enhance aggressive dominance interactions; indeed, the drug produced a sizable increase in submissive behaviors (Fig. 2). Bizarre stereotyped behaviors developed with the higher doses of methamphetamine, and the drug also

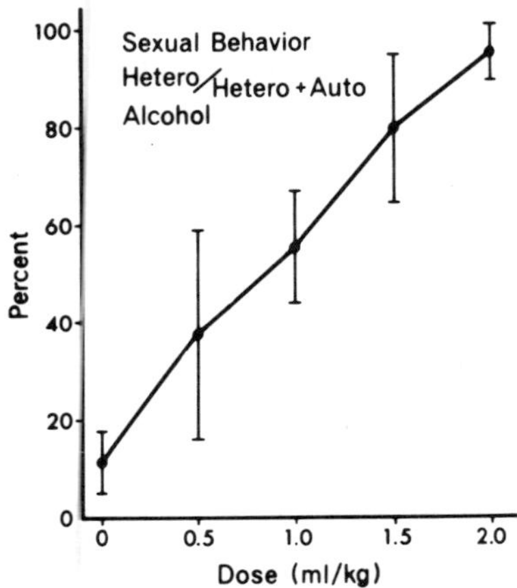

Fig. 4. Mean (± s.e.m.) percentage of heterosexual behavior in total of heterosexual and autosexual (masturbatory) behavior after ethanol, five male *M. nemestrina*. (Reprinted with permission from Arch Gen Psychiatr 31:829–838, 1974.)

suppressed food foraging while increasing spontaneous motility. The only effects produced by morphine in this study were the previously mentioned reductions (Fig. 1) of both autosexual and heterosexual behaviors.

This study was unique in that different drugs were given in several doses to the same animals while the occurrence of many social behaviors was quantified. The study emphasized the differential effects of different drugs, suggesting that abusers might sometimes choose a drug because it facilitated particular behaviors which would be reinforced in that user's particular environment. With this study completed, we had good evidence that drugs differed in their effects upon animal social behavior, that different doses produced different effects, and that duration of administration was also important in determining the social effects of drugs.

We next turned our attention to an animal model of methadone maintenance treatment (Crowley et al., 1975, 1977). When administered once daily to heroin addicts, this opioid agonist dramatically reduces heroin self-administration while blocking heroin withdrawal symptoms.

But might such a long-acting opioid drug produce some adverse behavioral side effects? For 6 weeks we gave a daily dose of fruit juice to a group of five *M. radiata* monkeys. Then, for 10 weeks we gave methadone in the fruit juice each day to each of the animals, and finally, for 3 weeks, we again gave only fruit juice. The doses produced blood levels of methadone comparable to those obtained in methadone maintenance clinics.

As noted earlier, methadone administration produced a sharp increase in spontaneous motility for several hours following each morning's drug dose, and there was a decline in motility on the nights following methadone administration (Fig. 3). These large changes in motility altered the form of the circadian wave of motor activity, advancing its phase by about 84 min while significantly expanding its amplitude.

It would seem probable that such dramatic changes in spontaneous motility might also change some important social behaviors. *M. radiata* frequently sit together in close physical contact, often clasping and embracing one another. Such associative behaviors including proximity, grooming, contact, and clasping, were significantly less frequent during the period of methadone administration (Fig. 5). Associative behavior occurred most often in the morning, and that was the time of greatest methadone-induced motility. It appeared that the animals simply engaged in so much motion that they had little time for normal social intercourse. It certainly is tempting to relate such changes to the hyperactive and seemingly disorganized "hustling" which often replaces normal social behavior in many opioid addicts, even during methadone maintenance treatment.

This study of methadone clearly indicated that the drug could disrupt normal social behavior when given in a maintenance regimen. Such an observation would not necessarily militate against the use of the drug, for heroin addiction also changes behavior and methdone has many advantages over heroin (Crowley and Rhine, 1981). But when informed about the

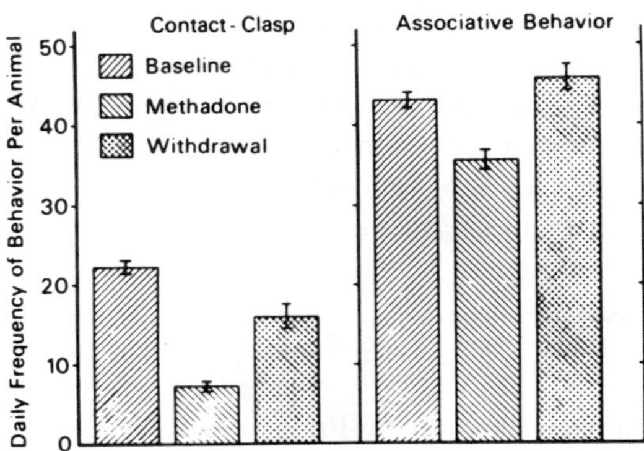

Fig. 5. Daily mean (± s.e.m.) of contact-clasp behavior, and of all associative behaviors, during 6 baseline weeks of daily placebo administration, 10 weeks of daily methadone administration, and 3 withdrawal weeks of daily placebo administration to five *M. radiata*. (Reprinted with permission from Psychopharmacol (Berl) 43:135–144, 1975.)

treatment's effects upon social behavior, both therapists and patients can make more rational choices about dosing and duration in such treatment.

Having shown that methadone significantly altered spontaneous motility and patterns of normal social behavior in monkeys, we then asked whether methadone or related drugs might have similar effects in human beings. About 80,000 former heroin addicts are maintained on such drugs in American methadone clinics, and it seemed important to determine whether these drugs might produce adverse behavioral effects in these patients. For several hours after each dose of methadone, our monkeys had been stimulated, and we then observed a reduction in motility in the hours just preceding the next daily dose. Unfortunately, we could not similarly study the effects of methadone itself in outpatients, since such patients provide no drug-free baseline period, as our monkeys did; these patients proceed directly from street heroin to methadone maintenance, and they experience no drug-free period for comparison with a period of methadone administration. But another comparison could be made with the methadone-like drug, l-alpha-acetylmethadol (LAAM). LAAM acts longer than methadone, so that patients take it every 2 or 3 days, rather than daily. If patients taking the drug every second day experienced effects like those which methadone produced in monkeys (early stimulation and later sedation following each dose), we might expect stimulation during the first day following a dose, with reduced activity on the second day.

Twelve former users of opioids who were in chronic LAAM maintenance treatment, wore a motility monitor for 48 hours, receiving LAAM on one of the experimental days. The subjects were about 50% more active (Fig. 6) on days of drug administration than on between-dose days (Crowley et al., 1979). This study demonstrated that, as with monkeys treated with methadone, human beings treated with LAAM were much more active early in the interval between doses than later in that interval. Following clues derived in the primate laboratory, we now had shown a drug side effect of potential clinical importance in a patient group.

CURRENT PROJECTS

LAAM in Monkeys

Following the Monday-Wednesday-Friday dosing regimen used in addiction treatment clinics, we now have administered LAAM to five male *M. radiata* living in a social group of about a dozen animals. We briefly withdrew the animals from their pen each Monday, Wednesday, and Friday morning during the course of 19 weeks; the animals were given a fruit-

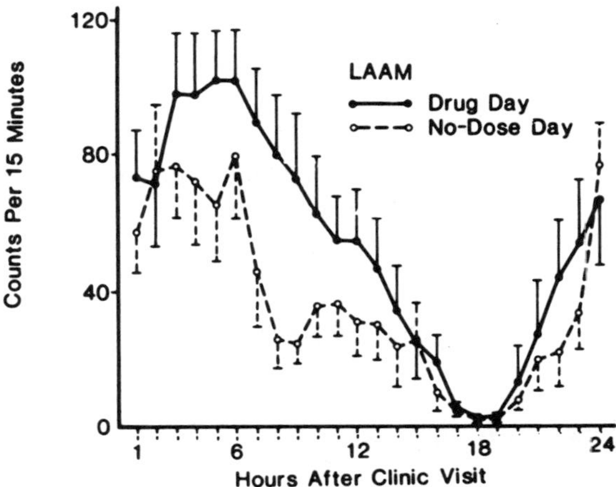

Fig. 6. Circadian curve of spontaneous motility, 12 LAAM-treated patients, on day of drug administration and on between-dose day. (Reprinted with permission from Psychopharmacol 62:151–155, 1979.)

flavored drink at this time. In weeks 7–17, the drink contained LAAM (mean dose, 1.2 mg/kg). As in our prior studies, backpack FM transmitters reported motility, and a trained observer recorded the occurrence of social behaviors. We hoped to demonstrate that acetylmethadol in monkeys would produce the same alternation of active and inactive days which we had observed in our human patients, and in addition, we hoped to identify exactly which social behaviors occurred more (or less) often on days of drug administration vs. between-dose days. Moreover, we expected to determine whether the daily alternation in motility represented stimulation on days of LAAM administration, or sedation on between-dose days, in comparison to drug-free baseline days.

Analyses of this project are still in progress, but even casual observation made it clear that the animals were much more active on days of drug administration than on between-dose days. Figure 7 plots the amount of Upright Rest, i.e., sitting quietly with eyes open, observed in each of the five animals throughout the study on dosing days and on between-dose days. During LAAM administration, all five animals spend much more time in Upright Rest on between-dose days than on dosing days. Clearly, the monkeys had the same alternation of active and inactive days which we had observed in LAAM-treated patients. Moreover, the graph makes it clear that these are not simply changes in automatically measured motility; day-to-day changes in specific behaviors (such as Upright Rest) result from the administration of this drug. Thus, this study further illuminates aspects of our earlier studies of LAAM effects in man, replicating the motor effects and showing effects on specific details of social intercourse.

Alcohol Drinking in Monkey Social Groups

The studies reviewed to this point involved examination of drug effects on social behavior in primate social groups. But, also, among human beings social influences affect drug self-administration. In a simple example, a

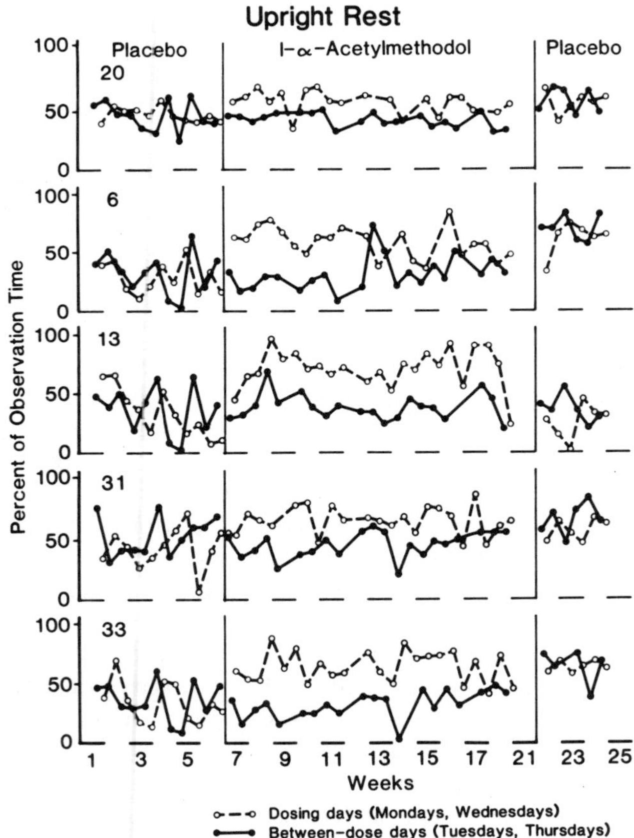

Fig. 7. Duration of Upright Rest, as percent of total observation time, five male *M. radiata*. Fruit-flavored drink given each Monday, Wednesday, and Friday contained LAAM during indicated weeks. Upright Rest record shown for Mondays and Wednesdays (dose days), and for Tuesdays and Thursdays (no-dose days); no observations on Fridays, Saturdays, or Sundays.

heroin abuser is less likely to inject himself if a policeman stands nearby. The efforts of Thompson et al. (1971) to examine social influences on drug self-administration by monkeys apparently were hampered by technical difficulties, and we know of only one other brief report assessing the effect of social influences on drug self-administration in primate social groups (Bowden and Jones, 1980). Our group recently has attempted to develop high-dose alcohol drinking among monkeys in a social group, utilizing techniques which Richard Meisch and his colleagues used to secure high-dose drinking among individually housed monkeys (Meisch and Henningfield, 1977; Henningfield and Meisch, 1978, 1979). Monkeys usually refuse intoxicating doses of alcohol solutions; alcohol's taste apparently is aversive to monkeys. But with modifications of the Meisch techniques, we have produced high-dose drinking among group-living *M. nemestrina*; during one period of daily sessions of alcohol availability, the animals consumed a mean of about 1.6 ml/kg/2 hr of absolute alcohol in an aqueous solution, showing clear signs of physical dependence. Fig. 8 plots the variability in the group's mean daily alcohol consumption, apparently related to such factors as feeding schedules, the occurrence of high-dose intoxications (which tended to suppress drinking on subsequent days), and social setting at the time of alcohol availability (Crowley et al., 1983). We hope in further studies to clarify factors which lead to variability in daily drinking, because controlling such factors may help to reduce the drinking of human alcoholics. After further development of the technique for inducing alcoholic-like drinking in monkey social groups, we plan to vary social situations systematically to determine their effect on drinking behavior.

CONCLUSIONS

For more than a decade, our group has been studying the effects of abused drugs, and of drugs used in the treatment of drug abuse, upon social and

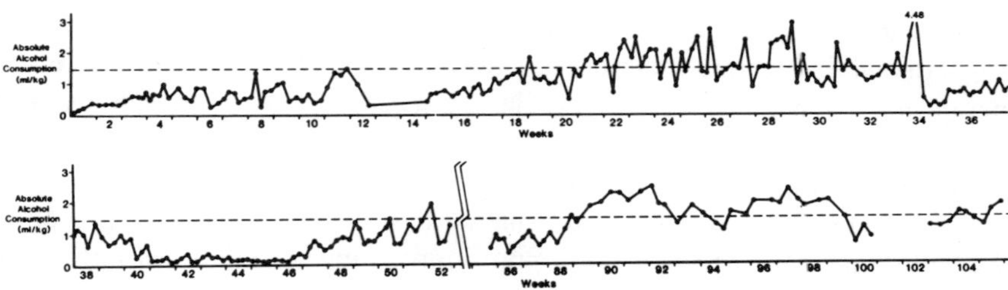

Fig. 8. Alcohol consumption by two to five group-living *M. nemestrina* during daily 2-hour sessions of availability of aqueous ethanol solutions. Dashed line indicates consumption required to produce mean blood levels of approximately 100 mg/dl.

motor behavior. We have conducted parallel studies in monkey social groups and in human beings.

Our experience emphasizes an obvious point which seems to be forgotten in the testing of new drugs (such as methadone or LAAM) for the treatment of drug abuse: behaviorally active drugs affect behavior. Enthusiasm for the important observation that a drug such as LAAM alters a target behavior, such as heroin self-administration, may inhibit examination of important behavioral side effects of the drug. Protocols for testing new psychotropic drugs require great attention to potential organ toxicity of the drugs, with very little attention to possible effects of the drugs on sexual, aggressive, submissive, associative, or resting behaviors. Although very gross effects of drugs on such behaviors may be detected in clinical drug trials, free-ranging outpatient subjects often may be unaware of profound drug-induced changes in their behavior (Crowley and Hydinger-Macdonald, 1979; Crowley et al., 1979). We have shown that the quantitative observation of social and motor behaviors in drug-treated, group-living primates is useful in assessing clinically relevant behavioral side effects from behaviorally active drugs.

Of course, we recognize that a drug's capacity to alter some target behavior (such as heroin self-administration) may outweigh its side effects on other aspects of behavior. But, we argued, "There is a need for careful research into the effects of any new psychotropic drug on animal and human social behavior before the drug's introduction into wide clinical use, so that the drug's 'cost' in altering normal social behaviors can be rationally weighed against its beneficial effects on symptomatic behaviors. As psychiatric researchers, we are convinced that a drug's toxicity on social behaviors is as important as its toxicity on organ systems, and we are concerned that these effects are inadequately emphasized in preclinical and early clinical drug evaluations" (Crowley and Simpson, 1978). Clinicians and their patients need to know a behaviorally active drug's possible adverse effects on social functioning, so that they can weigh the risk/benefit ratio of a particular drug in treating a particular patient. Inattention to the effects of behaviorally active drugs on subtle but important aspects of social and motor behavior deprives therapists and patients of this crucial information. Our research team is convinced that such research in primate social groups can inform clinical decisions and improve the lives of substance-abusing patients.

Further, we believe that basic behavioral science is approaching a new, clincially important threshold: the opportunity to investigate social influences upon drug self-administration in animal groups. Our preliminary studies with alcohol drinking in monkey social groups (Crowley et al., 1983) did produce severe intoxication, allowing future studies of how the behavior of other animals in the group may facilitate or suppress drinking by "alcoholic" monkeys. Moreover, it may become possible to assess social factors which contribute to the development of alcoholic-like drinking in monkeys; ethics prevent experiments designed to induce high-dose drinking among non-alcoholic human subjects, but an understanding of the development of high-dose drinking among monkeys could illuminate efforts at preventing the development of such drinking among human beings. This could be another important contribution from drug studies in primate social groups.

ACKNOWLEDGMENTS

The more recent work reported here was supported in part by grant DA02386 from the National Institute on Drug Abuse; by grant AA04926 from the National Institute on Alcohol Abuse and Alcoholism, U.S. Public Health Service; and by grant BRSG-05357 to the University of Colorado School of Medicine from Biomedical Research Grant Program, Division of Research Resources, National Institutes of Health. In addition to other participants named in our various publications, Patricia Okubo provided skilled technical assistance in our recent studies.

REFERENCES

Anker AL, Crowley TJ (1982) Use of contingency contracts in specialty clinics for cocaine abuse. In: Harris LS (ed) Problems of Drug Dependence, 1981. National Institute on Drug Abuse Research Monograph Series, 41. Washington DC, pp 452–459

Balster RL, Johanson CE, Harris RT, Schuster CR (1973) Phencyclidine self-administration in the rhesus monkey. Pharmacol Biochem Behav 1:167–172

Bowden DM, Jones RJ (1980) Social density and dominance status influence alcohol intake in pig-tailed macaques (abstr). Proc Am Society Primatologists

Crowley TJ (1972a) The reinforcers for drug abuse: Why people take drugs. Comp Psychiatr 13:51–62

Crowley TJ (1972b) Dose-dependent facilitation or suppression of rat fighting by methamphetamine, phenobarbital, or imipramine. Psychopharmacol (Berl) 27:213–222

Crowley TJ (1983) Contingency contracting treatment of drug-abusing physicians, nurses, and dentists. In: Grabowski J, Stitzer M (eds) Behavioral Interventions in Drug Abuse, National Institute on Drug Abuse Research Monograph Series (In Press)

Crowley TJ, Hydinger-Macdonald MJ (1979) Bedtime flurazepam and the human circadian rhythm of spontaneous motility. Psychopharmacol 62:157–161

Crowley TJ, Hydinger-Macdonald MJ, Stynes AJ, Feiger A (1975) Monkey motor stimulation and altered social behavior during chronic methadone administration. Psychopharmacol (Berl) 43:135–144

Crowley TJ, Jones RH, Hydinger-Macdonald MJ, Lingle JR, Wagner JE, Egan DJ (1979) Every-other-day acetylmethadol disturbs circadian cycles of human motility. Psychopharmacol 62:151–155

Crowley TJ, Lubanovic W, Halberg F, Hydinger M (1977) Daily oral methadone alters circadian activity rhythm of monkeys. In: (no editor) Twelfth International Conference Proceedings of the International Society for Chronobiology. Il Ponte, Milan, pp 395–402

Crowley TJ, Rhine MW (1981) Abuse of alcohol and other drugs. In: Simons RC, Pardes H (eds) Understanding Human Behavior in Health and Illness. Williams and Wilkins, Baltimore, pp 657–670

Crowley TJ, Rutledge CO (1974) Chronic methamphetamine, imipramine, and phenobarbital effects on shock-induced fighting in rats. In: Singh J, Lal H (eds) Drug Addiction, Vol 3: Neurobiology and Influences on Behavior. Miami Symposium Specialists, pp 65–80

Crowley TJ, Simpson R (1978) Methadone dose and human sexual behavior. Intl. J Addictions 13:285–295

Crowley TJ, Stynes AJ, Hydinger M, Kaufman IC (1974) Ethanol, methamphetamine, pentobarbital, morphine, and monkey social behavior. Arch Gen Psychiatr 31:829–838

Crowley TJ, Weisbard C, Hydinger-Macdonald MJ (1983) Progress toward high-dose alcohol drinking in monkey social groups. J Stud Alc (In press)

Deneau G, Yanagita T, Seevers MH (1969) Self-administration of psychoactive substances by the monkey. Psychopharmacol 16:30–48

Elton RH, Greaves DA, Bunger DR, Pyle TW (1976) Drinking patterns of pigtailed macaques. J Stud Alc 37:1548–1555

Goldberg SR, Hoffmeister F, Schlichting UU, Wuttke W (1971) A comparison of pentobarbital and cocaine self-administration in rhesus monkeys. J Pharmacol Exper Ther 179:277–283

Halberg F, Johnson E, Nelson W, Runge W, Sothern R (1972) Autorhythmometry procedures for physiologic self-measurements and their analyses. Physiol Teacher 1:1–10

Harringan SE, Downs DA (1978) Self-administration of heroin, acetylmethadol, morphine, and methadone in rhesus monkeys. Life Sci 22:619–624

Henningfield JE, Meisch RA (1978) Ethanol drinking by rhesus monkeys as a function of concentration. Psychopharmacol 57:133–136

Henningfield JE, Meisch RA (1979) Ethanol drinking by rhesus monkeys with concurrent access to water. Pharmacol Biochem Behav 10:777–782

Hoffmeister F, Schlichting UU (1972) Reinforcing properties of some opiates and opioids in rhesus monkeys with histories of cocaine and codeine self-administration. Psychopharmacol 23:55–74

Jones RJ, Bowden DM (1980) Social factors influencing alcohol consumption: a primate model. In: Eriksson K (ed) Animal Models in Alcohol Research. Academic Press, London, pp 185–189

Kaufman IC, Rosenblum LA (1966) A behavioral taxonomy for *macaca nemestrina* and *Macaca radiata*: based on longitudinal observations of family groups in the laboratory. Primates 7:205–258

Knight RP (1937) The psychodynamics of chronic alcoholism. J Nerv Ment Dis 86:538–548

Mast RT, Hydinger-Macdonald MJ, Crowley TJ (1982) Data acquisition system used in studying naltrexone and behavior in primates. Biomed Sci Instrum 18:37–44

Maxim PE (1978) Quantification of social behavior in pigtail monkeys. J Exper Psychol: Animal Behav Processes 4(1):50–67

Meisch RA, Henningfield JE (1977) Drinking of ethanol by rhesus monkeys: experimental strategies for establishing ethanol as a reinforcer. In: Gross MM (ed) Alcohol Intoxication and Withdrawal, Vol 3B. Plenum Press, New York, pp 443–463

Mello N, Mendelson J (1970) Experimentally induced intoxication in alcoholics: a comparison between programmed and spontaneous drinking. J Pharmacol Exper Ther 173:101–116

Mello N, Mendelson J (1971) A quantitative anlaysis of drinking patterns in alcoholics. Arch Gen Psychiatr 25:527–539

Meyer RE, Mirin SM (1979) The Heroin Stimulus. Plenum Press, New York, p 254

Thompson T, Bigelow G, Pickens R (1971) Environmental variables influencing drug self-administration. In: Thompson T, Pickens R (eds) Stimulus Properties of Drugs. Appleton-Century-Crofts, New York, pp 193–207

Thompson T, Pickens R (1975) An experimental analysis of behavioral factors in drug dependence. Fed Proc 34:1759–1770

Tinklenberg JR, Murphy PL, Murphy P, Darley CF, Roth WT, Kopell BS (1974) Drug involvement in criminal assaults by adolescents. Arch Gen Psychiatr 30:685–689

Walker S, Reite M (1975) Computer correlation of telemetered physiological data with behavior. Biomed Sci Instrum 11:1975–1978

Wallen K (1982) Influence of female hormonal state on rhesus monkey sexual behavior varies with space for social interaction. Sci 217:375–377

Wieder H, Kaplan EH (1969) Drug use in adolescents. Psychoanal Stud Child 24:399–431

Woods JH, Winger GD (1974) Alcoholism and animals. Prev Med 3:49–60

Young AM, Woods JH (1980) Behavior maintained by intravenous injection of codeine, cocaine, and etorphine in the rhesus macaque and the pigtail macaque. Psychopharmacol 70:163–271

Ethopharmacology: Primate Models of Neuropsychiatric Disorders,
pages 277–291

Assessment of Acute Versus Long-Term Effects of Delta-9-Tetrahydrocannabinol on Social Behavior and Adaptability in Group-Living Macaques

E.N. Sassenrath

Behavioral Sciences Laboratory, Department of Psychiatry, School of Medicine, University of California, Davis, California 95616

INTRODUCTION

The utility of primate models for predicting potential long-term drug effects in humans has yet to be fully assessed. This is an area of increasing importance in an era in which long-term or life-span drug usage is becoming more common. In particular, the issue of continued use of drugs of abuse from youth through adulthood is of concern when drugs such as marihuana and cocaine attain widespread popularity without a background of experience with these drugs in urbanized Western cultures.

The efficacy of a primate model for characterizing long-term effects of marihuana on social behavior and affect was tested in our laboratories over a 3-year period. At the time the study was initiated, the primary issues to be addressed were: 1) Does continued long-term use of marihuana lead to behavioral and personality changes; or is continuing heavy use of marihuana a function of underlying behavioral or personality characteristics? 2) Does psychological or social environmental stress play a role in the effects, if any, of long-term use of the drug?

This report will summarize the findings of this study and examine some of the interpretive problems in evaluating such a drug in such a test system.

EXPERIMENTAL CONDITIONS

Animals and Cage Groups

The data to be evaluated here were obtained from two four-membered caged groups of macaques, each composed of two males and two females aged 2 to 4 years at the start of the study. These groups were part of a larger experimental design which included seven mixed-sex groups: five four-membered groups and two six-membered groups (Sassenrath and Chapman,

1975). Two of the smaller groups were crab macaques *(M. fascicularis)*; all other groups were rhesus macaques *(M. mulatta)*. All groups had established social dominance structures with highly reproducible baseline behavior patterns. Group compositions of the two groups to be reported are specified in Table I.

Ranks within cage groups were determined from the direction of dominant-subordinate interactions within each dyad or pair of cagemates during spontaneous and competitive interaction. For all dyads in the four-membered cage groups in this study, the polarity of such interactions was consistent and remained unchanged throughout the study.

Drug Administration

The drug given was delta-9-tetrahydrocannabinol (THC), the principal psychoactive component of marihuana. THC was selected as the drug to be tested because of its availability in pure form and because of the extreme variation in cannabinoid content of marihuana from different sources. It was also assumed that effects observed with THC alone would represent a minimum effect to be expected from marihuana, per se, with comparable THC content.

THC was given orally daily 7 days per week on preferred food in late afternoon after all scheduled observations for that day, and 18 to 20 hours before observations on the following day. Since peak drug effect time was 2–3 hours after oral intake, and since intragroup interaction was minimal in early evening, the behavioral data represented "residual" drug effects free of immediate postdrug "intoxication" and its effect on ongoing overall group interaction patterns.

The drug was given daily on food at a level of 2.4 mg/kg body weight. This level was chosen as a dose which produced a reproducible state of tranquilization ("high") without ataxia or slowed responses to stimulation.

TABLE I. Composition of Prototype Cage Groups

Group	Species	Rank	Sex	Age*
A	Crab	1	F	3–7
	Macaque	2	M	3–7
		3	M	3–4
		4	F	3–7
B	Rhesus	1	M	2–7
	Macaque	2	M	3–8
		3	F	2–6
		4	F	2–4

*Age as years and months.

In each group of four members, one subject was drugged. In the overall experimental design, drugged subjects were selected to represent both males and females, dominants and subordinates. In all, there were 34 subjects in all cage groups, of which ten were drugged.

Behavioral Observations

Each group was observed a total of 4 hours on 4 different days within a 1-week period which constituted one behavioral assessment period (BAP). This was repeated at 1-month intervals prior to and throughout drug administration. Behavioral data was subsequently averaged over 3-month intervals to assess significant changes from predrug levels over long-term drug administration.

Social interaction behaviors and noninteractive behaviors were recorded for each animal and summarized as frequencies and/or durations for each BAP. For the present purposes, selected behaviors have been grouped into categories and total occurrences (frequencies) or total time spent (durations) in that behavioral category are reported. Behavioral categories are specified in Table II.

Neuroendocrine Measures

Urinary and plasma levels of stress-response hormones were determined during the predrug period and during the course of THC treatment. Urinary

TABLE II. Primate Behaviors for Assessing Drug Effects

Category	Behaviors
Interaction behaviors	
Agression: Mild	Stare, threat, huff, hit
Intense	Lunge, chase, bite, attack
Submission: Mild	Avoid, avert gaze, yield, leave
Intense	Flee, cringe
Affiliation	Embrace, huddle, groom
Play	Play
Watch	Watch or stare at cagemate
Noninteractive behaviors	
Self-directed	Self-groom, self-examine, self-mouth, self-bite
Exploration	Active investigation of inanimate cage environment
Disturbance	Cage shake (directed outside cage)
Stereotypy	Repetitive motor patterns such as pacing, head flipping, circling cage

levels of epinephrine, norepinephrine, cortisol, and creatine were determined for 24-hour urine collections from each group member during a 24-hour period immediately following removal from the home cage group. This procedure had been shown previously to provide characteristic reproducible excretion levels of each hormone for each individual which were representative of the ongoing level of activation of that system for that individual in adaptation to the group environment (Sassenrath et al., 1969).

After each baseline 24-hour collection, a second 24-hour collection was made after an ACTH challenge (4 μ/kg IM) to assess the maximum response potential of the adrenal cortex. The ACTH challenge test measures directly the adaptation of the adrenal cortex to the ongoing level of stimulation mediated by psychosocial stress to that individual in the cage group environment (Sassenrath, 1970).

This 2-day urine collection procedure was carried out on each member of each cage group three times during the predrug period and twice during each 3-month interval during drugging. In addition, at monthly intervals during the study, blood samples were taken at 9:00 a.m. from each subject for determination of circulating plasma cortisol levels.

RESULTS

Summary of Previously Reported Findings

We have previously reported distinct differences in behavioral effects comparing acute or short-term chronic THC administration (during days or weeks) with long-term chronic administration for 2 or more years (Chapman et al., 1979; Sassenrath and Chapman, 1975, 1976). In general, the sequence of drug action proceeds through three stages: 1) an early transient intoxication following drug intake characterized by increased sedation and a general decrease in active behavior, including all active interactions with cagemates (aggression, submission, play); 2) the gradual development of tolerance to these tranquilizing effects; and 3) the emergence of an increased irritability which resulted in increased aggression in most drugged dominant group members, especially under conditions of social stress. One index of this change in basic affect of chronically drugged subjects was the observation of increasing submission and avoidance behaviors of undrugged subordinate cagemates toward drugged animals of higher rank, especially in the two crab macaque cage groups. In other situations of extreme social stress, drugged subordinates in rhesus macaque groups were observed to initiate hierarchical shifts resulting in their rising in rank (Chapman et al., 1979).

However, there were paradoxical exceptions to this overall pattern of drug action. Following acute drug administration, a few subjects showed increased, rather than decreased, activity and aggression, whereas active stereotypic behaviors were increased in some and decreased in other subjects (Chapman et al., 1979). During long-term chronic drugging, one of four drugged dominants showed no increase in aggression, and, among all four, the observation of increased aggression varied in latency to behavioral change and in the social situation eliciting it (i.e., spontaneous group interaction vs. food competition).

These apparently conflicting observations of individual differences in drug responses suggested three possibilities: 1) that the primate cage-group model was too unstructured and unpredictable to function as a appropriate test system for characterization of drug-induced changes in social and affective behavior; 2) that social and affective behavior in naturalistic group situations could not be measured reliably; and/or 3) conversely, that the primate social group model was a highly sensitive system in which careful evaluation of observed behavioral correlates and contradictions might shed new insight into psychoactive drug action.

Our own data tended to support the latter possibility, but with reservations.

Variability in Drug Responses as a Function of Basic Individual Differences

In addressing the issue of interindividual differences in response to psychoactive drugs, two variables can be postulated to be proximal influences on drug effects on social behavior: i.e, qualitative and quantitative differences in 1) undrugged behavioral profiles and 2) autonomic and neuroendocrine profiles of each group member, both of which reflect the adaptation of that individual to its unique role in group interaction (Sassenrath, 1969, 1982).

A comparison of two similar cage groups from our study of long-term THC effects is a case in point. Cage A was a group of crab macaques composed of two males and two females; cage B was a group of rhesus macaques of similar composition. In both cage groups, the No. 2 male received long-term daily THC treatment. However, rank ordering by sex was different for the two groups: cage A—No. 1 female, No. 2 male, No. 3 male, No. 4 female; cage B—No. 1 male, No. 2 male, No. 3 female, No. 4 female.

A comparison of selected indices of the baseline (predrug) behavioral profiles of the No. 2 males in each group is shown in Fig. 1. From this it is apparent that the No. 2 male in cage A showed more interaction with subordinate cagemates No. 3 and No. 4—i.e., more aggression and play as well as more time spent in close proximity to them. Conversely, the No. 2 male in cage B showed much less interaction with subordinates, more submission to the dominant (No. 1) animal, and higher levels of noninteractive

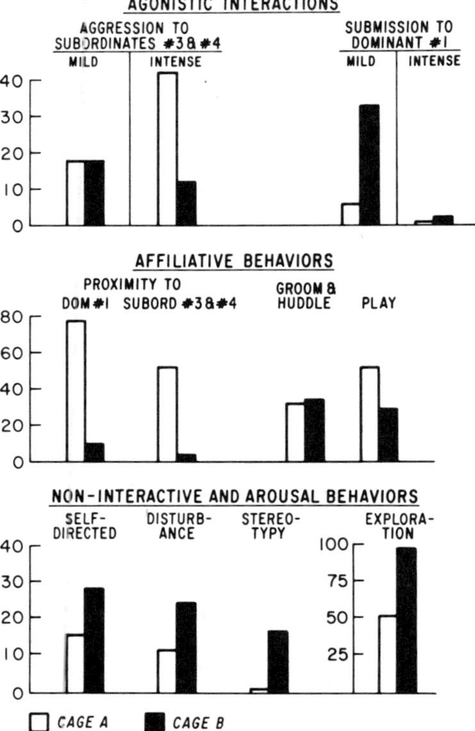

Fig. 1. Predrug behavioral profiles for No. 2–ranked males in cages A and B.

self-directed and cage exploration behaviors as well as disturbance (cage shaking) and motor stereotypy. Overall, the No. 2 male in cage B exhibited a pattern of social adaptation characterized by less interaction with cagemates and more nonsocial activity.

Since the No. 1–ranked dominant in each group performs a key role in shaping the characteristic social milieu of the group, including the interaction potential of subordinate members, it is of interest also to compare these roles in the two cage groups. As shown in Fig. 2, the behavioral profile of the No. 1 female in cage A contrasts sharply with the profile of the No. 1 male in cage B.

Although both dominants show low levels of aggression toward all subordinates, the No. 1 male in cage B receives much more submission, especially from the lowest ranking females No. 3 and No. 4. Conversely, the No. 1 female in cage A engages in more affiliative grooming and huddle behaviors

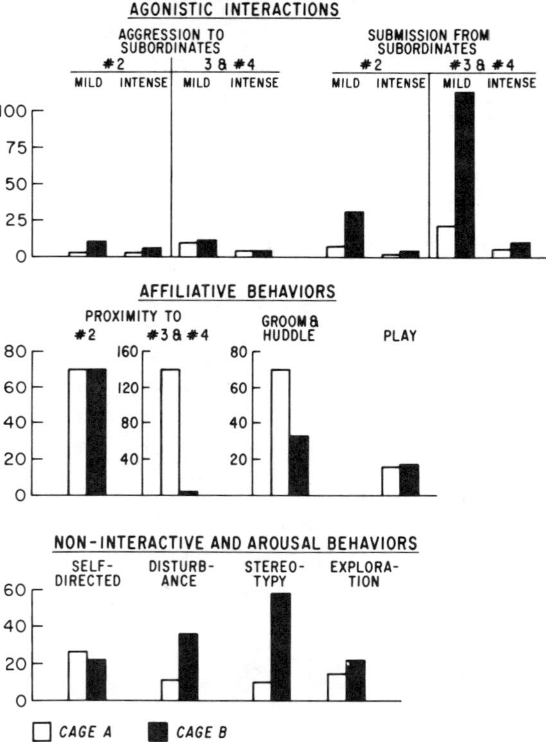

Fig. 2. Behavioral profile of the first-ranked dominants in cages A and B prior to THC treatment of second-ranked males in each cage group.

with subordinates and spends much more time in close proximity to her lowest ranking No. 3 and No. 4 cagemates. Appropriately, the No. 1 male in cage B exhibits higher levels of activity manifest as disturbance and stereotypy behavior.

Taken together, the behavioral comparison of No. 1– and No. 2–ranked animals in cages A and B suggests less aggressive control of group interaction by the No. 1 dominant female in cage A, permitting more aggression by the No. 2 male relative to cage B. Both No. 1 and No. 2 males in cage B show higher levels of disturbance and stereotypy behaviors.

The differences in baseline behaviors of the No. 2–ranking males can now be compared to the differences in their responses to long-term daily treatment with THC. Table III summarizes the behavioral changes in these two males during the course of daily drugging. The No. 2 male in cage B who was

TABLE III. Comparison of Behavioral Changes of No. 2–Ranked Males in Cage Groups A and B During 9 Months of Daily THC Administration

Behaviors[a]	Cage group	Predrug frequency[b] (means ± SD)	Behavioral changes: Months of drugging		
			1–3	4–6	7–9
Aggression					
Threat	A	18 ± 12	0	0	0
	B	18 ± 4	+	+	⊕
Active	A	43 ± 30	0	0	0
	B	12 ± 4	(+)	+	⊕
Submission					
Avoid	A	6 ± 1.5	0	0	0
	B	33 ± 6	−	(−)	0
Escape	A	0.3 ± 0.6	0	0	0
	B	1.7 ± 0.6	−	0	0
Affiliation					
Groom/huddle	A	26 ± 4	0	0	0
	B	27 ± 8	+	⊕	0
Play	A	52 ± 53	⊖	⊖	(−)
	B	29 ± 19	⊖	(−)	−
Watch/stare					
	A	42 ± 30	+	+	+
	B	35 ± 9	+	+	+
Noninteractive					
Self-directed	A	15 ± 3.5	+	+	+
	B	28 ± 8	+	+	(+)
Explore	A	51 ± 18	0	0	0
	B	93 ± 52	(−)	0	0
Disturbance	A	8 ± 5	0	0	0
	B	24 ± 17	0	0	0
Stereotypy	A	0.7 ± 1.1	0	0	0
	B	16 ± 12	−	(−)	(−)

[a]See text for specific behaviors in each category.
[b]Behavioral changes expressed as direction of change from predrug frequency: 0: no change; + or −: significant increase or decrease at $P < 0.05$; (+) or (−): change approaching significance at $P < 0.10$; ⊕ or ⊖: change approaching significance at $P < 0.15$.

normally less aggressive to subordinates No. 3 and No. 4 and more submissive to No. 1 showed an increase in aggression and a decrease in submission. His normally high frequency of stereotypy was also decreased. In contrast, the No. 2 male in cage A showed no change in agonistic behavior or stereotypy.

The behavioral changes which were parallel for both males were decreased play, increased watch/stare, and increased self-directed behaviors. In no case were there opposite changes in behavioral frequency for these two drugged males.

In an attempt to characterize stress response neuroendocrine systems as possible mediators of drug response, 24-hour excretion levels of epinephrine, norepinephrine, and cortisol as well as circulating levels of cortisol were monitored before and during long-term drugging. Individual differences in predrug profiles supported expectations; i.e., all hormones studied tended to be higher in the lower-ranking group members, reflecting the higher stress-activation of these systems in these subjects (Sassenrath, 1970; Sassenrath et al., 1969).

However, drugged group members did not show a consistent change in any of these neuroendocrine measures which would suggest drug action on these neuroendocrine systems. Where changes in neuroendocrine indices were observed during the course of chronic THC administration, there was no apparent correlation with either predrug baseline neuroendocrine profiles or with behavioral changes during drugging. As shown in Table IV, comparing the second-ranked males in cages A and B, predrug baseline excretion levels of the hormones studied differed only in the cortisol measures. The greatest difference was in cortisol response to ACTH challenge, where the cage A male was higher, suggesting much higher levels of chronic response of the pituitary-adrenal axis to the stimulation of psychosocial stress in his cage group environment. As shown in Fig. 3, during the 9-month course of THC administration, this same male showed increases in both excretion levels of norepinephrine and circulating levels of cortisol. The No. 2 male in cage B showed low baseline ACTH response and no change in any measure during drugging. The significance of the endocrine changes in the drugged male in cage A in the absence of changes in agonistic behavior and of the behavioral changes in the drugged male in cage B without endocrine changes is difficult to explain. The endocrine data suggest some subtle changes in

TABLE IV. Predrug Excretion Levels of Catecholamines and Cortisol in No. 2–Ranked Males in Cages A and B

Urine component	No. 2 male cage A (μg per mg creatinine)	No. 2 male cage B
Epineprine	20 ± 4.5[a]	19 ± 1.2[a]
Norepinephrine	27 ± 4.3	32 ± 5.3
Cortisol	24 ± 11.5	17 ± 1.9
Cortisol response to ACTH challenge	242 ± 143	62 ± 17

[a]Values expressed as means ± SD for triplicate determinations on 24-hour urine collections.

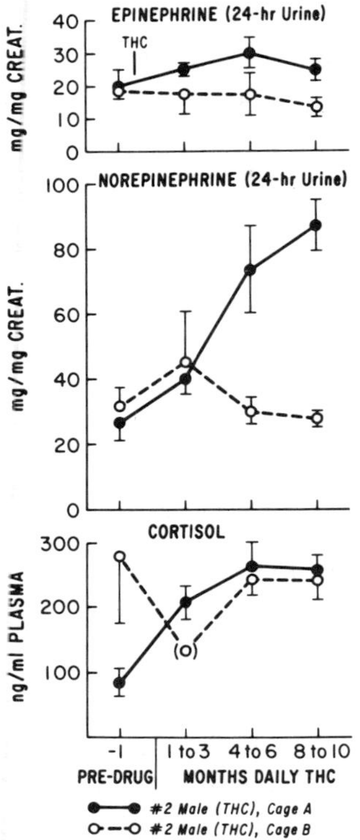

Fig. 3. Excretion and circulating levels of stress response hormones for second-ranked males cages A and B during 9 months of treatment with THC.

cage A social structure which were not apparent in the observed group behavior, but a logical connection between this and a drug action in the No. 2 male is not apparent.

DISCUSSION

Interpretation of Social Behavioral Data

In assessing the significance of drug-induced behavioral changes in a group setting, several considerations are critical to interpretation of the data. One consideration is the differentiation of primary from secondary drug-induced effects. Primary effects can be viewed as those resulting from a direct action of the drug on the drugged subject, altering that individual's responses to the social environment. Such behavioral changes must also be further differentiated from altered responses which are a function of drug-induced decrements in neuromuscular function or arousal state. Secondary drug effects are those reflecting altered dynamics of group interaction, resulting in altered behavior of nondrugged group members in response to behavioral changes in the drugged member. In such cases, behavioral changes of all group members would reflect each individuals's adaptation to the altered environment.

A second major consideration concerns individual differences among group members in "behavioral response potential." This has been demonstrated in the baseline, predrug profiles for cages A and B presented in Figs. 1 and 2. Thus, a group member normally at a maximally elevated behavioral frequency or at a minimally detectable frequency cannot show significant drug-induced increases or decreases, respectively, in that behavior. Further, since social behaviors and their utilization are primarily learned responses, it is not to be expected that a drug can induce a behavioral response that is not normally in that individual's repertoire at some level of frequency.

From this it is clear that all statistically significant changes in behavior frequencies after or during drug treatment must logically be assessed for their behavioral significance in the context of each individual's undrugged profile in interaction with each other group member. Where drug-induced behavioral changes are both subtle and variable among individuals—as with THC—it is a formidable task to extract generalities regarding specific drug effects on social behavior, per se.

Validity and Relevance of Behavioral Changes Observed During Long-Term Chronic Administration of THC to Monkeys

Generality of drug effects. Of the three behavioral indices in which the No. 2 males of cages A and B showed similar changes with long-term drugging, only one represented true social interaction behavior. This was the observed frequencies of "play" behavior which decreased for both of these subjects as well as for the drugged subjects in all other groups studied (not reported here). The reduction of "play" behavior in the absence of reduction in other interactive behaviors suggests an underlying change in positive affect characteristic of play. Such decrements in positive affect have been reported by some marihuana users, who also report loss of interest in the drug as a pleasure-enhancing experience (private communications).

The increases in both watch and self-directed behaviors may be manifestations in monkeys of commonly observed effects of marihuana intoxication in humans. Altered visual attending or "narrowed attention" is a frequent effect of the marihuana "high" which may be related to sustained watching or staring at cagemates. Altered attention has also been reported in very young monkeys chronically exposed to THC during early development in utero and throughout lactation from mothers treated daily with THC (Golub, 1979; Golub et al., 1982). Similarly, the increased "self-directed" behavior may be related to the introspective nature of marihuana intoxication in man, which has been contrasted to that of alcohol, which is characterized as a "social" drug.

Of particular relevance here is the fact that these behavioral effects, which have correlates in the human marihuana "high," were observed in monkeys that were past the state of immediate postdrug intoxication. In monkeys with long-term regular exposure to THC, then, these appear to be residual drug effects, which suggest a direct and persistent drug action on central pathways influencing expression of these behaviors.

It is of interest to note here that the same long-term THC-treated monkeys which demonstrated a high degree of tolerance to the immediate postdrug tranquilizing effects of daily THC doses of 2.4 mg/kg/day again showed the initial postdrug effects of sedation and reduced activity and competition when the daily dose was increased to 3.6 or 4.8 mg/kg. Such immediate postdrug intoxication effects appear to predominate whenever drug blood levels exceed the level of acquired tolerance. This tolerance, then, appears to be centrally mediated, and may be one aspect of long-term drug effects on central mechanisms influencing behavior.

Individual differences in drug response. The interindividual differences in monkey behavioral responses to long-term THC treatment, where the variables of sex and social rank are held constant, also have some parallel in the wide range of sensitivity to marihuana in humans. While much of the variability in human responses to the drug is clearly a function of differences in drug potency and frequency and duration of drug exposure—with resultant differences in levels of acquired tolerance to the drug—the concept of underlying differences in basic sensitivity to the drug is a generally accepted phenomenon. Similar to the increased aggression observed in some THC-treated monkeys, a hostile, defensive affective responsivity to challenge or threat is a reported observation in heavy marihuana users (Kolansky and Moore, 1972).

This type of drug effect has also been noted and studied for another psychoactive drug prescribed for its tranquilizing or anxiolytic action, namely chlordiazepoxide (CDE) or Librium. This drug has been reported to give "paradoxical" side effects of rage, hostility, aggression, or excitability in some psychiatric patients. In animal studies, CDE had been observed to have a calming effect on individually caged subjects, but caused increased aggression in group-caged subjects (Fox et al., 1970). In a clinical study of healthy male volunteers in a small group interaction setting, chronic CDE administration significantly elevated self-ratings of affective hostility, but only in the subset of subjects rating high and mid-anxious on the Taylor Manifest Anxiety Scale. Under conditions of superimposed frustration in the group setting, the behavior of these same high-anxious subjects was rated as more hostile in group interaction by their fellow group members, as well as by raters assessing verbal hostility (Salzman et al., 1974).

These observations, together with our own primate data, support the concept of individual differences in affective and behavioral responsivity to chronic administration of a psychoactive drug, which can be directly related to a basic psychological or personality trait. Further, such differences in drug effects are manifest primarily in interactive processes involving concurrent activation of stress response pathways, e.g., frustration or challenge. Increased irritable aggression in long-term THC treated group-living primates, then, can be viewed as a primary drug effect which becomes apparent only in the appropriate combination of subject and setting.

Proposed Functional Level of THC Action

Our observations of behavioral changes during long-term chronic THC administration show only few and subtle behavioral changes which are consistent across all or most drugged subjects; these include play, "watch," and "self-directed" behaviors. Further, the more dramatic changes in agonistic behavior (aggression, submission) are not observed in all drugged subjects, and this variability in drug response cannot be related directly to individual differences in baseline frequencies of these behaviors or to rank or role of that individual in the group.

One tenable concept of long-term chronic THC action which accomodates such individual differences proposes a drug-induced alteration of perception and processing of psychosocial stimuli, resulting in interference with appropriate learned adaptive responses (Chapman et al., 1979). Such drug-induced alteration of stimuli processing could be mediated by direct drug alteration of receptor sensitivity, especially noradrenergic receptors known to modulate aggressive behavior (Segal et al., 1975; Thoa et al., 1972). THC has been shown to potentiate the stressor response to epinephrine and norepinephrine (Zitko et al., 1972). If one postulates a similar enhancement of central receptors modulating behavior under conditions of chronic drugging, the release of catecholamines during a stress response could result in hyperactivation of a system involved in control of affect and aggression.

It has been reported that noradrenergic neuronal degeneration induced by 6-hydroxydopa results in an initial hypersensitivity of central noradrenergic receptors to endogenous amines which can be manifest as increased aggression under stress (Thoa et al., 1972). The possibility of such a degenerative action resulting from long-term exposure to THC is suggested by recent observations of McGahan et al. (1981) on our own THC-treated monkeys. Using computerized tomographic techniques, he has observed significant ventricular enlargement in the forebrain area in long-term THC-treated monkeys (i.e., THC daily for 2 to 5 years). This effect was significant compared to either short-term THC-treated monkeys (i.e., THC daily for 2 to 10 months) or to undrugged controls, which were not significantly different from each other.

These recent observations on long-term THC-treated monkeys which had been drug-free for at least 2 years at the time of evaluation suggest an irreversible drug action resulting in cerebral atrophy. If atrophy is substantianted by further proposed studies on these subjects, then the observed changes in social behavior in long-term THC-treated monkeys may have been the early manifestations of a drug action which resulted ultimately in cell death. In view of the many correlates between our findings on THC behavioral effects in a primate model and those of marihuana in man, these recent observations of brain changes suggest a reevaluation of the possibility of such sequelae of long-term marihuana use in man, previously reported in a controversial study by Campbell et al. (1971).

CONCLUSIONS

The data generated from a study of behavioral effects of long-term THC administration in a group-living primate model suggest drug-induced subtle changes in social behavior and affect, manifest as decreased play behavior, increased nonsocial and self-directed behavior, and increased irritability associated with stress. In this test system, these effects are shown to be "residual" drug effects not associated with the immediate intoxication following drug intake.

The drug-related increases in irritable aggression is variable across drugged individuals, but is not a function of sex, social rank, or baseline behavioral profiles per se. Although apparently triggered or enhanced by stress, it is not paralleled or mediated by concurrent changes in either the sympathetic adrenomedullar or pituitary adrenocortical stress response systems.

The types of behavioral changes and individual differences observed in response to long-term THC exposure are consistent with a mechanism of a drug action on central noradrenergic receptors resulting in a hypersensitivity to stress-generated catecholamines as well as more subtle changes in affect.

The initial impetus for this study of potential long-term effects of THC on social behavior in a group-living primate model was to generate data with optimum relevance to man. Ironically, the effectiveness of the primate model in demonstrating such subtle variable effects as those reported can now be assessed only in light of observations of comparable effects in man.

REFERENCES

Campbell AMG, Evans M, Thomson JLG, Williams MJ (1971) Cerebral atrophy in young cannabis smokers. Lancet 2: 1219–1225

Chapman LF, Sassenrath EN, Goo GP (1979) Social behavior of rhesus monkeys chronically exposed to moderate amounts of delta-9-tetrahydrocannabinol. In: Nahas GG, Paton WDM (eds) Marihuana: Biological Effects. Pergamon Press, Oxford, pp 693–712

Fox KA, Tuckosh JR, Wilcox AH (1970) Increased aggression among grouped male mice fed chlordiazepoxide. Eur J Pharmacol 11: 119–121

Golub MS (1979) A primate model for detecting behavioral impairment in offspring after chronic parental drug exposure. Pharmacol Biochem Behav 11(Suppl): 47–50

Golub MS, Sassenrath EN, Chapman LF (1982) An analysis of altered attention in monkeys exposed to delta-9-tetrahydrocannabinol during development. Neurobehav Toxicol Teratol 4: 469–472

Kolansky H, Moore WT (1972) Toxic effects of chronic marihuana use. J Am Med Assn 222(1): 35–41

McGahan JB, Dublin AB, Sassenrath EN (1981) Computerized tomography of the brain on long-term THC treated rhesus monkeys. Proc 67th An Meeting Radiology Society North Am Chicago

Salzman C, Kochansky GE, Shader RI, Porrino LJ, Harmatz JS, Swett CP Jr (1974) Chlordiazepoxide-induced hostility in a small group setting. Arch Gen Psychol 31: 401–405

Sassenrath EN (1969) Neuroendocrine adaptation to the stress of group caging in M. mulatta. Physiologist 12(3): 348

Sassenrath EN (1970) Increased adrenal responsiveness related to social stress in rhesus monkeys. Hormones Behav 1: 283–298

Sassenrath EN (1982) Studies in adaptability: experimental, environmental and pharmacological influences. In: Steklis H, Kling A (eds) Hormones, Drugs and Social Behavior. Spectrum Publ, New York

Sassenrath EN, Chapman LF (1975) Tetrahydrocannabinol-induced manifestations of the "marihuana syndrome" in group-living macaques. Fed Proc 34(8): 1666–1670

Sassenrath EN, Chapman LF (1976) Primate and social behavior as a method of analysis of drug action: studies with THC in monkeys. Fed Proc 35(11): 2238–2244

Sassenrath EN, Hein LJ, Kaita AA (1969) Social behavior and corticoid correlates in Macaca mulatta. Proc 2nd Int Congr Primat Atlanta Georgia 1968 Vol 1 Karger/Basel, New York, pp 219–231

Segal DS, Geyer MA, Weiner BE (1975) Strain differences during intraventricular infusion of norepinephrine: possible role of the receptor sensitivity. Sci 189: 301–303

Thoa NB, Eichelman B, Richardson JS, Jacobwitz D (1972) 6-Hydroxydopa depletion of brain norepinephrine and facilitation of aggressive behavior. Sci 178: 75–77

Zitko BA, Howes JF, Razdan RK, Dalzell BC, Dalzell HC, Sheehan JC, Pars HG (1972) Water soluable derivatives of delta-9-tetrahydrocannabinol. Sci 177: 441–444

Ethopharmacology: Primate Models of Neuropsychiatric Disorders,
pages 293–305

Effects of Subacute Administration of Amphetamine on Food Competition in Primates

Marvin C. Wilson, Lillian Bailey, and John A. Bedford

Department of Pharmacology and the Research Institute of Pharmaceutical Sciences, School of Pharmacy, University of Mississippi, University, Mississippi 38677

INTRODUCTION

One particular aspect of the effect of drugs on nonhuman primate social behavior is their ability to alter competitive behaviors. Such an effect may be demonstrated as a change in the differential access of treated subjects to desired objects such as food, water, and proximity to subjects of the opposite sex. It has been argued that the relative success of each member of a group of subjects in competitive situations may be a valid index of the dominance relationships among these subjects (Farres and Haude, 1976; Richards, 1974; Syme, 1974). Therefore, a drug-induced alteration in competitive behavior may suggest that the substance has altered the dominance relationships among the participants. This change in dominance relationships would then be demonstrated by changes in the success of the treated subjects in competitive situations. Alternatively, it could be hypothesized that as a result of selective drug-induced changes in competitive situations, the dominance relationships within the test group may change.

This laboratory has reported the results of several studies in which the effects of the acute administration of d-amphetamine on food competition were determined (Bellarosa et al., 1980; Lovell et al., 1980; Wilson et al., 1982). In both heterosexual and isosexual grouped and paired competition situations in which amphetamine was concurrently administered to all participants, there appeared to be a differential drug effect based on the relative dominance position of the subjects in the control situation. In general, subjects which had been rarely successful in obtaining food under control conditions obtained the majority of fruit or biscuits following amphetamine treatment. Amphetamine appeared to differentially improve the success of these subjects in the competitive situation at the expense of the most dominant subjects. This effect has been observed in three totally different groups of *Macaca arctoides* and in one group of *Macaca mulatta*.

These data do not appear to result from drug-induced change in the dominance relationships among the participants. Even though the least dominant subjects were now successful in obtaining the food, these same subjects did not demonstrate either a decrease in submissive behaviors or an increase in dominance behaviors as measured by the frequency of presenting, relinquishing of space, etc. In fact, increased expression of submissive behavior by the "winners" directed toward the more dominant "losers" generally resulted. Schlemmer and Davis (1981) have suggested that this increase in submissive behaviors is mediated by activation of dopaminergic pathways.

A similar effect of converting "losers" into "winners" has been reported following administration of amphetamine and other dopamine agonists to rats in a food-competition paradigm (Masur et al., 1974; Terada and Masur, 1973). It is indeed interesting, in view of the well-known anorectic effect of these substances in these species, that their administration would result in an increase in food consumption. One could speculate that the differential sensitivity to the anorectic effects of these drugs might result from differences in the same neurochemical or hormonal processes which might also be responsible for the expression of "dominance" behaviors.

The present studies were conducted in order to determine whether these acute actions of amphetamine on grouped food competition are altered as a result of prior administration of the substance. These effects were assessed using both concurrent and individual dosing regimens in an attempt to ascertain whether the effects observed in a particular subject during concurrent treatment resulted primarily from that subject receiving amphetamine or from the other subjects being treated with amphetamine.

METHODS

Subjects

Three feral-born sexually mature male (Levi, 13.7 kg; Warjoe, 12.9 kg; Ernie, 8.3 kg) and three feral-born sexually mature female (Minnie, 8.3 kg; Susan, 6.4 kg; Birdie, 6.9 kg) *Macaca arctoides* served as subjects. These animals were housed in a cage which measured 3.13 m × 1.19 m × 2.44 m (height × width × depth). The back and one side wall of the chamber were covered with Formica, and the other side wall and ceiling were constructed of 5 × 15 cm, 4-gauge wire (Behlan Manufacturing Co., Columbus, NE). The front wall was constructed of 6.4-mm Plexiglas, framed in 5 cm angle iron. A watering device (Lixit, Ancare Corp., Manhasset, NY) was located on one side wall, 0.76 m from the floor and directly adjacent to the front wall. A food hopper (Hoeltge, Cincinnati, OH) was centered on the opposite side wall, 0.38 m from the floor. A standard stainless steel primate cage measuring 75 cm × 61 cm × 71 cm (height × width × depth; Hoeltge, Cincinnati, OH) was mounted on the outside of the wire side wall, 0.86 m from the floor and adjacent to the back wall of the enclosure. One side of this cage was fitted with a Plexiglas sliding door (30 cm × 30 cm) which faced into the social cage. The social cage also contained several perches of various sizes located on the back wall, as well as one centered 30 cm under the watering device. Unless otherwise indicated, 75 pieces of food (Purina Monkey Chow, Ralston-Purina Co., St. Louis, MO) were provided to the group twice daily, at 10:00 and 16:30 hours. Water was available ad libitum. A chewable multiple vitamin was provided daily to each subject. Subject weights were recorded weekly. Temperature was maintained at 21 ± 2°C and humidity at 50 ± 5%. The cage was illuminated between the hours of 8:30 and 17:00.

Procedure

Testing occurred in the home cage described above. A given session consisted of injecting all subjects in the group with either saline (0.5 ml) or d-amphetamine (AMP) 1.0 mg/kg IM (concurrent dosing) or injecting five of the subjects with saline and the remaining subject with AMP (individual dosing). Fifteen minutes later, a test session began. Thus dose and pretreatment time were chosen based on the previously reported results of acute AMP treatment (Bellarosa et al., 1980; Lovell et al., 1980; Wilson et al., 1982). The onset of the session was indicated by a technician simultaneously placing 72 pieces of food (Purina Monkey Chow) into the common hopper. The order in which the pieces of food were removed from the hopper was recorded. This part of the session was terminated 15 min later and any remaining food was removed. The number of biscuits retrieved by each subject was calculated. Water was available ad libitum during testing. A 50-min behavioral session then commenced during which the frequency, duration, and dyadic nature of various social and solitary behaviors were recorded. For purposes of this chapter, only the data on two of these behaviors—i.e., presenting and yielding (displacement, supplanting)—will be included. Presenting is defined as the directing of the hindquarters of one subject to another subject with head and shoulders lowered and the buttocks raised. Yielding is defined as abandonment (never all extremities simultaneously off the surface) of a cage area or perch in response to the approach or facial threat of another subject.

The control values for these parameters were determined by analyzing the data from the five consecutive sessions immediately preceding AMP dosing, during which saline was administered to all subjects. The concurrent AMP phase of the study was then initiated during which AMP 1.0 mg/kg was administered as a pretreatment to each subject daily for 21 consecutive days. During this period, behavioral sessions were conducted Monday through Friday. Following this 21-day sequence, saline was again administered to each subject for 7 consecutive days. Behavioral assessments were conducted during five of these sessions. On those days in which no behavioral observations were taken, the group received 75 biscuits at 10:00 and again at 16:30 hours. On days on which behavioral sessions were conducted, the morning feeding was omitted, and 100 biscuits were provided at the afternoon feeding. This was done to insure a state of approximately 18 hours of food deprivation at the time of competition testing. These feeding parameters also provided for growth and adequate nutrition of all subjects in the group.

Three months after completion of the concurrent study, the individual subacute dosing regimens commenced. The procedure was identical to that above with the exception that rather than all subjects being simultaneously treated with AMP for 21 days, only a single subject was so treated. The other five subjects received daily saline injections. Four (Susan, Warjoe, Minnie, and Levi) of the six subjects were tested in this manner. It had been initially decided to test all subjects; however, one subject (Ernie) became ill before either he or Birdie could be tested. Ernie had to be removed from the group environment, which precluded completion of the entire project. A 30-day period was interspersed between the end of treatment of one subject and the initiation of treatment with another monkey.

In each test situation, the treatment effects were compared to the control data obtained immediately prior to the onset of each 21-day dosing regimen.

RESULTS

Table I illustrates the suggested control dominance relationships among the six subjects in the treatment group. This proposed dominance hierarchy was developed from the results of both the food-competition tests and the number and dyadic identity of presenting and yielding behaviors. It seems apparent that Levi is the most dominant subject in the group and Birdie is the least dominant. Ernie is the least dominant male, but is dominant over Birdie. Susan is the most dominant female and is more dominant than Warjoe, the middle-ranking male. The relative dominance relationship between Warjoe and Minnie, the middle-ranking female, is not apparent since reciprocal submissive gestures of similar frequency were emitted by these two subjects. These animals also obtained essentially equivalent amounts of food in the competition tests.

TABLE I. Suggested Dominance Relationships Among Subject Group as Assessed by Results of Food Competition Tests and Dyadic Identity of Submissive Behaviors[a]

	Number of food biscuits retrieved	Submissive behaviors[b] emitted	Submissive behaviors[b] received
Levi	54.0 ± 4.6	1.8 ± 1.1 Susan	12.8 ± 3.1 Warjoe Susan Ernie Birdie
Susan	11.8 ± 4.1	6.8 ± 3.1 Levi Warjoe	4.0 ± 2.6 Ernie Minnie Birdie
Minnie	2.2 ± 1.3	2.0 ± 0.3 Susan Levi	2.2 ± 1.2 Warjoe Ernie Birdie
Warjoe	0.8 ± 0.4	4.8 ± 2.3 Levi Minnie	13.6 ± 4.5 Ernie Birdie Susan
Ernie	0.2 ± 0.2	7.2 ± 2.6 Levi Warjoe Minnie Susan	1.4 ± 0.7 Birdie
Birdie	0.2 ± 0.2	11.8 ± 6.7 All	0.4 ± 0.3

[a]Values represent the mean (± SEM) obtained from five saline control sessions conducted prior to the onset of concurrent AMP dosing.
[b]Submissive behaviors refers to "presents" plus "yields." Subjects named are those either to whom submissive behaviors were directed or from whom these were received.

The effects of concurrent subacute administration of AMP in the competition test are illustrated in Table II. Amphetamine increased food retrieval in three of the four least dominant subjects—Warjoe, Ernie, and Birdie. This increase was seen during both the second and third weeks of treatment in all three subjects. During the initial week of AMP dosing, this result was demonstrated in Ernie and Birdie, but not in Warjoe. This treatment reduced food retrieval by Levi and Susan, the two most dominant subjects. Partial tolerance appeared to be developing to the suppressant effects in both of these subjects during the dosing regimen. The increases seen in Ernie and Birdie were still present during the initial week of saline dosing after cessation of AMP treatment, whereas food retrieval by Levi and Susan had returned to pre-AMP baseline values. Total food retrieval by the entire group was decreased during each of the 3 weeks of treatment. Tolerance developed to this effect during the treatment period. Retrieval returned to baseline values during the post-AMP control week.

TABLE II. Amphetamine Effects on Grouped Food Competition[a]

	Levi	Warjoe	Ernie	Minnie	Susan	Birdie
Pre-AMP week	54.0 (41.1–66.9)	0.8 (0–2.2)	0.2 (0–0.8)	4.2 (0–10.8)	11.8 (0.3–23.3)	0.2 (0–0.8)
AMP week 1	2.8 ± 1.9[b]	0	3.0 ± 2.1[b]	0.6 ± 0.6	0[b]	4.0 ± 4.0[b]
AMP week 2	9.2 ± 3.3[b]	5.8 ± 5.8[b]	1.6 ± 1.6[b]	4.4 ± 4.4	0[b]	4.2 ± 2.8[b]
AMP week 3	19.8 ± 3.9[b]	8.4 ± 4.0[b]	4.2 ± 1.9[b]	0	2.6 ± 1.6	14.2 ± 4.4[b]
Post-AMP week	43.4 ± 2.9	1.4 ± 0.9	4.2 ± 1.4[b]	2.4 ± 1.1	15.6 ± 1.2	3.2 ± 0.7[b]

	Total (2 dominant subjects)	Total (4 least dominant subjects)	Total
Pre-AMP week	65.8 (59.1–72)	5.4 (0–12.1)	71.2 (69.0–72.0)
AMP week 1	2.8 ± 2.0[b]	7.6 ± 3.8	10.4 ± 5.2[b]
AMP week 2	9.2 ± 3.3[b]	16.0 ± 9.9[b]	25.2 ± 7.9[b]
AMP week 3	22.4 ± 5.5[b]	26.8 ± 7.8[b]	49.2 ± 10.7[b]
Post-AMP week	59.0 ± 2.1	11.2 ± 1.7	70.2 ± 0.9

[a]Except for the pre-AMP control values which represent the mean and 95% confidence interval, numbers represent the mean (± SEM) of the number of food biscuits retrieved daily by specific subjects following IM treatment of all subjects for 21 consecutive sessions with 1.0 mg/kg of d-amphetamine.

[b]Mean values which are outside the pre-AMP control 95% confidence interval.

In addition to the effects on food competition, concurrent AMP treatment altered the frequency of submissive behaviors (Table V). Amphetamine increased the number of submissive behaviors emitted by Minnie and Susan. This effect was demonstrated during the initial 2 weeks of treatment in Minnie, but only during the third week in Susan. These behaviors were almost exclusively directed toward Levi, but owing to daily intersubject variability, appeared most prominent in the third week of treatment. AMP treatment reduced the occurrence of these submissive behaviors in the other four subjects. Furthermore, all subjects with the exception of Levi were the recipients of fewer submissive gestures. Most of these parameters returned to control values during the week following AMP dosing. However, there was a rebound decrease below control values in the number of submissive gestures directed toward Levi by both Minnie and Susan.

The effects of subacute AMP treatment of just the dominant subject, Levi, are illustrated in Tables III and V. Food retrieval by Levi was reduced during each of the 3 weeks; partial tolerance appeared to develop to this effect as had occurred during concurrent dosing. Food retrieval by some of the other subjects, which had received saline injections, increased during this time. Greater amounts of food were obtained by Warjoe, Minnie, Birdie, and Susan during the initial week of AMP treatment of Levi. This effect was present during all 3 weeks in Minnie and Birdie and also during the second week of dosing in Warjoe. A similar increase in food retrieval by Ernie also occurred during the second and third weeks of treatment. Levi showed a dramatic increase in the frequency of submissive behaviors emitted during the initial 2 weeks of treatment. This effect did not occur during concurrent dosing. These were primarily directed toward Warjoe and Susan. At the

TABLE III. Alterations in Grouped Food Competition Induced by AMP Treatment of the Dominant Male (Levi)[a]

	Levi	Warjoe	Ernie	Minnie	Susan	Birdie
Pre-AMP week	51.3 (36.0–66.6)	0.3 (0–1.1)	0	2.8 (0–7.7)	16.5 (5.0–28.0)	0
AMP week 1	0.8 ± 0.8^b	6.5 ± 4.9^b	1.3 ± 1.3	25.8 ± 7.4^b	29.5 ± 4.4^b	1.3 ± 0.8^b
AMP week 2	4.6 ± 1.9^b	7.0 ± 3.2^b	3.8 ± 2.7^b	16.0 ± 3.4^b	17.2 ± 2.0	6.6 ± 2.4^b
AMP week3	12.6 ± 2.2^b	0.8 ± 0.8	10.2 ± 2.9^b	19.2 ± 4.7^b	10.0 ± 1.5	7.0 ± 2.3^b
Post-AMP week	47.5 ± 4.6	0	1.2 ± 0.8	7.2 ± 3.5	15.2 ± 3.2	1.0 ± 1.0

[a]Except for the pre-AMP control values which represent the mean and 95% confidence interval, numbers represent the mean (± SEM) of the number of food biscuits retrieved daily by specific subjects following daily administration of 1.0 mg/kg of AMP to Levi and 0.5 ml of saline to the other subjects for 21 consecutive days.

[b]Mean values which are outside the pre-AMP control 95% confidence interval.

same time, there was no decrease in the frequency at which submissive behaviors were directed toward Levi by each of the other five subjects. However, once treatment of Levi was discontinued, the number of these behaviors directed toward Levi decreased below control values.

Individual AMP treatment of the middle-ranking male, Warjoe, essentially resulted in no change in the food-competition data. The number of submissive behaviors directed to Warjoe during this treatment period was reduced and remained low during the week after dosing was terminated (Table V). No decrease occurred in the frequency at which Warjoe emitted submissive behaviors, an effect which had been seen during concurrent AMP treatment.

The effects of subacute AMP dosing of the dominant female, Susan, in the competition test, are presented in Table IV. Food retrieval was reduced during each week of AMP treatment. During the initial week of dosing, Warjoe obtained more food, and during the second and third weeks, Levi retrieved more food. The number of submissive behaviors emitted by Susan during all 3 weeks of treatment was dramatically increased (Table V). These were initially directed only toward Levi, but during the second and third weeks were also directed toward Warjoe and Minnie. A similar effect had occurred during the third week of concurrent dosing. There was no change in the frequency of behaviors directed toward Susan during treatment.

Individual AMP treatment of Minnie, the middle-ranking female, did not dramatically alter the results of the food-competition tests. There was a slight increase in the number of biscuits retrieved by the two lower-ranking males, with the primary effect seen during the third week in Warjoe. Since baseline retrieval for Minnie was zero, no suppressant action of AMP could have been detected. Baseline values (pre-AMP week) for Minnie varied from 2 to 10; post-AMP week values for Minnie were within this range. The number

TABLE IV. Alterations in Grouped Food Competition Induced by AMP Treatment of the Dominant Female (Susan)[a]

	Levi	Warjoe	Minnie	Susan	Birdie
Pre-AMP week	40.3 (25.8–54.8)	0.8 (0–2.8)	10.2 (1.9–18.5)	17.6 (9.8–26.2)	2.3 (0–7.1)
AMP week 1	47.0 ± 3.5	5.3 ± 1.7[b]	12.0 ± 2.7	1.0 ± 1.0[b]	6.0 ± 2.0
AMP week 2	57.0 ± 6.0[b]	0.5 ± 0.5	12.5 ± 6.5	0[b]	2.0
AMP week 3	60.8 ± 1.9[b]	1.0 ± 0.6	6.0 ± 2.0	1.5 ± 1.5[b]	2.8 ± 1.3
Post-AMP week	38.2 ± 2.2	1.0 ± 1.0	10.8 ± 2.5	19.0 ± 2.1	2.8 ± 1.2

[a]Except for the pre-AMP control values which represent the mean and 95% confidence interval, numbers represent the mean (± SEM) of the number of food biscuits retrieved daily by specific subjects following daily administration of 1.0 mg/kg of AMP to Susan and 0.5 ml of saline to the other subjects for 21 consecutive days.

[b]Mean values which are outside the pre-AMP control 95% confidence interval.

TABLE V. Effects of Subacute Amphetamine Administration on the Frequency of Expression of Submissive Behaviors (SB)[a]

	Pre-AMP week (saline)	AMP week 1	AMP week 2	AMP week 3	Post-AMP week (saline)
Levi					
SB received (C)	12.8 ± 3.1	29.4 ± 27.2	10.7 ± 4.8	52.0 ± 32.9[b]	3.6 ± 1.3[b]
SB emitted (C)	1.8 ± 1.1	0[b]	0[b]	0[b]	0.7 ± 0.7
SB received (I)	23.6 ± 5.1	30.8 ± 7.8	15.2 ± 4.5	23.4 ± 6.8	5.9 ± 0.7[b]
SB emitted (I)	1.5 ± 0.3	244.3 ± 48.7[b]	16.6 ± 6.9[b]	2.0 ± 1.5	0.8 ± 0.5
Warjoe					
SB received (C)	13.6 ± 4.5	2.2 ± 1.9[b]	9.2 ± 7.5	0.6 ± 0.2[b]	12.4 ± 2.7
SB emitted (C)	4.8 ± 2.3	1.0 ± 1.0[b]	0[b]	0.2 ± 0.2[b]	1.4 ± 0.5[b]
SB received (I)	11.0 ± 3.2	0.8 ± 0.5[b]	1.0 ± 0.4[b]	0[b]	4.1 ± 0.6[b]
SB emitted (I)	7.2 ± 4.1	4.5 ± 1.3	5.0 ± 1.9	6.3 ± 2.8	5.5 ± 1.1
Ernie					
SB received (C)	1.4 ± 0.7	0[b]	0[b]	1.4 ± 1.4	1.4 ± 0.2
SB emitted (C)	7.2 ± 2.6	0.2 ± 0.2[b]	0.6 ± 0.4[b]	0.4 ± 0.3[b]	7.2 ± 2.4
Minnie					
SB received (C)	2.2 ± 1.2	0[b]	0[b]	0.2 ± 0.2[b]	1.4 ± 0.5
SB emitted (C)	2.0 ± 0.3	29.8 ± 28.3[b]	13.0 ± 7.5[b]	3.6 ± 2.1	0.8 ± 0.4[b]
SB received (I)	4.0 ± 1.6	1.5 ± 1.2	1.0 ± 0.7[b]	1.4 ± 0.7[b]	3.4 ± 1.4
SB emitted (I)	3.0 ± 0.8	25.0 ± 19.1	19.5 ± 6.2[b]	40.2 ± 20.7[b]	4.1 ± 0.6
Susan					
SB received (C)	4.0 ± 2.6	0[b]	0[b]	0[b]	3.0 ± 0.7
SB emitted (C)	6.8 ± 3.1	0.6 ± 0.4[b]	8.0 ± 5.4	48.6 ± 32.7[b]	1.4 ± 0.7[b]
SB received (I)	3.0 ± 1.6	1.3 ± 0.5	2.5 ± 0.5	2.3 ± 0.6	6.5 ± 0.5[b]
SB emitted (I)	3.0 ± 2.7	70.3 ± 37.5[b]	43.3 ± 12.5[b]	30.3 ± 6.3[b]	7.0 ± 0[b]
Birdie					
SB received (C)	0.4 ± 0.3	0[b]	0[b]	0.2 ± 0.2	0[b]
SB emitted (C)	11.8 ± 6.7	0[b]	0[b]	1.2 ± 0.6[b]	10.2 ± 0.6

[a]Numbers represent the daily mean ± SEM of the total number of occurrences of submissive behaviors (presenting + yielding) either emitted or received by specific subjects when pretreated either concurrently (C) or individually (I) with 1.0 mg/kg of d-amphetamine (AMP) IM for 21 consecutive sessions.

[b]Values (mean ± SEM) which do not overlap the mean ± SEM for that subject during the pre-AMP control week.

of submissive gestures directed toward Minnie decreased, whereas, more submissive behaviors were emitted by Minnie (Table V). Similar effects had occurred with concurrent treatment. As was true in most other situations in which the number of submissive behaviors was altered, the dyadic identity of these interactions was not changed from that seen during baseline control sessions.

DISCUSSION

The results of subacute concurrent dosing with AMP are in agreement with previous reports of the effects of acute concurrent treatment with AMP in this competition test (Bellarosa et al., 1980; Lovell et al., 1980; Wilson et al., 1982). Food retrieval was reduced in the most dominant subjects, whereas the least dominant subjects demonstrated an increase in the number of biscuits obtained. There was no evidence of the development of tolerance to this effect in the less dominant subjects. However, the suppressant effect on the dominant animal, Levi, was considerably less during the final week than in the initial 2 weeks of treatment. Furthermore, food retrieval by the entire group demonstrated an increasing trend toward control values, during the treatment period. Therefore, tolerance appeared to develop to the disruptive action of AMP, but not to its facilitative effect in the less dominant subjects.

The increase in food retrieval by lower-ranking subjects was correlated with a decrease in the number of submissive behaviors directed toward more dominant subjects by these animals. This suggests that concurrent AMP treatment may have resulted in an elevation in the dominance rank of these subjects. However, these same subjects—Ernie, Birdie, and Warjoe—did not become the recipients of submissive gestures by more dominant animals, which would have been expected if a shift in dominance status had occurred.

Two subjects, Minnie and Susan, did demonstrate an increase in the frequency at which they emitted submissive behaviors; these were directed to the dominant subject, Levi. This effect was associated with a reduction in food retrieval by Susan. There was no consistent effect of time on this enhancement of submissive behaviors across subjects. This is in agreement with a previous report by Schlemmer and Davis (1981). In one case, the effect was most prominent at the beginning of treatment (Minnie), whereas with Susan the greatest effect was seen during the final week of dosing. Similar increases in submissive behaviors engendered by AMP treatment have been previously reported (Bellarosa et al., 1980; Haber et al., 1977, 1981). Schlemmer and Davis (1981) reported that chronic treatment with amphetamine increased the number of submissive behaviors emitted by treated females. This effect was observed only in more dominant females, which was also the case in the present study. These alterations in both submissive behavior and food retrieval were essentially absent 1 week following AMP treatment. Therefore, if concurrent AMP treatment did alter the dominance hierarchy, the change was only of a temporary nature. Previous reports have suggested that chronic AMP treatment may result in a loss (Schlemmer et al., 1976) or temporary increase (Machiyama et al., 1974; Utena et al., 1975) in the dominance status of treated subjects.

The effects of AMP treatment in a particular subject appeared to be partly dependent on the nature of the treatment administered to the remaining subjects in the group. For example, during the concurrent dosing, Levi did not emit any submissive behaviors. In contrast, when Levi was the only subject dosed, a dramatic increase in submissive behaviors resulted. This relationship suggests that the treatment of a subject, as well as the identity of the treatment of the remaining animals, can determine the effects of a given drug on social behaviors. Perhaps untreated subjects appeared to be more threatening to the treated animal than were untreated subjects. Similarly, both Susan and Minnie demonstrated a greater increase in the frequency of submissive behavior following individual, rather than concurrent dosing. This same relationship has also been reported when the effects of concurrent and individual acute AMP treatments were compared (Bellarosa et al., 1980).

In general, treated subjects, with the exception of Levi, did not receive more submissive behaviors. This suggests that AMP did not generally increase attack or threatening behaviors in the treated subjects. In fact, these subjects may have appeared less threatening since the number of submissive behaviors directed toward them decreased. Concurrent dosing only resulted in Levi's receiving more submissive gestures. This again suggests that he appeared more threatening only to other treated subjects. When Levi alone was dosed, no change occurred in the frequency at which submissive behaviors were directed toward him. It had been previously reported that chronic AMP treatment of a dominant Japanese macaque resulted in fewer submissive gestures being directed toward him by untreated males (Machiyama et al., 1974; Utena et al., 1975). Unlike in the present study, the alpha male did not emit more submissive gestures toward these untreated males. Threatening behavior decreased in this dominant male; however, agonistic behavior was increased in a treated middle-ranking male. Furthermore, there were some indications that the treated dominant male lost his alpha position to the untreated second-ranking male as a result of chronic AMP treatment.

Haber et al. (1977, 1981), using rhesus monkeys, reported that the effect of chronic AMP treatment on agonistic behaviors was dependent on the dominance position of the treated subject. Submissive behaviors were increased in subordinant males, whereas threat behavior was increased in the treated alpha male. No changes in aggressive or submissive behavior occurred in untreated subjects as a result of these effects. Therefore, as previously suggested, the effects of AMP on social behavior are dependent on dose, duration of treatment, dominance status of treated subject, and whether other subjects are treated with AMP.

Data from the current study in the competition test indicate that the facilitative effect of AMP on food retrieval occurs only if more dominant subjects are treated with AMP. Therefore, with respect to the competition test, the behavior of more dominant subjects greatly dictates the qualitative nature of the effect of AMP in subordinate subjects. Although concurrent AMP treatment resulted in an increase in food retrieval by Warjoe, Ernie, and Birdie, a similar effect did not occur when only Warjoe was dosed. When Levi alone was treated, retrieval by all other subjects was increased. Therefore, the facilitative effect of AMP was greatly dependent on the behavior of more dominant animals and also the dominance status of the animal being treated. Furthermore, AMP-induced changes in the results of food-competition tests do not necessarily reflect changes in the dominance relationship of the participants. In the current study, there was no indication that AMP had in fact altered the dominance status of the alpha male. Even though he emitted inappropriate submissive gestures, no other subject was treated as being dominant by the other animals. Perhaps if the group composition had been different, a more aggressive beta male would have obtained the most dominant position in the hierarchy.

These results, which are in agreement with those of others (Haber et al., 1977, 1981; Machiyama et al., 1974; Schlemmer et al., 1976; Schlemmer and Davis, 1981; Utena et al., 1975), illustrate the complexity involved in analyzing the actions of drugs on social behavior. However, the realization of these intricacies attests to the rapid expansion of interest and methodologies in the study of drug action on social behavior.

ACKNOWLEDGMENTS

This work was supported by the Research Institute of Pharmaceutical Sciences and by NIDA grant 5Ro1DA01764.

REFERENCES

Bellarosa A, Bedford JA, Wilson MC (1980) The sociopharmacology of d-amphetamine in *Macaca arctoides*. Pharmacol Biochem Behav 13:221–228

Farres AG, Haude R (1976) Dominance testing in rhesus monkeys: Comparison of competitive food-getting, competitive avoidance, and competitive drinking procedures. Psychol Rep 38: 127–134

Haber S, Barchas PR, Barchas JD (1977) Effects of amphetamine on social behaviors of rhesus macaques; an animal model of paranoia. In: Hanin I, Usdin E (eds) Animal Models in Psychiatry and Neurology. Pergamon, Oxford, pp 107–115

Haber S, Barchas PR, Barchas JD (1981) A primate analogue of amphetamine-induced behavior in humans. Biol Psychiatr 16: 181–196

Lovell DK, Bedford JA, Grove L, Wilson MC (1980) Effects of d-amphetamine and diazepam on paired and grouped primate food competition. Pharmacol Biochem Behav 13: 177–181

Machiyama Y, Hsu SC, Utena H, Katagiri M, Hirata A (1974) Aberrant social behavior induced in monkeys by chronic methamphetamine administration as a model for schizophrenia. In: Mitsuda H, Fukuda T (eds) Biological Mechanisms of Schizophrenia and Schizophrenia-Like Psychoses. Igoku Shoin Ltd., Tokyo, pp 97–106

Masur J, Czeresmia S, Skitnevsky H, Carlini EA (1974) Brain amine levels and competitive behavior between rats in a straight runway. Pharmacol Biochem Behav 2: 55–62

Richards SM (1974) The concept of dominance and methods of assessment. Animal Behav 22: 914–930

Schlemmer RF, Casper RC, Siemsen FK, Garver DL, Davis JM (1976) Behavioral changes in a juvenile primate social colony with chronic administration of d-amphetamine. Psychopharmacol Comm 2: 49–59

Schlemmer RF, Davis JM (1981) Evidence for dopamine mediation of submissive gestures in the stumptail macaque monkey. Pharmacol Biochem Behav 14(Suppl. 1): 95–102

Syme GJ (1974) Competitive orders as measures of social dominance. Animal Behav 22: 931–940

Terada C, Masur J (1973) Amphetamine- and apomorphine-induced alteration of the behavior of rats submitted to a competitive situation in a straight runway. Eur J Pharmacol 24: 375–380

Utena H, Machiyama Y, Hsu SC, Katagiri M, Hirata A (1975) A monkey model for schizophrenia produced by methamphetamine. In: Kondo S, Kawai M, Ehara A (eds) Contemporary Primatology. Basel, Karger, pp 502–507

Wilson MC, Nail G, Bedford JA (1982) Alterations in non-human primate food competition induced by d-amphetamine. Res Comm Sub Abuse 3:467–482

Ethopharmacology: Primate Models of Neuropsychiatric Disorders, pages 307–312

Are Primate Models of Neuropsychiatric Disorders Useful to the Pharmaceutical Industry?

James L. Howard and Gerald T. Pollard

Department of Pharmacology, Wellcome Research Laboratories, Research Triangle Park, North Carolina 27709

INTRODUCTION

The question posed by the title has not been considered formally in print, to the best of our knowledge, and the more general question whether infrahuman primates are superior to lower animals as model subjects in neuropsychiatric research has received insufficient attention. We shall address briefly the issue of primate superiority in terms of model validity, then the specific issue of the appropriateness of primates in the commercial development of neuropsychiatric drugs. The guiding principle will be that if the cost of obtaining a given amount of information from primates is greater than the cost of obtaining it from members of lower orders, then the information from primates should be qualitatively superior. Our conclusion is that primate models are rarely desirable or cost-effective for industrial psychopharmacology.

THE NATURE OF AN ANIMAL MODEL

An animal model is an attempt to create in an infrahuman a representation of some aspects of a human disease state. Models vary along a continuum of approximation to the disease (Thompson and Schuster, 1968). A model can very nearly replicate the human condition—e.g., poliomyelitis in *Macaca fascicularis*, in which the cause and gross symptoms are the same as in human (Mitruka and Bonner, 1976). At the other end of the spectrum are models which bear little if any obvious resemblance to the disease in terms of etiology or symptomatology—e.g., the DOPA potentiation model of depression (Howard et al., 1981)—but yield useful information about the disease and its treatment.

The assumption that a model which is demonstrably homologous with the disease is better than one which is less so has not received sufficient scrutiny. A researcher using a model to investigate a disease process will probably wish to work at the highest feasible level of face validity. However, because most neuropsychiatric disorders are not precisely defined, they cannot now be precisely modeled. Therefore if a researcher wishes to use a model, especially a researcher in the pharmaceutical industry, then in most cases he must accept one with little face validity.

THE NATURE OF DRUG DEVELOPMENT RESEARCH

The objective of pharmaceutical research is to identify therapeutic compounds which are more effective than those currently available, or compounds which are as effective but have fewer side effects. In the field of neuropsychiatric pharmacology, we are searching for drugs to treat schizophrenia, depression, anxiety, senility, convulsive states, and some other disorders. Pursuant to this objective, we define a model empirically as any test procedure which predicts whether a compound will be clinically useful against a specific disease (Howard et al., 1981). A model so defined is quite different from the ideals proposed in the research literature (e.g., McKinney, 1977; Kornetsky, 1977). Most statements of the characteristics of a good animal model emphasize homology with the human disorder; that is, animal symptoms should resemble human symptoms and the etiologies should be similar. In the pharmaceutical industry, on the other hand, elegance and homology are irrelevant if the model does not identify which members of a large set of compounds will be clinically useful. Some commentators have set as one requirement of a good model that it show a positive response to known therapeutic agents; from our perspective in industry, this requirement is the sine qua non.

Most neuropsychiatric models used in industry function at a level called empirical (Howard et al., 1981) or standard drug correlational (Thompson and Schuster, 1968). An empirical or correlational model can be any procedure in which clinically active drugs in a therapeutic class produce effects which drugs not belonging to that class do not produce. Routine use of empirical models has yielded many new therapeutic agents. Primate models need to be measured against this background of success. To be competitive with the economical empirical tests, a primate model must show a positive reaction to drugs known to be effective against a specific human disease, and it must provide superior prediction of efficacy or of side effects, pharmacokintetics, metabolism, and the like.

COMPARISON OF PRIMATE AND NONPRIMATE MODELS

Table I lists some neuropsychiatric conditions along with proposed primate and corresponding nonprimate models. We feel that, with the possible excep-

TABLE I. Primate and Nonprimate Models of Neuropsychiatric Disorders

Neuropsychiatric disorder	Primate model	Nonprimate model
Depression	Separation/isolation Drug-induced	Muricide Drug-induced
Schizophrenia	Drug-induced	Drug-induced CAR
Anxiety	Conflict	Conflict
Epilepsy	Photo-induced Drug-induced	Electroschock-induced Drug-induced
Cognitive deficits/senility	Delayed matching, other "learning" tasks	Passive avoidance, other "learning" tasks
Drug psychoses	Acute or chronic drug adminstration	Acute or chronic drug administration
Drug abuse	Self-administration	Self-administration

tion of the delayed matching and similar models of cognitive deficit, there is no instance in which an industrial researcher should choose primates over nonprimates. Antidepressant research may be used to illustrate this proposition. A recent review of empirical models of antidepressant action (Howard et al., 1981) concluded that at least three of the available tests are very good at identifying known agents—viz., tetrabenazine antagonism, muricide, and the Porsolt swimming test. The tetrabenazine-antagonism test, for example, correctly identifies all first-generation antidepressants (tricyclics, monamine oxidase inhibitors) and, with the exception of mianserin, all second-generation antidepressants (e.g., iprindole, bupropion, trazedone). The test is specific in that very few compounds outside the antidepressant class show activity. In addition, it is reliable, easy to use, and can handle the screening of a large number of compounds.

A primate procedure said to have features which reflect aspects of human depression is the separation model, either mother-infant (Seay and Harlow, 1965) or peer-peer (Suomi et al., 1970). Although McKinney (1977) has been careful not to claim great face validity for the separation model, he and others have pointed out similarities between primate symptoms and human symptoms (see chapters by Reite and Short; Kraemer, Ebert, Lake and McKinney). One argument in favor of face validity is that drugs which reverse human depression also reduce the behavioral symptoms which follow separation in the model (Suomi et al., 1978; Hrdina et al., 1979). However, to date only a few antidepressants have been tested, all of them tricyclics. Clearly, then, this model at its current stage of development would be inappropriate as a primary screen to identify new antidepressants.

If most known clinically active antidepressants had been shown to work in the separation procedure—that is, if the primate model had been demonstrated to be as valid as the rodent tetrabenazine-antagonism model—the separation model would still not meet the needs of industry. It could be argued that the primate model is better since it has greater face validity, the implication being that it would offer a higher probability of identifying a substantively new therapeutic entity, not just a compound similar to those used as positive controls in an empirical model, the basis of which could be a similarity of side effects as well as of therapeutic effect. But this argument would be opposed by the finding that empirical models have in fact led to the discovery of new drugs. For example, bupropion (Soroko et al, 1977), which appears to have a mechanism of action different from that of other known antidepressants (Cooper et al., 1980; Ferris et al., 1981), was identified by the tetrabenazine-antagonism test.

Primate models have been proposed as preclinical screening methods for behavioral side effects (e.g., chapters by Crowley; Schlemmer and Davis). These models are subject to the same objections as models of therapeutic action: Few standard compounds have been tested, cost is high, and face validity is a matter of interpretation. In some cases, existing rodent models could serve the same purpose; e.g., rats have been trained to discriminate hallucinogens from non-hallucinogens (see Seiden and Dykstra, 1977, for examples).

In addition to the conceptual and historical arguments in favor of empirical models using infraprimates, there is the matter of economics. The cost of purchase, maintenance, and testing of a primate is at least ten times that of a rat (J.R. Pick, personal communication; J. Wagner, personal communication). Each year at Wellcome Research Laboratories approximately 1,500 compounds are screened for antidepressant activity. Even if this number were an order of magnitude lower, the primate separation model would remain far too expensive for routine screening.

It has been suggested that primate models might be useful for validation purposes following an empirical screen. There are at least two objections to this idea. A two-stage screen would not answer the question whether a proposed compound is new or is similar to standard drugs. And if a compound were novel and non-toxic and had good activity in the rodent models, then, regardless of results in a primate model, that compound would be tested in man.

CONCLUSION

The effort to develop infrahuman primate models of neuropsychiatric disease should certainly continue. As diseases are better understood, models will improve. However, the assumption that infrahuman primates are inherently better than lower animals as model subjects is based upon little formal evidence; there is no evidence that primate models, in comparison with rodent models, yield better information about how a novel compound might act therapeutically in man; and primates are too expensive to be used in routine drug screening. Therefore, except for specific, limited purposes, the use of primates in neuropsychiatric drug development would be inappropriate and not cost-effective.

REFERENCES

Cooper BR, Hester T, Maxwell RA (1980) Behavioral and biochemical effects of the antidepressant bupropion (Wellbutrin): Evidence for selective blockade of dopamine uptake in vivo. J Pharmacol Exp Therap 215:127–134

Ferris RM, White HL, Cooper BR, Maxwell RA, Tang FLM, Beaman OJ, Russell A (1981) Some neurochemical properties of a new antidepressant, bupropion hydrochloride (Wellbutrin TM). Drug Develop Res 1: 21–35

Howard JL, Soroko FE, Cooper BR (1981) Empirical behavioral models of depression with emphasis on tetrabenazine antagonism. In Enna SJ, Malick JB, Richelson E (Eds) Antidepressants: Neurochemical, Behavioral, and Clinical Perspectives. Raven Press, New York

Hrdina PD, von Kulmiz P, Stretch R (1979) Pharmacological modification of experimental depression in infant macaques. Psychopharmacol 64:89–92

Kornetsky C (1977) Animal models: Promises and problems. In Hanin I, Usdin E (Eds) Animal Models in Psychiatry and Neurology. Pergamon Press, Elmsford New York

McKinney WT (1977) Biobehavioral models of depression in monkeys. In Hanin I, Usdin E (Eds) Animal Models in Psychiatry and Neurology. Pergamon Press, Elmsford New York

Mitruka BM, Bonner MJ (1976) Uniquely useful animal species for biomedical research. In Mitruka BM, Rawnsley HM, Vadehra DV (Eds) Animals for Medical Research. Wiley, New York

Seay B, Harlow HF, (1965) Maternal separation in the rhesus monkey. J Nerv Ment Dis 140:434–441

Seiden LS, Dykstra LA (1977) Psychopharmacology: A Biochemical and Behavioral Approach. Ch. 12, Van Nostrand Reinhold, New York

Soroko, FE, Mehta NB, Maxwell RA, Ferris RM, Schroeder DH (1977) Bupropion hydrochloride (+ −) alpha-t-butylamino-3-chloropropiophenome HCl): A novel antidepressant agent. J Pharm Pharmacol 29:767–770

Suomi SJ, Harlow HF, Domek CJ (1970) Effects of repetitive infant-infant separation of young monkeys. J Abnorm Psychol 76:161–170

Suomi SJ, Seaman SF, Lewis JK, DeLizio RD, McKinney WT (1978) Effects of imipramine treatment of separation-induced social disorders in rehesus monkeys. Arch Gen Psychiat 35:321–325

Thompson T, Schuster CR (1968) Behavioral Pharmacology. Prentice-Hall, Englewood Cliffs New Jersey, pp 208–214

Ethopharmacology: Primate Models of Neuropsychiatric Disorders, pages 313–328

Animal Models: Are They Useful in the Study of Psychiatric Disorders?

M.T. McGuire, G.L. Brammer, and M.J. Raleigh

Neurochemistry Laboratory, Veterans Administration Brentwood Medical Center, Los Angeles, California 90073 (G.L.B., M.J.R.); Nonhuman Primate Research Laboratory, Veterans Administration Medical Center, Sepulveda, California 91343 (M.T.M., G.L.B., M.J.R.); and Department of Psychiatry, University of California Los Angeles, School of Medicine, Los Angeles, California 90024 (M.T.M., G.L.B., M.J.R.)

INTRODUCTION

The chapter builds on three ideas: (1) There are different kinds of animal models of psychiatric disorders; (2) the utility of specific models varies as a function of the type of research question; and (3) there are bidirectional relationships between animal models and human models in that both kinds of models inform research of other species. We will illustrate these points using primarily examples from earlier chapters in this book and from the symposium out of which the book developed. We emphasize that we are neither summarizing nor critically evaluating findings presented in the preceding chapters. Although we focus on nervous system–behavior relationships, the dominant themes developed below should apply to animal models of other systems.

We begin by describing basic considerations applicable to all animal models of human psychiatric disorders; we continue by examining five particular types of animal models including homologous, analogous, survey, mathematical, and outcome models; and we conclude by discussing the implications of animal models for psychiatric research.

BASIC CONSIDERATIONS APPLICABLE TO ALL TYPES OF ANIMAL MODELS

We propose the following working definition of animal models used in psychiatric research: Animal models are hypothetical constructs (e.g., patterns, exemplars, ideas, representations) of events occurring within or to animals that may be used to increase our understanding of psychiatric disorders in humans. Such models have been developed from animal studies of social interactions, mother-infant separations, behavioral-physiological responses to pharmacological agents, and gene-environment interactions. With varying degrees of success, findings from each of these areas have been generalized to humans.

When studies of animals are used to increase our understanding of human physiology and behavior, it is implicit that the nonhuman species being studied is in some way similar to humans. This assumption has at least three implications: First, an understanding of the general principles and the organizational framework of evolutionary biology is critical for determining how species are similar; second, postulated cross-species similarities both direct and constrain ways in which different kinds of models may be helpful in addressing specific research questions; and third, the kind of model being used will influence data interpretation. It is, we suggest, far from an easy task to be certain that two species share similar characteristics, to select a model appropriate to a given research question, and to be certain that one has correctly interpreted findings. These points are illustrated in the discussion which follows.

TYPES OF ANIMAL MODELS

Homologous Models

Homologous models build on the assumption that those aspects of the species being studied are similar because of the shared phylogenetic histories (i.e., descended from a common ancestor). An obvious advantage of studying cross-specific commonalities due to common descent is that findings derived from the study of one species apply to the second species (Fairbanks, 1977). A potential difficulty with homologous models is that species differentiate themselves from their common ancestor and, generally, the greater the differentiation, the less likely species will be homologous with respect to particular physiological processes or behavioral functions. In closely related species this "loss of homology" is not necessarily the consequence of once shared processes having changed. Rather, additions of new anatomical characteristics and/or physiological mechanisms influence processes and functions once shared in common. The relative importance of the frontal cortex in humans compared to that of monkeys is an obvious case in point.

While space precludes a thorough review of the history and use of homologous models in psychiatric research, it is our impression that this type of model has been most compelling when phylogenetically old physiological mechanisms have been investigated in species closely related to man (e.g., blood platelet properties in great apes and man). The case has been least compelling (e.g., plagued with troublesome research design and data interpretation problems) in studies focusing on possible external causes of psychiatric disorders (e.g., "stress" models). And, homologous models have been moderately compelling in investigations of physiology-behavior relationships. These impressions are not surprising. The number of possible intervening variables and the potential importance of cross-species differences increases rapidly as one moves from the study of discrete, phylogenetically old mechanisms to the study of possibly external effects on physiological systems and behavioral functions.

Because of the many interesting and unresolved issues associated with homologous models, this kind of model will be discussed at some length. In referring to previous chapters, we emphasize that none of the authors claimed that he or she was using homologous models and that our motive in selecting examples is to illustrate particular points.

None of the investigators report research which focuses solely on physiological mechanisms in the sense we will use the term—sequences of interrelated physiological events leading to a physiological endpoint. Thus an evaluation of findings where homologies are most likely to hold is precluded. However, a number of investigators reported combined physiology-behavior findings. From the perspective of homology, perhaps the least ambiguous research is that reported by Raleigh et al. (this volume), who examine relationships between social behavior and the serotonin system(s) in vervet monkeys. The lack of ambiguity has several sources. First, three different pharmacological agents, selected because each agent increases available central nervous system serotonin at the synaptic patch, were used as experimental treatments. Because each of these agents resulted in essentially similar behavioral responses, the serotoninergic systems are implicated in the mediation of the reported behaviors. Second, the behavioral effects of pharmacological treatments were measured in identical ways across all experimental and control groups. Third, all control and experimental subjects live in stable groups with similar age-sex social compositions and in the same physical environment. Fourth, studies were controlled for physiological state differences (see below). And fifth, the behaviors measured were those in which animals frequently engage (e.g., groom, approach, eat, etc.) rather than infrequent or atypical behaviors. These methods reduced possible alternate interpretations of findings which could have resulted—for example, had group composition or physical characteristics of the environment varied (e.g., available space per animal; see McGuire et al., 1983). While these authors did not suggest that their findings are applicable to humans, they are clearly interested in the generalizability of their findings and have developed their model to improve understanding of human physiology-behavior relationships.

The Raleigh et al. chapter can be profitably compared with studies reported by Ridley and Baker (this volume). Monkeys were given a variety of drugs affecting the central nervous system which not only alter the frequency of observed behaviors but also increase the probability of atypical behaviors such as cognitive inflexibility and behavioral stereotypy. Ridley and Baker addressed a broader set of questions in their attempt to assess the effects of drug treatments on behavioral tasks designed to simulate human behaviors (e.g., visual discrimination and learning tasks) which are atypical in certain psychiatric disorders (e.g., infantile autism).

Can the findings from either of these studies be said to apply to humans? This question of course cannot be unambiguously answered. The findings reported both by Raleigh et al. and Ridley and Baker may not be homologous with human physiology at the level of discrete physiological mechanisms, at any one of the intervening points between drug-induced physiological changes and observable behavior or physiological responses, and the measured behaviors may not have cross-species equivalents (e.g., there may not be a human counterpart equivalent for nonhuman primate grooming). Because these issues cannot now be resolved, one can approach the interpretative issue in another way, namely: Does regarding the findings of these studies as if they were examples of homologous models have potential value for human research? The answer to this question is clearly yes. Both groups of data suggest a new set of research questions relevant to humans. The Raleigh et al. findings point to the possibility that serotonin may be involved in the mediation of a wider array of behaviors than has been previously thought. The Ridley and Baker findings suggest that alteration of neurotransmitter-mediated functions is only partially a function of drug parameters. Moreover, their findings potentially serve to focus human research with greater specificity than the Raleigh et al. findings, because Ridley and Baker attempt explicit cross-species interpretations.

Homologous features are not necessarily limited to anatomical or physiological characteristics. Social behavior also may be relevant to this type of model, although, as we have suggested, studies of nonhuman social behavior, in which findings have been interpreted as homologous with humans, have often left many unanswered questions. Social behavior was discussed by a number of investigators. For example, Smith and Byrd (this volume) present data which demonstrate that nonhuman primates living in social groups behave differently when compared to animals matched for age and sex housed alone. Such differences are to be expected because socially isolated animals lack the opportunity to interact with other animals and necessarily have a limited behavioral repertoire. However, more is implied in Smith and Byrd's work. Presumably, different social compositions as well as within-group social relationships (e.g., social dominance relationships) affect physiological variables one result of which is that animals develop different physiological profiles. In turn, such physiological differences are associated with different behavioral probabilities as well as metabolic and behavioral responses to drugs. Physiological changes are of course known to occur during breeding season and these changes differ across both sex and species. With few exceptions (see Raleigh and McGuire, 1980), however, nonextreme social composition differences have not been thought to have significant and lasting physiological effects.

The theme emphasized in the Smith and Byrd chapter—different types of social conditions and/or social relationships impact physiological states—is implicit throughout this book. In addition to these investigators, Wilson (this volume), Miczek and Gold (this volume), and Raleigh et al. report that animals of different social status respond differently to weight-equated doses of particular drugs. Thus, issues relating to homology may have to be extended to details of the social characteristics of groups. An interesting potential implication of these findings is that two animals from two different species living in groups with similar social composition may in certain ways be more homologous than two animals of the same species living in different social groups with different social compositions.

Observable drug effects may occur in both group and individual settings. For example, Wilson, studying the effects of amphetamine on the behavior of rats, presents data showing that some drug effects are dependent on housing conditions while other effects are observed both in group-living and isolated individuals. Miczek and Gold, working with squirrel monkeys, also studying the effects of amphetamine treatment, present similar results: Some drug effects appear independent of whether or not animals are in social groups. Recognizing these differences does not make establishing homologies easier, however. To claim homology in either individual-individual or social-social comparisons requires a behavior by behavior comparison across species. For example, elevation of serotonin levels through the administration of L-tryptophan appears to affect social living adult male vervet monkeys and normal adult male humans in noticeably different ways. Vervets increase the frequency of a variety of social interactions whereas humans tend to become sleepy, mentally confused, and do not increase the frequency of social behaviors (Brammer et al., unpublished data). The potential heuristic value of such findings again requires emphasis. The fact that certain drug-induced behavioral changes appear among animals living in social groups but not among animals living in isolation points to the need to conduct ethopharmacological studies in humans living in a wide variety of conditions.

Yet other findings bear on the issue of homology as, for example, those presented by Nielsen et al. (this volume). These investigators have demonstrated that the slow release of amphetamine from subcutaneous capsules results in within-animal behavioral frequency changes over time. A host of possible intervening variables must be considered in interpreting such findings, including compensatory physiological mechanisms, the relationship of primarily altered systems to systems which are minimally affected, physiological habituation to drugs, possible pharmacokinetic changes over time, alteration in the number of receptor sites in response to changes in neurotransmitter concentrations, and "feedback" and/or inhibitory effects resulting from drug-induced changes on the system(s) drugs are targeted to change. Given these many possibilities, the greater the number of intervening variables the less likely findings in one species will be homologous with those in another species. Both Nielsen et al. and Wilson address the difficulties inherent in studying one species while thinking of another. Their concerns are particularly relevant to chronic drug treatment studies. The possibility that chronic treatment may result in irreversable physiological alterations is underscored by Sassenrath (this volume), who showed that the repeated use of delta-9-tetrahydrocannabinol produces anatomical changes in the ventricles of rhesus monkeys. Not unexpectedly, these changes are associated with alterations in the normal psychosocial processing of social stimuli. However, the question remains: Are such findings applicable to humans?

A related set of problems are addressed by Kraemer et al. (this volume), who found that early rearing experience is an important factor in explaining much of the variance in behavioral responses to drugs among adult animals. Animals that have had atypical early experiences compared with animals with normal upbringing experiences respond differently to selected drugs. Moreover, when such animals are in social settings, and not receiving medications, they are behaviorally indistinguishable from age- and sex-matched peers that have had normal upbringings. While the impact of different developmental settings on adult behavioral and physiological relationships has been postulated for nearly a century, the work of Kraemer and his colleagues begins to specify the kinds of experiences that have long-term consequences. These findings have obvious implications for claims of homology.

Reite and Short (this volume) review data dealing with a related point: Among many nonhuman primate species certain types of early mother-infant separation have physiological and immunological consequences. An important feature of this work is that of identifying the time frames in which physiological and behavioral changes occur. Changes that are closely correlated in time suggest the possibility of direct physiological-behavioral interdependence whereas changes that occur in different time frames suggest indirect interdependence (i.e., the presence of intervening variables). (Sensitive therapeutic interventions among humans would take such differences into account.) The preceding points notwithstanding, the problem of determining what is homologous and what is not remains. As Reite and Short point out, cross-species comparisons are not possible until comprehensive studies of the effects of mother-infant separation in one species have been conducted. Observed species differences in behavioral responses to separation pose interpretative problems as does observed within-species variance to separation. Evidence is available to suggest that both within- and cross-species differences in response to separation may in part result from the environmental and social conditions in which animals are studied (Coe et al., 1983; McGuire and Essock-Vitale, 1983). Presumably, these differences would exert their effects through different physiological mechanisms. Similar themes are discussed by Crowley (this volume), who reviews the effects of substance abuse research among monkeys living under different social conditions and compares these findings to humans who have used similar drugs. He emphasizes the importance of testing drugs in different social settings in order to document the full array of behavioral responses and side effects. He further emphasizes a point that undoubtedly applies to all the studies reported in the preceding chapters: namely, if one observes behavior and/or measures physiological variables in individual monkeys, even those not being treated with drugs, baseline measures vary. This means that when conducting either within-animal or cross-species studies one must attend to baseline measures in order to assess drug metabolism and drug effects.

The review of physiological models of psychoses presented by Schlemmer and Davis (this volume) illustrates a number of the preceding points. Three models of psychosis were discussed (amphetamine, phencyclidine, and hallucinogen induced) along with evidence from nonhuman primate studies testing these models. In Schlemmer and Davis's view, none of the models appear to qualify as fully homologous to human psychoses, although available evidence suggests to them that each model may be homologous to some aspect of human psychoses. A variety of reasons underlie their conclusion but a more detailed consideration of these reasons must await the discussion of other models.

One related model should be mentioned—the within-animal homologous model. This model is frequently used when peripheral tissue (e.g., platelets) are studied on the assumption that the properties of such tissues resemble those of other tissues (e.g., brain cells). Such models have obvious value in investigating detailed questions (e.g., characteristics of receptor sites), especially when tissues of interest are difficult to obtain. However, they also carry with them certain dangers if homologous characteristics are assumed. For example, brain-receptor sites for specific neurotransmitters are part of a highly integrated and complex set of neurochemical systems, each of which influences the other. Isolation of a single system, while often necessary for research purposes, may lose sight of the integration. It is at the integration level, however, that assumed homologies begin to breakdown.

Analogous Models

Analogous models assume that two or more species share the same functions as a result of parallel evolution. Although the concept of analogy is usually applied to physiological and anatomical features, it may also be useful in evaluating animal models of human behavior. Determining how one species manages certain problems in living may inform us about how other species manage similar problems (Fairbanks, 1977). Behaviors that are analogous need not be equivalent in form, provided functions are similar. For example, different animals utilize different behaviors while eating, but the cross-species functions are in all probability quite similar. All the papers presented at the symposium which emphasized behavioral findings could be viewed as possible examples of analogous models.

Analogous models have had a long association with clinical psychiatry (McKinney and Bunney, 1969). Despite this history a number of critical questions remain unresolved. One of these concerns "layering" or the progressive use of new behaviors when an attempted behavior is unsuccessful as a consequence of parallel processing. For example, a bird may escalate threats to drive a potential predator away from young offspring. A human may do likewise, but also attempt at the same time to gain information about what it is that attracted the predator. For a bird, these might be: "divert the predator's attention," "scare the predator," and "attack him directly." For the human, the same sequence of behaviors might occur, but, in addition, the human may attempt to "determine what attracted the predator" and "develop new behaviors which reduce the probability of future predation." Though elements of the preceding responses appear to be analogous, they differ in their complexity, the number of functions involved, and the consequences of these functions. Because of these differences, an important question for research concerns whether or not common functions can be studied independent of the influence of nonshared functions. Further, while the term "layers" suggests a hierarchical arrangement of functions, the details of such arrangements are far from clear (see Dawkins, 1976, for a helpful discussion on this point, and McGuire and Essock-Vitale, 1983, for a recent discussion). The findings presented by Raleigh et al., Wilson, Smith and Byrd, and Miczek and Gold suggest that hierarchical arrangements change as a function of an animal's social status and/or physiological state. Differential drug responses in high- and low-status animals may in part reflect these changes.

The most difficult problems one encounters using analogous models have to do with the interpretation of findings. For example, while functional similarity often is assumed, the specific behaviors associated with possible equivalent functions may differ to such a degree that assumptions of functional equivalence must be questioned. Precopulatory behavior provides an interesting example. In some species it is highly ritualized. In other species it appears to be almost nonexistent (in vervet monkeys, for example). In yet other species (e.g., humans) there are significant variances in its length, intensity, and in the array of observed behaviors. How is one to interpret such differences? The usual practice is to search for common elements across species and to disregard differences in form and complexity. But such practices are as likely to perpetuate the assumption of functional equivalence as they are to lead to the experimental exploration of possible analogous or nonanalogous behaviors.

The animal model which probably has been most extensively studied is that of mother-infant separation. Numerous studies reported in the preceding chapters and elsewhere demonstrate that in a variety of primate species separation affects behavioral, physiological, and maturational variables. Disregarding for the moment previously mentioned points about within-species variance, we can ask: Is the separation model more compelling as a homologous or an analogous model? The answer to this question is contingent on the research question being asked. For example, selected physiological changes in rhesus infants following separation may be similar (homologous) to those seen in human infants following separation, while a number of the behavioral responses (e.g., protest and despair) may be more appropriately thought of as analogous, since they differ in forms, complexity, and duration across these two species.

An issue we have delayed discussing until this point concerns the implications of studies discussed by Dubach and Bowden (this volume). Oral, intramuscular, or intraperitoneal administration of pharmacological agents is far from optimal. Sites other than the central nervous system are usually affected and, within the central nervous system, areas other than those most immediately involved with behaviors under study may be affected. In principle, discrete intracerebral injection of either drugs or natural substances overcomes these methodological limitations. Yet even here one must be cautious, primarily because responses to injections at single sites, while perhaps resulting in dramatic behavioral effects, are probably insufficient to explain any complex behavior let alone psychiatric disorders. A significant behavioral effect following a single-site injection of a drug may represent the last point in a long succession of events many of which began in different parts of the brain.

Survey Models

Another type of model may be called a survey model. Survey models use data from a wide range of species in order to detect general tendencies which otherwise might go unnoticed (Fairbanks, 1977). A comparative review of separation studies would so qualify, as would perhaps a similar review of amphetamine effects on the physiology and behavior of primates. Of the preceding chapters, the findings presented by Reite and Short and by Crowley are closest to this type of model.

While survey models have limitations—important pieces of data are missing and reasoning is post hoc—these limitations do not gravely affect these models. It is simply a truism to say that similar characteristics across seven related species provide a more compelling story for both homologous and analogous hypotheses than do similar characteristics across two species.

Outcome Models

One model, sometimes implied by the findings presented in the preceding chapters, deserves discussion because of its continuing use in psychiatric research. We will refer to this model as the outcome model. Outcome models are independent-dependent variable models in which little may be known about intervening variables (e.g., physiological mechanisms) causing specific responses to drugs. Most clinical drug research of the last two decades has been outcome research.

Outcome models are neither scientifically nor aesthetically pleasing, primarily because of the uncertainty about the events that occur between the administration of a drug and behavioral responses. That knowledge of these events is essential to our understanding of human physiology is underscored by the high rate of side effects of many psychopharmacological agents. Academic investigators thus often are in opposition to the practices of clinicians and the pharmaceutical industry where the outcome model often prevails (Howard, this volume). But even when intervening mechanisms are partially known, problems remain. As an illustration, the early clinical trials of chlorpromazine reduced many of the troublesome symptoms associated with psychoses. One by-product of such reduction was often that of rendering patients socially ineffective. Thus, as Crowley points out, there are gains and losses depending on where one chooses to look. Moreover, the decision to give chlorpromazine was often dictated by conditions that were not directly relevant to optimal patient care. For example, in situations where a hospital ward was minimally staffed but housed many psychotic and difficult patients, the probability of chlorpromazine treatment increased. These points are not to be taken as a criticism of chlorpromazine. Rather, they are introduced to direct attention to the kinds of difficulties that exist independent of our knowledge of mechanisms and issues concerning the appropriateness of models.

Mathematical Models

The last type of model to be considered is mathematical. Although mathematical models are seldom used in psychiatric research, we mention this type of model for completeness. Such models posit general relationships which are assumed to apply across a wide variety of species (Fairbanks, 1977). Examples from fields where such models have been used suggest that there are two advantages to these models: They direct attention to possible general relationships, and they are useful paradigms in which to design research (e.g., critical research questions can be deduced from the model). But there are also disadvantages. Perhaps the most troublesome one is that revisions of once-established models often are slow in coming even though research findings do not support the model from which hypotheses and research are developed (see Brown, 1982, for an interesting discussion of this point with regard to the MacArthur-Wilson model of island biogeography).

The points raised in the previous paragraph deserve special emphasis. Research findings which are explained post hoc using existing models often serve to perpetuate models that deserve revision. An example in the area of behavioral research is the interpretation of findings in terms of a territory model. Models implicating norepinephrine destabilization as a major cause in severe depression also may be a case in point. For example, newer drugs that have little or no effect on the norepinephrine system appear to clinically cure depression with the same frequency as the older tricyclic drugs; yet this fact seems to have had minimal impact on the life of the norepinephrine model. Models might therefore have greater utility when thought of as hypotheses and the research designed accordingly.

IMPLICATIONS OF ANIMAL MODELS FOR PSYCHIATRIC RESEARCH

Before turning to a discussion of the models described above, some points peculiar to research in psychiatry should be mentioned. A frequent oversight is that psychiatry is a branch of medicine. Medicine has pragmatic goals (e.g., reduction of suffering), and these goals are not necessarily central themes in animal research (we are not referring here to humane treatment of animals) where physiological mechanisms or mechanism-behavior relationships may be a more immediate research focus. Thus clinicians, because they have different objectives from those of investigators, will sometimes use a new drug before nonclinician investigators believe they should. A second point is that in psychiatry one often treats signs and symptoms and investigates issues that are not normally found in nature. For example, the authors have probably spent over 20,000 hours observing vervet monkeys in quasi-natural environments and we have never seen behavior suggestive of schizophrenia, mania, agitiated depression, or involutional depression. Moreover, to develop depression-like or schizophrenia-like syndromes in animals often requires that animals be treated in extreme fashion (e.g., complete and prolonged deprivation, extreme doses of drugs, etc.). Humans, on the other hand, often develop these disorders in nonextreme settings. Thus, one is faced with the possibility that there may be no animal models directly applicable to certain characteristics observed in humans. Current evidence suggests that this may be in part due to genetic contributions to psychiatric disorders, for which there are no well-established counterparts among non-human primates.

Where does the preceding discussion leave us? Or, can a reasonable justification be made for the use of animal models in psychiatric research? In attempting to answer this question we will restrict our remarks to scientific matters. This restriction should not be taken as an indication that undiscussed issues, such as the aesthetic preferability of first studying drug effects in animals before administering drugs to humans, are unimportant.

In our view, perhaps the point that needs greatest emphasis concerns our uncertainty about what it is in humans that animal models are modeling. Decisions are still being made as to the taxonomy, etiology, consequences, behavioral characteristics, and meaning of psychiatric disorders (Colby and McGuire, 1981; McGuire and Essock-Vitale, 1983). Thus, as Schlemmer and Davis point out, an investigator using animals to model psychiatric disorders can only approximate what he or she is attempting to model. There is of course a generally accepted body of signs and symptoms which are taken as indicating the presence of psychiatric disorders. But in everyday clinical practice one rarely sees the same cluster of signs and symptoms twice. Thus, what exactly constitutes psychiatric disorders still remains an unresolved issue despite recent advances in taxonomic classification (e.g., DSM-III). Even greater uncertainty prevails concerning when disorders begin and end.

Since models may not be as precise as one might hope, the focus of this discussion changes to the following question: Are not advances in our understanding of psychiatric disorders and their underlying mechanisms the result of animal and human studies each informing the other? It is our view that the answer to this question is yes. The preceding chapters provide excellent support for this view. For example, several participants emphasized the importance of observing pharmacological effects in both social and nonsocial settings. Their recommendations derive from evidence suggesting that different social compositions and/or environmental conditions have physiological consequences. These consequences are thought to affect drug metabolism, information processing, macro- and microbehavioral responses, and so on. What is implied in these studies of animals is still at a rudimentary stage in human research. Thus, human research is informed by suggesting a variety of new human-relevant research questions. In turn, studies of humans inform animal research. It is simply reiterating the obvious to say that the recognition of the effects of marijuana, cocaine, amphetamine, alcohol, and many other "drugs" in humans led to new sets of questions being asked of animals, and that resulting investigations have probably taught us more about animals than about humans.

A second major point concerns the number of factors that can affect behavior. Arguments were made by Kraemer et al., Reite and Short, and Crowley in support of this point. Different upbringing and social conditions result in animals that are different behaviorally, physiologically, immunologically, and, probably, psychologically. In turn, physiological mechanisms and responses to drugs may differ. Such findings will undoubtedly inform both clinical and nonclinical human research studies in the future, primarily by providing examples of the number of variables that can affect drug actions and response. Yet findings in humans originally inspired the animal studies. These preceding points hold for physiologically focused studies. The work of Raleigh et al., Ridley and Baker, Wilson, Miczek and Gold, and Nielsen et al. indicate that it is possible to make relatively precise statements about physiological-behavior relationships by using multiple approaches to similar questions and standardizing outcome measures. These studies are logically extended by the work of Dubach and Bowden (this volume), who reported findings from intracerebral injections of dopamine. Again, it is our understanding of animals that increases, and in most instances far more rapidly than our understanding of humans.

An interesting point is suggested by Miczek and Gold. In their chapter they reviewed their own and others' findings on amphetamine effects in several species of nonhuman primates. They concluded that no particular nonhuman primate species has emerged as the preferred species with which to model human behavior. This view raises obvious questions in terms of the preceding discussion: In particular, how would one come to such a conclusion? Several findings appear to have influenced their reasoning. Briefly, amphetamine effects often differ among animals of different age, status, and sex as well as across study conditions. Moreover, species response differences exist. The variety of variables that influence these effects have presented a more compelling picture of species differences than direct leads to understanding human behavior. But can we take Miczek and Gold's suggestion seriously if we are uncertain than their findings were developed on species often thought to be homologous with *Homo sapiens*? Perhaps, though not for reasons of failed homology, just the opposite is true, because they could not satisfy themselves that they had identified a homologous model. Schlemmer and Davis encountered the same problem and drew the same conclusion.

Finally, we ask ourselves the question: "What will be the relationship between animal models and psychiatric research in the year 2000?" One answer occurs to us. Different models will become progressively refined as to their utility for directing research in different areas. As a result, a particular disorder, such as schizophrenia, might be studied using a variety of different models, each applicable to a specific aspect of the disorder(s). Such studies may require the use of many different species, many different models, and a host of new uncertainties not even envisioned in this paper. But animal models may represent our only choice for many relevant studies.

ACKNOWLEDGMENTS

The work of the authors reported in this paper was in part supported by grant H80606 from the Harry Frank Guggenheim Foundation and in part by the research service of the Veterans Administration.

REFERENCES

Brown JH (1982) Two decades of homage to Santa Rosalia: Toward a general theory of diversity. Amer Zool 21: 877–888

Coe CL, Smith ER, Mendoza SP, Levine S (1983) Varying influence of social status on hormone levels in male squirrel monkeys. In: Steklis HD, Kling A (eds) Hormones, Drugs and Social Behavior in Primates. New York, Spectrum, pp 7–32

Colby K, McGuire MT (1981) The core problem in psychiatry: Uncertainty of diagnosis. Sci 21: 21–23

Crowley T (1983) Substance abuse research in monkey social groups. In: Miczek KA (ed) Ethopharmacology: Primate Models of Neuropsychiatric Disorders. Alan R. Liss, New York

Dawkins R (1976) Hierarchical organization: A candidate principle for ethology. In: Bateson PPG, Hinde RA (eds) Growing Points in Ethology. Cambridge University Press, Cambridge, pp 7–54

Dubach MF, Bowden, DM (1983) Response to intracerebral dopamine injection as a model of schizophrenic symptomatology. In: Miczek KA (ed) Ethopharmacology: Primate Models of Neuropsychiatric Disorders. Alan R. Liss, New York

Esler M, Turbot J, Schwartz R, Leonard P, Bobik A, Skews H, Jackman G (1982) The peripheral kinetics of norepinephrine in depressive illness. Arch Gen Psychiatr 39: 295–300

Fairbanks LA (1977) Animal and human behavior: Guidelines for generalizations across species. In: McGuire MT, Fairbanks LA (eds) Ethological Psychiatry. Grune and Stratton, New York, pp 87–110

Howard JL, Pollard GT (1983) Are primate models of neuropsychiatric disorders useful to the pharmaceutical industry? In: Miczek KA (ed) Ethopharmacology: Primate Models of Neuropsychiatric Disorders. Alan R. Liss, New York

Kraemer G, Ebert MH, Lake CR, McKinney W (1983) Amphetamine challenge: Effects in previously isolated rhesus monkeys and implications for animal models of schizophrenia. In: Miczek KA (ed) Ethopharmacology: Primate Models of Neuropsychiatric Disorders. Alan R. Liss, New York

McGuire MT, Essock-Vitale SM (1983) Psychiatric disorders in the context of evolutionary biology: A functional classification of behavior. J Nerve Ment Dis 169: 672–686

McGuire MT, Raleigh MJ, Johnson C (1983) Social dominance in adult male vervet monkeys. I: General considerations. Soc Sci Info. 22:89–124

McKinney WR, Bunney WE (1969) Animal models of depression. Arch Gen Psychiat 21:240–248

Miczek KA, Gold LH (1983) Ethological analysis of amphetamine action on social behavior in squirrel monkeys (*Saimiri sciureus*). In: Miczek KA (ed) Ethopharmacology: Primate Models of Neuropsychiatric Disorders. Alan R. Liss, New York

Nielsen E, Eison MS, Lyon M, Iversen SD (1983) Hallucinatory behaviors in primates produced by around-the-clock amphetamine treatment for several days via implanted capsules. In: Miczek KA (ed) Ethopharmacology: Primate Models of Neuropsychiatric Disorders. Alan R. Liss, New York

Raleigh M, Brammer G, McGuire MT (1983) Male dominance, serotonergic systems, and the behavioral and physiological effects of drugs in vervet monkeys (*Cercopithecus aethiops sabaeus*). In: Miczek KA (ed) Ethopharmacology: Primate Models of Neuropsychiatric Disorders. Alan R. Liss, New York

Raleigh MJ, McGuire MT (1980) Biosocialpharmacology. McLean Hosp J 2:73–84

Reite M, Short R (1983) Maternal separation studies: Rationale and methodological considerations. In: Miczek KA (ed) Ethopharmacology: Primate Models of Neuropsychiatric Disorders. Alan R. Liss, New York

Ridley RM, Baker HF (1983) Is there a relationship between social isolation, cognitive inflexibility and behavioral stereotypy? An analysis of the effects of amphetamine in the marmoset. In: Miczek KA (ed) Ethopharmacology: Primate Models of Neuropsychiatric Disorders. Alan R. Liss, New York

Sassenrath EN (1983) Assessment of acute vs. long-term effects of delta-9-tetrahydrocannabinol on social behavior and adaptability in group-living macaques. In: Miczek KA (ed) Ethopharmacology: Primate Models of Neuropsychiatric Disorders. Alan R. Liss, New York

Schlemmer FR, Davis JM (1983) A comparison of three psychotomimetic-induced models of psychosis in non-human primate social colonies. In: Miczek KA (ed) Ethopharmacology: Primate Models of Neuropsychiatric Disorders. Alan R. Liss, New York

Smith EO, Byrd LD (1983) Studying the behavioral effects of drugs in group-living nonhuman primates. In: Miczek KA (ed) Ethopharmacology: Primate Models of Neuropsychiatric Disorders. Alan R. Liss, New York

Wilson MC, Bailey L, Bedford JA (1983) Effects of subacute adminstration of amphetamine on food competition in primates. In: Miczek KA (ed) Ethopharmacology: Primate Models of Neuropsychiatric Disorders. Alan R. Liss, New York

Index

PROGRESS IN CLINICAL AND BIOLOGICAL RESEARCH

Vol 1: **Erythrocyte Structure and Function,** George J. Brewer, *Editor*

Vol 2: **Preventability of Perinatal Injury,** Karlis Adamsons, Howard A. Fox, *Editors*

Vol 3: **Infections of the Fetus and the Newborn Infant,** Saul Krugman, Anne A. Gershon, *Editors*

Vol 4: **Conflicts in Childhood Cancer: An Evaluation of Current Management,** Lucius F. Sinks, John O. Godden, *Editors*

Vol 5: **Trace Components of Plasma: Isolation and Clinical Significance,** G.A. Jamieson, T.J. Greenwalt, *Editors*

Vol 6: **Prostatic Disease,** H. Marberger, H. Haschek, H.K.A. Schirmer, J.A.C. Colston, E. Witkin, *Editors*

Vol 7: **Blood Pressure, Edema and Proteinuria in Pregnancy,** Emanuel A. Friedman, *Editor*

Vol 8: **Cell Surface Receptors,** Garth L. Nicolson, Michael A. Raftery, Martin Rodbell, C. Fred Fox, *Editors*

Vol 9: **Membranes and Neoplasia: New Approaches and Strategies,** Vincent T. Marchesi, *Editor*

Vol 10: **Diabetes and Other Endocrine Disorders During Pregnancy and in the Newborn,** Maria I. New, Robert H. Fiser, *Editors*

Vol 11: **Clinical Uses of Frozen-Thawed Red Blood Cells,** John A. Griep, *Editor*

Vol 12: **Breast Cancer,** Albert C.W. Montague, Geary L. Stonesifer, Jr., Edward F. Lewison, *Editors*

Vol 13: **The Granulocyte: Function and Clinical Utilization,** Tibor J. Greenwalt, G.A. Jamieson, *Editors*

Vol 14: **Zinc Metabolism: Current Aspects in Health and Disease,** George J. Brewer, Ananda S. Prasad, *Editors*

Vol 15: **Cellular Neurobiology,** Zach Hall, Regis Kelly, C. Fred Fox, *Editors*

Vol 16: **HLA and Malignancy,** Gerald P. Murphy, *Editor*

Vol 17: **Cell Shape and Surface Architecture,** Jean Paul Revel, Ulf Henning, C. Fred Fox, *Editors*

Vol 18: **Tay-Sachs Disease: Screening and Prevention,** Michael M. Kaback, *Editor*

Vol 19: **Blood Substitutes and Plasma Expanders,** G.A. Jamieson, T.J. Greenwalt, *Editors*

Vol 20: **Erythrocyte Membranes: Recent Clinical and Experimental Advances,** Walter C. Kruckeberg, John W. Eaton, George J. Brewer, *Editors*

Vol 21: **The Red Cell,** George J. Brewer, *Editor*

Vol 22: **Molecular Aspects of Membrane Transport,** Dale Oxender, C. Fred Fox, *Editors*

Vol 23: **Cell Surface Carbohydrates and Biological Recognition,** Vincent T. Marchesi, Victor Ginsburg, Phillips W. Robbins, C. Fred Fox, *Editors*

Vol 24: **Twin Research, Proceedings of the Second International Congress on Twin Studies,** Walter E. Nance, *Editor* Published in 3 volumes: Part A: **Psychology and Methodology** Part B: **Biology and Epidemiology** Part C: **Clinical Studies**

Vol 25: **Recent Advances in Clinical Oncology,** Tapan A. Hazra, Michael C. Beachley, *Editors*

Vol 26: **Origin and Natural History of Cell Lines,** Claudio Barigozzi, *Editor*

Vol 27: **Membrane Mechanisms of Drugs of Abuse,** Charles W. Sharp, Leo G. Abood, *Editors*

Vol 28: **The Blood Platelet in Transfusion Therapy,** G.A. Jamieson, Tibor J. Greenwalt, *Editors*

Vol 29: **Biomedical Applications of the Horseshoe Crab (Limulidae),** Elias Cohen, *Editor-in-Chief*

Vol 30: **Normal and Abnormal Red Cell Membranes,** Samuel E. Lux, Vincent T. Marchesi, C. Fred Fox, *Editors*

Vol 31: **Transmembrane Signaling,** Mark Bitensky, R. John Collier, Donald F. Steiner, C. Fred Fox, *Editors*

Vol 32: **Genetic Analysis of Common Diseases: Applications to Predictive Factors in Coronary Disease,** Charles F. Sing, Mark Skolnick, *Editors*

Vol 33: **Prostate Cancer and Hormone Receptors,** Gerald P. Murphy, Avery A. Sandberg, *Editors*

Vol 34: **The Management of Genetic Disorders,** Constantine J. Papadatos, Christos S. Bartsocas, *Editors*

Vol 35: **Antibiotics and Hospitals,** Carlo Grassi, Giuseppe Ostino, *Editors*

Vol 36: **Drug and Chemical Risks to the Fetus, Newborn,** Richard H. Schwarz, Sumner J. Yaffe, *Editors*

Vol 37: **Models for Prostate Cancer,** Gerald P. Murphy, *Editor*

Vol 38: **Ethics, Humanism, and Medicine,** Marc D. Basson, *Editor*

Vol 39: **Neurochemistry and Clinical Neurology,** Leontino Battistin, George Hashim, Abel Lajtha, *Editors*

Vol 40: **Biological Recognition and Assembly,** David S. Eisenberg, James A. Lake, C. Fred Fox, *Editors*

Vol 41: **Tumor Cell Surfaces and Malignancy,** Richard O. Hynes, C. Fred Fox, *Editors*

Vol 42: **Membranes, Receptors, and the Immune Response: 80 Years After Ehrlich's Side Chain Theory,** Edward P. Cohen, Heinz Köhler, *Editors*

Vol 43: **Immunobiology of the Erythrocyte,** S. Gerald Sandler, Jacob Nusbacher, Moses S. Schanfield, *Editors*

Vol 44: **Perinatal Medicine Today,** Bruce K. Young, *Editor*

Vol 45: **Mammalian Genetics and Cancer: The Jackson Laboratory Fiftieth Anniversary Symposium,** Elizabeth S. Russell, *Editor*

Vol 46: **Etiology of Cleft Lip and Cleft Palate,** Michael Melnick, David Bixler, Edward D. Shields, *Editors*

Vol 47: **New Developments With Human and Veterinary Vaccines,** A. Mizrahi, I. Hertman, M.A. Klingberg, A. Kohn, *Editors*

Vol 48: **Cloning of Human Tumor Stem Cells,** Sidney E. Salmon, *Editor*

Vol 49: **Myelin: Chemistry and Biology,** George A. Hashim, *Editor*

Vol 50: **Rights and Responsibilities in Modern Medicine: The Second Volume in a Series on Ethics, Humanism, and Medicine,** Marc D. Basson, *Editor*

Vol 51: **The Function of Red Blood Cells: Erythrocyte Pathobiology,** Donald F. H. Wallach, *Editor*

Vol 52: **Conduction Velocity Distributions: A Population Approach to Electrophysiology of Nerve,** Leslie J. Dorfman, Kenneth L. Cummins, Lary J. Leifer, *Editors*

Vol 53: **Cancer Among Black Populations,** Curtis Mettlin, Gerald P. Murphy, *Editors*

Vol 54: **Connective Tissue Research: Chemistry, Biology, and Physiology,** Zdenek Deyl, Milan Adam, *Editors*

Vol 55: **The Red Cell: Fifth Ann Arbor Conference,** George J. Brewer, *Editor*

Vol 56: **Erythrocyte Membranes 2: Recent Clinical and Experimental Advances,** Walter C. Kruckeberg, John W. Eaton, George J. Brewer, *Editors*

Vol 57: **Progress in Cancer Control,** Curtis Mettlin, Gerald P. Murphy, *Editors*

Vol 58: **The Lymphocyte,** Kenneth W. Sell, William V. Miller, *Editors*

Vol 59: **Eleventh International Congress of Anatomy,** Enrique Acosta Vidrio, *Editor-in-Chief.* Published in 3 volumes: Part A: **Glial and Neuronal Cell Biology,** Sergey Fedoroff, *Editor* Part B: **Advances in the Morphology of Cells and Tissues,** Miguel A. Galina, *Editor* Part C: **Biological Rhythms in Structure and Function,** Heinz von Mayersbach, Lawrence E. Scheving, John E. Pauly, *Editors*

Vol 60: **Advances in Hemoglobin Analysis,** Samir M. Hanash, George J. Brewer, *Editors*

Vol 61: **Nutrition and Child Health: Perspectives for the 1980s,** Reginald C. Tsang, Buford Lee Nichols, Jr., *Editors*

Vol 62: **Pathophysiological Effects of Endotoxins at the Cellular Level,** Jeannine A. Majde, Robert J. Person, *Editors*

Vol 63: **Membrane Transport and Neuroreceptors,** Dale Oxender, Arthur Blume, Ivan Diamond, C. Fred Fox, *Editors*

Vol 64: **Bacteriophage Assembly,** Michael S. DuBow, *Editor*

Vol 65: **Apheresis: Development, Applications, and Collection Procedures,** C. Harold Mielke, Jr., *Editor*

Vol 66: **Control of Cellular Division and Development,** Dennis Cunningham, Eugene Goldwasser, James Watson, C. Fred Fox, *Editors.* Published in 2 volumes.

Vol 67: **Nutrition in the 1980s: Contraints on Our Knowledge,** Nancy Selvey, Philip L. White, *Editors*

Vol 68: **The Role of Peptides and Amino Acids as Neurotransmitters,** J. Barry Lombardini, Alexander D. Kenny, *Editors*

Vol 69: **Twin Research 3, Proceedings of the Third International Congress on Twin Studies,** Ligi Gedda, Paolo Parisi, Walter E. Nance, *Editors.* Published in 3 volumes: Part A: **Twin Biology and Multiple Pregnancy** Part B: **Intelligence, Personality, and Development** Part C: **Epidemiological and Clinical Studies**

Vol 70: **Reproductive Immunology,** Norbert Gleicher, *Editor*

Vol 71: **Psychopharmacology of Clonidine,** Harbans Lal, Stuart Fielding, *Editors*

Vol 72: **Hemophilia and Hemostasis,** Doris Ménaché, D. MacN. Surgenor, Harlan D. Anderson, *Editors*

Vol 73: **Membrane Biophysics: Structure and Function in Epithelia,** Mumtaz A. Dinno, Arthur B. Callahan, *Editors*

Vol 74: **Physiopathology of Endocrine Diseases and Mechanisms of Hormone Action,** Roberto J. Soto, Alejandro De Nicola, Jorge Blaquier, *Editors*

Vol 75: **The Prostatic Cell: Structure and Function,** Gerald P. Murphy, Avery A. Sandberg, James P. Karr, *Editors.* Published in 2 volumes: Part A: **Morphologic, Secretory, and Biochemical Aspects** Part B: **Prolactin, Carcinogenesis, and Clinical Aspects**

Vol 76: **Troubling Problems in Medical Ethics: The Third Volume in a Series on Ethics, Humanism, and Medicine,** Marc D. Basson, Rachel E. Lipson, Doreen L. Ganos, *Editors*

Vol 77: **Nutrition in Health and Disease and International Development: Symposia From the XII International Congress of Nutrition,** Alfred E. Harper, George K. Davis *Editors*

Vol 78: **Female Incontinence,** Norman R. Zinner, Arthur M. Sterling, *Editors*

Vol 79: **Proteins in the Nervous System: Structure and Function,** Bernard Haber, Jose Regino Perez-Polo, Joe Dan Coulter, *Editors*

Vol 80: **Mechanism and Control of Ciliary Movement,** Charles J. Brokaw, Pedro Verdugo, *Editors*

Vol 81: **Physiology and Biology of Horseshoe Crabs: Studies on Normal and Environmentally Stressed Animals,** Joseph Bonaventura, Celia Bonaventura, Shirley Tesh, *Editors*

Vol 82: **Clinical, Structural, and Biochemical Advances in Hereditary Eye Disorders,** Donna L. Daentl, *Editor*

Vol 83: **Issues in Cancer Screening and Communications,** Curtis Mettlin, Gerald P. Murphy, *Editors*

Vol 84: **Progress in Dermatoglyphic Research,** Christos S. Bartsocas, *Editor*

Vol 85: **Embryonic Development,** Max M. Burger, Rudolf Weber, *Editors.* Published in 2 volumes: Part A: **Genetic Aspects** Part B: **Cellular Aspects**

Vol 86: **The Interaction of Acoustical and Electromagnetic Fields With Biological Systems,** Shiro Takashima, Elliot Postow, *Editors*

Vol 87: **Physiopathology of Hypophysial Disturbances and Diseases of Reproduction,** Alejandro De Nicola, Jorge Blaquier, Roberto J. Soto, *Editors*

Vol 88: **Cytapheresis and Plasma Exchange: Clinical Indications,** W.R. Vogler, *Editor*

Vol 89: **Interaction of Platelets and Tumor Cells,** G.A. Jamieson, *Editor*

Vol 90: **Beta-Carbolines and Tetrahydroisoquinolines,** Floyd Bloom, Jack Barchas, Merton Sandler, Earl Usdin, *Organizers*

Vol 91: **Membranes in Growth and Development,** Joseph F. Hoffman, Gerhard H. Giebisch, Liana Bolis, *Editors*

Vol 92: **The Pineal and Its Hormones,** Russel J. Reiter, *Editor*

Vol 93: **Endotoxins and Their Detection With the Limulus Amebocyte Lysate Test,** Stanley W. Watson, Jack Levin, Thomas J. Novitsky, *Editors*

Vol 94: **Animal Models of Inherited Metabolic Diseases,** Robert J. Desnick, Donald F. Patterson, Dante G. Scarpelli, *Editors*

Vol 95: **Gaucher Disease: A Century of Delineation and Research,** Robert J. Desnick, Shimon Gatt, Gregory A. Grabowski, *Editors*

Vol 96: **Mechanisms of Speciation,** Claudio Barigozzi, *Editor*

Vol 97: **Membranes and Genetic Disease,** John R. Sheppard, V. Elving Anderson, John W. Eaton, *Editors*

Vol 98: **Advances in the Pathophysiology, Diagnosis, and Treatment of Sickle Cell Disease,** Roland B. Scott, *Editor*

Vol 99: **Osteosarcoma: New Trends in Diagnosis and Treatment,** Alexander Katznelson, Jacobo Nerubay, *Editors*

Vol 100: **Renal Tumors: Proceedings of the First International Symposium on Kidney Tumors,** René Küss, Gerald P. Murphy, Saad Khoury, James P. Karr, *Editors*

Vol 101: **Factors and Mechanisms Influencing Bone Growth,** Andrew D. Dixon, Bernard G. Sarnat, *Editors*

Vol 102: **Cell Function and Differentiation,** G. Akoyunoglou, A.E. Evangelopoulos, J. Georgatsos, G. Palaiologos, A. Trakatellis, C.P. Tsiganos, *Editors.* Published in 3 volumes. Part A: **Erythroid Differentiation, Hormone-Gene Interaction, Glycoconjugates, Liposomes, Cell Growth, and Cell-Cell Interaction.** Part B: **Biogenesis of Energy Transducing Membranes and Membrane and Protein Energetics.** Part C: **Enzyme Structure—Mechanism, Metabolic Regulations, and Phosphorylation-Dephosphorylation Processes**

Vol 103: **Human Genetics,** Batsheva Bonné-Tamir, *Editor,* Tirza Cohen, Richard M. Goodman, *Associate Editors.* Published in 2 volumes. Part A: **The Unfolding Genome.** Part B: **Medical Aspects**

Vol 104: **Skeletal Dysplasias,** C.J. Papadatos, C.S. Bartsocas, *Editors*

Vol 105: **Polyomaviruses and Human Neurological Diseases,** John L. Sever, David L. Madden, *Editors*

Vol 106: **Therapeutic Apheresis and Plasma Perfusion,** Richard S.A. Tindall, *Editor*

Vol 107: **Biomedical Thermology,** Michel Gautherie, Ernest Albert, *Editors*

Vol 108: **Massive Transfusion in Surgery and Trauma,** John A. Collins, Kris Murawski, A. William Shafer, *Editors*

Vol 109: **Mutagens in Our Environment,** Marja Sorsa, Harri Vainio, *Editors*

Vol 110: **Limb Development and Regeneration.** Published in 2 volumes. **Part A,** John F. Fallon, Arnold I. Caplan, *Editors.* **Part B,** Robert O. Kelley, Paul F. Goetinck, Jeffrey A. MacCabe, *Editors*

Vol 111: **Molecular and Cellular Aspects of Shock and Trauma,** Allan M. Lefer, William Schumer, *Editors*

Vol 112: **Recent Advances in Fertility Research,** Thomas G. Muldoon, Virendra B. Mahesh, Bautista Pérez-Ballester, *Editors.* Published in two volumes. Part A: **Developments in Reproductive Endocrinology.** Part B: **Developments in the Management of Reproductive Disorders**

Vol 113: **The S-Potential,** Boris D. Drujan, Miguel Laufer, *Editors*

Vol 114: **Enzymology of Carbonyl Metabolism: Aldehyde Dehydrogenase and Aldo/Keto Reductase,** Henry Weiner, Bendicht Wermuth, *Editors*